SPORTS AND AGING

SPORTS
& AGING

A Prescription for Longevity

EDITED AND WITH AN INTRODUCTION

BY GERALD R. GEMS

University of Nebraska Press
LINCOLN

Chapter 15 by Gertrud Pfister previously appeared as "Fit,
Fun . . . Forever Young? The Physical Activities of Ageing
Women" in *Gérontologie et société* 40, no. 156 (2018): 181–96.

The University of Nebraska Press is part of a land-grant institution
with campuses and programs on the past, present, and future
homelands of the Pawnee, Ponca, Otoe-Missouria, Omaha,
Dakota, Lakota, Kaw, Cheyenne, and Arapaho Peoples, as well as
those of the relocated Ho-Chunk, Sac and Fox, and Iowa Peoples.

Library of Congress Cataloging-in-Publication Data
Names: Gems, Gerald R., editor.
Title: Sports and aging : a prescription for longevity /
edited and with an introduction by Gerald R. Gems.
Description: Lincoln : University of Nebraska Press, [2022] |
Includes bibliographical references and index.
Identifiers: LCCN 2021046863
ISBN 9781496226006 (Hardback)
ISBN 9781496231611 (Paperback)
ISBN 9781496232267 (Epub)
ISBN 9781496232274 (PDF)
Subjects: LCSH: Sports for older people. | Exercise for older
people. | Aging. | Longevity. | BISAC: SPORTS & RECREATION /
Cultural & Social Aspects | HEALTH & FITNESS / Longevity
Classification: LCC GV708.5 .S68 2022 |
DDC 796.084/6—dc23/eng/20220126
LC record available at https://lccn.loc.gov/2021046863

Set in Lyon by Laura Buis.
Designed by N. Putens.

CONTENTS

Acknowledgments   vii

Introduction   1
GERALD R. GEMS

1. A History of Aging   17
    GERALD R. GEMS

2. Life with a Purpose   35
    FRANCES GEMS

3. Looking Back   44
    TONY KALETH

4. It Was Not Easy!   56
    MAHA EBEID

5. My Life of Physical Activity and Fitness   72
    JAMES R. COATES JR.

6. Aging, Antiaging, and Infinite Youth in Taiwan   96
    CHIA-JU YEN

7. A Matter of Perspective   116
    SAMUEL O. REGALADO

8. Dance until the Music Stops 134
    TANSIN BENN

9. Carpe Diem 153
    LUCIANE LAUFFER

10. Aging as an Adventure 160
    M. ANN HALL

11. An Antiaging Sporting Life in an Aging Society 176
    KOHEI KAWASHIMA

12. Going Strong 191
    GARY OSMOND

13. On a Meaningful Life with Sport as a Permanent Companion 213
    ELSE TRANGBÆK

14. Making a Difference 229
    JANICE J. CROSSWHITE

15. Fit, Fun, Forever Young 246
    GERTRUD PFISTER

    Conclusion 277
    GERALD R. GEMS

    Appendix: Aging Project Survey 297

    Contributors 299

    Index 303

ACKNOWLEDGMENTS

In such an undertaking as this, there are many people to thank. First, I'd like to acknowledge Rob Taylor, who planted the seeds for such a study and supplied encouragement along the way. Courtney Ochsner's efforts and efficiency expedited the process. Haley Mendlik skillfully guided the manuscript through the sequence. Deb Oliver, Jennifer Comeau, and the diligent employees of the University of Nebraska Press helped to bring the project to fruition. Wayne Larsen's skills as copyeditor greatly enhanced the product. I offer sincere thanks to all the contributors, who generously shared the accounts of their lives and put up with my prodding for more information and greater introspection. Their patience and understanding in a long review process and the sluggishness imposed by the COVID-19 pandemic are truly appreciated. I especially thank Professor Shaoli Wang of the Northeast Normal University in China, who offered a visit to his institution that enabled me to gather a wealth of information for this study. He was a truly exceptional host and a fine scholar. Sincere thanks must also be extended to Professor Wang's graduate student Li Jiaqi (Dolores), whose excellent command of the English language provided indispensable help. It was her initiative and persistence that enabled the completion of twenty interviews with Chinese subjects. Her amiability and near constant care made the trip even more enjoyable for my wife and me.

SPORTS AND AGING

Introduction

GERALD R. GEMS

During the overlapping 2017–18 sport seasons, commentators often questioned the intention of New England Patriots quarterback Tom Brady to
continue to play beyond his fortieth birthday. Journalists marveled as he
began the 2019 season at the age of 42, and a year later he led his new team,
the Tampa Bay Buccaneers, to the Super Bowl. Others wondered how long
basketball star LeBron James could continue to maintain his elite status
and statistical production once he had reached the seemingly advanced
age of 33. Still others questioned Serena Williams's decision to return to
competitive tennis at the age of 36 after giving birth to a daughter. Such
questioners neglect to consider a long history of aged athletes who continued to play at elite levels. Such concerns belie a long history of continued
excellence by aging American athletes.

Early in the twentieth century, Bobby Marshall played end for three
different professional football teams into his forty-fifth year. Likewise,
John Nesser, one of the six Nesser brothers who manned the Columbus
Panhandles team, played as a lineman at 45. George Blanda not only played
but also starred as a quarterback and kicker for the Oakland Raiders at 48
in 1975.[1] More recently, Doug Flutie still quarterbacked the New England
Patriots at 43 in 2005, while Jerry Rice, the greatest pass receiver in National
Football League (NFL) history, continued to play at 42. Adam Vinatieri began
his twenty-fourth season in the NFL as a 46-year-old placekicker in 2019.

Darrell Green still played the position of cornerback, one that required great speed and agility in the NFL, at 42. He reportedly ran a forty-yard dash in 4.43 seconds on his fiftieth birthday.[2]

A host of Major League Baseball players have competed into their forties: Alex Rodriguez, 41; David Ortiz, 41; Randy Johnson, 43; Ichiro Suzuki, 44; Bartolo Colón, 44; Roger Clemens, 45; Nolan Ryan, 46; Julio Franco, 49; Jamie Moyer, 49; Hoyt Wilhelm, 49. And the seemingly ageless Satchel Paige began his major league career at 42, made the all-star team at 47, and pitched his last game at 59.[3] Minnie Miñoso played professional baseball across seven decades, getting his last hit in his fifties. He drew a walk in a minor league game at the age of 77.[4]

Similarly, the great Michael Jordan continued to play in the National Basketball Association at age 40, and many others competed well beyond that: for instance, Bob Cousy, John Stockton, Karl Malone, Kareem Abdul-Jabbar, Robert Parish, Dikembe Mutombo, Tim Duncan, Grant Hill, Steve Nash, Jason Kidd, and Vince Carter, who played until 2020 at age 43.[5]

In the National Hockey League, Chris Chelios was still on the ice at the age of 48, and Jaromír Jágr lasted until age 45. "Mr. Hockey," Gordie Howe, played into his fifty-second year alongside his sons. He came out of retirement to play in a minor league game at the age of 69. Such longevity is noticeable across sport forms. Karch Kiraly played pro volleyball at 46. Willie Shoemaker rode thoroughbreds for more than forty years, finally retiring at 54. George Foreman won a heavyweight championship at the age of 45. Roberto Duran battled in the boxing ring across five decades until the age of 50, and even he was surpassed by Saoul Mamby, who fought at 60. Gary Player still played in the Masters golf tournament and the British Open at 73. ESPN: The Magazine featured him in its body issue in 2013, when he was 77. The 2018 edition displayed a nude Greg Norman golfing at 63.

Men have no monopoly on athletic excellence or longevity. Eleanora Sears excelled at nineteen different sports, winning national championships and captaining an international squash team into her fifties.[6] Martina Navratilova won the 2006 US Open mixed doubles tennis championship at age 49. Nancy Lieberman played in the Women's National Basketball Association at age 50, and Diana Nyad swam from Cuba to Florida at the age of 64. Dara Torres swam on five Olympic teams, her last in 2008 as a 41-year-old, winning a total of twelve medals.

One might argue, rightfully so, that these are not average human beings. All are exceptionally gifted in their physical abilities. Physiologists and medical doctors continue to document the decline of one's physicality as we grow older. That loss of speed, strength, power, and VO_2 max (a measure of aerobic capacity), however, is relative. While such capabilities begin to decline about the age of 25 or 30, the rate of decline is much slower in active people. With the advent of the Masters Games in 1985, athletes beyond the age of 40 continued to compete against their peers in five-year age cohorts, that is, 40–45, 45–50, and so on, and even as centenarians.[7]

Such amateur athletes have recorded some amazing feats of their own. Canadian Betty "BJ" Mchugh, a skier, tennis player, and mother of four, worked as a nurse and cared for her husband, who suffered from dementia. She took up running at age 50 and cross-trained as a cyclist, with weight training and yoga. At age 85 she finished a marathon with a time of 5:12.03.[8] Another Canadian, Olga Kotelko, set twenty-six world records in her 90–95 age group. At five feet one-half inch and 130 pounds, she hardly figured to be an athletic wonder, but she competed in as many as eleven events. At the 2010 World Masters Indoor Championships she ran the sixty-meter dash against the men and finished a respectable third. A 92-year-old Italian, Ugo Sansonetti, set the world record of 11.57 seconds in the sixty-meter dash. Kotelko became one of the most studied elderly athletes in the world, subjecting herself to physiological, psychological, and cognitive examinations at various universities. Like Betty McHugh, she proved to be extremely resilient. A schoolteacher, she gave up smoking and her abusive marriage of ten years, which left her with two daughters, one of whom died of cancer in 1999. Kotelko began playing softball at 70 and took up track at 77, while painting, gardening, and training in her spare time.[9]

Australian Ruth Frith, born in 1909, initiated her track and field endeavors in her seventies. In addition to competing in the long jump and triple jump, she specialized in the weight throws, earning gold medals in the hammer throw, shot put, and javelin. At the World Masters Games in Sydney in 2009, she set six world records, amassing nine over her career.[10]

The male competitors in the World Masters Games are equally impressive. In addition to the sprinter Sansonetti, Ed Whitlock ran three marathons in less than three hours each after the age of 70, clocking a 2:54.48 time at age 73. He ran 2:59.12 at 72 in a pair of fifteen-year-old running shoes. Whitlock also held world age group records for five thousand meters and the half marathon.[11] In 2018 a 70-year-old Gene Dykes surpassed Whitlock's marathon time with 2:54.23. He did so after running a fifty-kilometer trail race and another marathon only two weeks before. Dykes did not take up competitive running until the age of 58.[12] That same year, 86-year-old Hiromu Inada completed the Ironman Triathlon in Hawaii, which consists of a 3.86-kilometer swim, followed by a 180.25-kilometer bike ride, and then a full marathon. Inada trains assiduously, sticking to a strict diet of balanced proteins and carbohydrates, and soup for breakfast. He considers these to be the best years of his life and serves as an inspiration for more youthful athletes.[13]

Like Ruth Frith, Fauja Singh continued to compete as a centenarian. Like Olga Kotelka, he had to overcome personal loss and tragedy, as his son was killed in an auto accident in 1999. He ran his first marathon at 89. It took him six hours and forty-one minutes to finish, but he reduced that time to 4:59 by age 94.[14] Stanislaus Kowalski still competed in the one hundred meters, shot put, and discus at the age of 105. Julia "Hurricane" Hawkins, a former schoolteacher, started as a cyclist at age 75 before turning to running at 100; she captured gold medals in the fifty- and hundred-meter races at the 2019 National Senior Games at the age of 103. She set a world record in the sixty-meter race in 2018. Philippa Raschker began competing in multiple events at age 33 in 1980 and continues her phenomenal career. At age 65 she held more than two hundred world and national age-group records in a variety of events, including the pole vault. In 2007 she was named the Masters female athlete of the year and was even a finalist for the Sullivan Award, presented to the greatest amateur athlete.[15]

Pam Reed won the Badwater Ultramarathon, a distance of 135 miles, at age 42, beating all male competitors in the process. Ann Trason also defeated all male runners to win the 1998 Western States Endurance Run of one hundred miles over the Sierra Nevada Mountains. She continued to compete in that race, and at age 41 she bettered the time she had achieved as a 29-year-old. At age 58 in 2018, she still ran more than twenty long-distance races. Lee Bergquist, in his study of aging athletes noted, "Speed and quickness are attributes of youth. But endurance sports favor older athletes."[16]

Ray Scharenbrock, a retired teacher, had run 506 marathons by the age of 72. Don McNelly, a retired business executive, ran his first marathon at age 48 and had completed 680 marathons by age 85. Jim Reeve, at age 48, finished sixty-three marathons in one year. Ed Barreto even surpassed that mark with eighty-four marathons over fifty-two weeks. Others, known as streakers, log miles daily in consecutive fashion, some for more than forty years straight. For them, running is a compulsive behavior that they refer to as a positive addiction. Bergquist claims, "Looking and feeling healthy are important parts of many older athletes' self-image." Emmanuelle Tulle, in her study of aging runners, found that the activity served as a means of resisting the aging process. Obsessions, however, are not healthy, and some marriages have resulted in divorce due to misplaced priorities.[17]

Runners are not the only healthy and engaged elders; walking was once considered a sport, one that most people can perform at any age. Edward Payson Weston, the great pedestrian, walked four thousand miles (6,437 km) from California to New York in seventy-seven days at the age of 71 in 1910. Three years later, in his seventy-fourth year, he covered 1,546 miles (2,488 km) from New York to Minneapolis in 1913.[18]

ESPN, the American sports media conglomerate, produced a documentary in 2018 on Mark Sertich, a 96-year-old ice hockey player, who still competes with much younger men throughout the season. Sertich is not an exception, as several senior hockey leagues and national tournaments offer competition for older players by age groups for people in their fifties, sixties, seventies, and older. One New York team has both men and women ranging in age from 59 to 95, including a female goalie and a player with prosthetic arms. Players tease their oldest member, 95-year-old Marsh Webster, that his Social Security card is numbered 1. The camaraderie of the group is a particular strength of the diverse members.[19]

The San Diego Women's Basketball Association sponsors a league for women 50 years of age and older. One of its teams, known as the Splash Sisters, is composed of members over 80, with some encroaching on centenarian status. The women play thirty-minute games, three on three, on a half court; but competition remains spirited.[20] Another spirited woman, African American Willie Murphy, is a competitive powerlifter at the age of 82. She took up the sport only a decade earlier. Although she weighs only 105 pounds, she holds New York state and national records. In her spare time, she volunteers to exercise with others at a local health clinic.[21]

Such athletes are perhaps more remarkable for their longevity than for their physical performances, and idolization can also be a form of ageism. The Masters athletes present a heroic model of aging, in which they fight against and defeat the process of aging, "while conversely giving in to ageing is regarded as a failure."[22] Top scholars of sport and aging state that "we must stop demonizing sedentary behavior in policy and the media, cease blaming inactivity for disease and increased health costs and begin by valuing and enabling all forms of leisure and lifestyles across the lifespan."[23] Nevertheless, active adults have shown that aging need not fit the stereotype of poor health, fragility, debility, dependency, and disengagement that can result in becoming a ward of the state and a burden on the health care system.[24] Such a perception has been labeled the deficit model of aging.[25] A recent Danish study that characterized the elderly as unproductive consumers whose illnesses were a drain on the national health care resources cited the need for activity centers.[26]

Most elderly persons are not invalids and should not be characterized as such. Historian Lawrence Samuel has asserted that "the very concept of aging remains a social taboo, eliciting fear and dread despite all the research showing that getting older is usually an enjoyable part of life."[27] This is especially true for those who have attained a middle-class status and the inherent privileges of whiteness in western societies. The global COVID-19 pandemic that exploded in 2019 more clearly exposed the deadly ramifications for the poor and people of color. In Asian societies elderly citizens enjoy greater respect for their wisdom and contributions to the society.[28]

Successful aging has become a contested concept in the United States. Such an optimistic characterization ignores not only differences in gender, ethnicity, social class, and age but also the systemic inequities that promote social inequalities, income disparities, and consequent health disparities.[29] While there is no consensus on the definition of successful aging, some studies have shown positive results among Masters athletes. David Geard and colleagues defined successful aging as late-life change via physical, psychological, cognitive, and social functioning, and determined that Masters swimmers fit that characterization.[30] Hirofumi Tanaka drew similar conclusions in a study of aging competitive athletes.[31]

One need not be athletic to enjoy a long, healthy, and happy life. Sport generally connotes competition, but in this study, sport is used generically to include any form of physical exertion, including dance, exercise to meet a level of fitness, and competitive games. The Centers for Disease Control and Prevention in the United States advocate thirty minutes of aerobic exercise five days per week with supplemental strength activities.[32] Inactivity is the cause of 9 percent of premature deaths and contributes to cardiorespiratory disease, type 2 diabetes, musculoskeletal disorders, sleep problems, and increases in the risks of cancer and obesity.[33]

Diet is also an important part of aging well. For nearly two decades researchers have been studying and analyzing five areas of the world known as blue zones, where an inordinate number of people live beyond one hundred years. On the Greek island of Ikaria, there is little dementia. Okinawa, the southernmost island in Japan, is the residence of the world's oldest women. In the mountains of Sardinia, an Italian island in the Mediterranean Sea, live the most centenarian men. In Loma Linda, California, a community consisting largely of Seventh Day Adventists, people live on average ten years longer than other Americans. Men living in the Nicoya Peninsula of Costa Rica have the second highest number of centenarians in the world.[34]

Despite their differences in geography and culture, the inhabitants of such areas have some common characteristics and lifestyles. Their diets are largely vegetarian, with a lot of fruits and nuts, and the Mediterranean diet includes substantial amounts of olive oil. Beans are an important and virtually daily component of meals. Water, coffee, tea, and red wine serve as daily liquids. All inhabitants of these areas remain physically active throughout their lives through working, walking, or exercise. Their relatively stress-free lives often include a strong social support network of family, friends, or a religious community. Despite their age, they are still valued members of the society and maintain a purpose in their lives.[35]

Conversely, Americans continue to follow a diet prone to obesity, heart disease, and cancer that lowers the average lifespan. "Today, the average American adult consumes 79 pounds of fat and 8,000 teaspoons of added sugar annually. And we wash it all down with 57 gallons of soda a year."[36] A recent U.S. government study showed that a third of American adults, both men and women, eat fast food daily, and the wealthier classes eat more fast food than lower income groups do.[37]

Americans are not the only ones who neglect their health. Modern life in industrialized countries tends to produce sedentary lifestyles that result in major health issues such as obesity and heart conditions that can result in debility or death.

Numerous studies have indicated the value of physical activity relative to aging. Sufficient physical activity in the form of sport or less competitive leisure pursuits can improve muscle mass and function, and can lower the chances of cancer, diabetes, and cardiovascular and heart diseases.[38] Other studies indicate a positive change in appearance, self-concept, and psychological well-being due to such activity.[39] Some studies show the benefit of physical activity for individuals with dementia, while others indicate that even informal team games promote greater sociability for aging populations.[40]

Aging has long been perceived as a negative culmination of life, and exercise considered a chore or a work-like and exhaustive means to health and fitness. That need not and should not be the case, as more recent perceptions of aging frame it as a period of renewal, discovery, and fulfillment; and physical activity can be a source of joy, pleasure, happiness, sensuality, amusement, mirth, tranquility, and fun as one ages.[41]

Studies of aging and the role of physical activity in that process have assumed greater importance as older populations increase around the world. Many studies have focused on privileged elderly white men from western capitalistic nations as subjects and beneficiaries of such research.

Scholars and policy makers have called for more research on women, ethnic and racial minorities, varied social classes and religious groups, people of diverse gender identities, and international studies to provide a more heterogeneous and cross-cultural perspective.[42]

This book contributes to that quest for new knowledge as it presents the lives of individuals from across the globe who have aged well. Successful aging has been defined as good health, life satisfaction, independence, a sense of purpose, and the support of family and friends.[43] The book covers various regions of the world, a variety of cultures and religious groups, and people with diverse gender identities as well as married, divorced, single, and widowed persons across different social classes with the intent to determine whether there are any common characteristics or strategies for aging well despite the diversity of the sample. While the concept of aging and what constitutes "elderly people" may differ across cultures, all participants are beyond 50 years of age, ranging from 51 to 96.

Contributors are drawn from all continents other than Antarctica. Contrary to previous studies, there are more women than men. In that sense, it is a diverse and international sample that provides a greater female voice and multiple perspectives on the aging process. Despite the attempt to be inclusive, this is not a scientific sample. Participants were chosen due to their recognized ability to age successfully. While an attempt was made to engage all major religious groups as well as nonreligious persons, all races, and a variety of ethnicities and varied socioeconomic classes, it failed to produce any Jewish contributors or African American female participants. Therefore, any conclusions must be considered tentative at this point. Nevertheless, the study points to promising questions for future study.

For purposes of the study, the World Health Organization's definition of *elderly* as older than 50 is used as a benchmark. Methodological procedures are derived from the Chicago School of Sociology, including ethnography, surveys, oral histories, biographical narratives, interpretation, and analysis with the intent to minimize western and Eurocentric biases prevalent in previous works.[44]

Autoethnography is a qualitative research process employed across numerous academic disciplines to promote self-reflection for producing a narrative that connects to wider cultural and social meanings and thus increases understanding.[45] It is a means for individuals to make sense of their own lives.[46] One disadvantage of the autoethnographic approach is that the researcher might misrepresent the subjects in his or her characterization.[47] This study provided a survey to participants in which each told his or her own story relative to a series of questions (see appendix) to avoid that possibility.

Participants were encouraged to use autoethnographic approaches that began to appear late in the twentieth century to tell their own stories of successful aging. Given the international nature of the contributors, this book might serve as an ethnographic social history, a way to discern how individuals developed within their own societies and diverse cultures over time. Such stories have proven to be "evocative, emotional, engaging, and meaningful" for the storytellers as well as the readers, who may find a personal and emotional attraction.[48] Some stories may inspire personal life changes that ultimately result in social change.[49] Autoethnography in the form of "narrative gerontology is now recognized as a discipline in itself."[50]

Such personal histories also provide healing value for some struggling with disability or the aging process. As Arthur Frank, author of *The Wounded Storyteller*, has stated, "people need a guidebook" for life with physical impairments. A similar guidebook is helpful for aging and unprepared adults facing or coping with lives in retirement, some of whom have a "fear of diminished lives."[51]

Positive stories of successful aging also counteract common narratives of aging as a period of decline. They "describe how cultures, subcultures, or family patterns are reflected in the life of the storyteller and how certain people adapt to or expand the possibilities and limits set by the historical time period in which they live."[52]

For many, successful aging means a change in one's identity that is a dynamic and unfinished process negotiated over time. Reminiscence can be of therapeutic value as people examine their past and future attitudes, values, and practices and thus make coherent sense of their lives.[53] Such investigation of one's identity is negotiated over time, as borne out by the reflections of the participants who have been drawn from generations that experienced different chronological, cultural, and social changes over the course of their lives. Yet all have persevered to overcome obstacles and setbacks to live successful and rewarding lives.[54]

NOTES

1. Bill Soliday, "Blanda of Old Ignites Raiders 27–23 Triumph," *Argus*, December 15, 1974, 17.

2. MJD, "The Only Thing Darrell Green Doesn't Do Quickly Is Age," *Yahoo Sports*, February 16, 2010.

3. Will Leitch, "MLB's Oldest Players for 2017," accessed January 2, 2018, www .sportsonearth.com/article/215862870/oldest-players-mlb-2017-season; Larry Tye, *Satchel: The Life and Times of an American Legend* (New York: Random House, 2009). This list of Major League Baseball players in their forties is not all-inclusive.

4. Baseball Reference, accessed January 2, 2018, https://www.baseball-reference .com/players/m/minosmi01.shtml; "Minoso Plays in 7 Decades," *Brainerd (Minnesota) Dispatch*, July 17, 2003, http://www.brainerddispatch.com/content/minoso -plays-7-decades.

5. Jason Alsher, "The 10 Oldest NBA Players of All Time," *Cheatsheet*, November 30, 2017, https://www.cheatsheet.com/sports/the-oldest-nba-players-of-all -time.html/?a=viewall.

6. *Harrisburg Telegraph*, February 10, 1934, 5.

7. "A Brief History of the World Masters Games," International Masters Games Association, July 14, 2020, https://imga.ch/2020/07/14/a-brief-history-of-the -world-masters-games/.

8. Roger Robinson, "New Research on Older Runners: The Whitlock Mystery May Soon Be Solved," *Runner's World*, March 20, 2003, https://www.runnersworld .com/website-only/new-research-on-older-runners; Jean Sorenson, "Running Up New Times for Seniors," seniorliving.com, January 2012, www.seniorliving .com/articles/running-up-new-times-for-seniors.

9. Bruce Grierson, *What Makes Olga Run? The Mystery of the 90-Something Track Star and What She Can Teach Us about Living Longer, Happier Lives* (New York: Henry Holt, 2014).

10. Kim Stephens, "Masters Athlete Ruth Frith Dies Aged 104," *Sydney Morning Herald*, May 11, 2014, http://www.smh.com.au/sport/masters-athlete-ruth-frith -dies-aged-104-20140311-34jtu.html; Beverley Hadgraft, "Two of Us: Ruth Frith and Helen Searle," *Sydney Morning Herald*, October 31, 2009, http://www

.smh.com.au/lifestyle/two-of-us-ruth-frith-and-helen-searle-20140806-3d7zm
.html.

11. Scott Douglas, "Masters Marathon Legend Ed Whitlock Dies at 86," *Runners World*, March 13, 2017, https://www.runnersworld.com/ed-whitlock/masters -marathon-legend-ed-whitlock-dies-at-86.

12. Katherine Turner, "70-Year-Old Gene Dykes Runs 2:54.23 Marathon World Record," Strava Stories, December 21, 2018, https://blog.strava.com/gene-dykes -marathon-world-record.

13. Ayana Shimizu, "For Hiromu Inada, an 86-Year-Old Ironman Athlete, Age Really Is Just a Number," *Japan Times*, December 21, 2018, https://www.japantimes.co .jp/life/2019/04/05/lifestyle/hiromu-inada-86-year-old-ironman-triathlete -age-really-just-number/#.XSSrEY97nv8.

14. Manpreet K. Singh, "At Almost 106 Years Old Fauja Singh Reveals the Secrets of His Youthfulness," SBS, March 30, 2017, https://www.sbs.com.au/yourlanguage /punjabi/en/article/2017/03/29/almost-106-years-old-fauja.

15. Lee Bergquist, *Second Wind: The Rise of the Ageless Athlete* (Champaign IL: Human Kinetics, 2009); National Senior Games Association, accessed September 25, 2018, http://nsga.com/news/2016-04-20-13-53-19/2017daily/the-games-daily-june -2-3-2017; Aishwarya Kumar, "103-Year-Old Runner Julia 'Hurricane' Hawkins on Bikes, Her Bucket List, and the Brooklyn Bridge," espnW.com, accessed June 28, 2019, https://www.espn.com/espnw/culture/story/_/id/27073873/; Daniel J. Levitin, *Successful Aging: A Neuroscientist Explores the Power and Potential of Our Lives* (Boston: Dutton, 2020), 22–23.

16. Results of search for "Ann Trason," UltraSignup, accessed October 3, 2018, https://ultrasignup.com/results_participant.aspx?fname=Ann&lname=Trason; Bergquist, *Second Wind*, 112, quote from 123.

17. Bergquist, *Second Wind*, 125–38, 171–94, quote from 121; Emmanuelle Tulle, *Ageing Science, the Body, and Social Change: Running in Later Life* (Basingstoke, UK: Palgrave Macmillan, 2008). Alexane Marinho, Adriana A. F. Viscardi, and Isabela M. Vieira, "Adventure Sports and the Perception of Being, or Not Being Elderly," paper presented at the European College of Sport Congress, Prague, Czech Republic, July 3, 2019. These researchers also found that in their study of Brazilian athletes over age 60 who engaged in adventure sports, the athletes did not feel old and did not like the connotation of being elderly. Their sport- ing activities provided sociability and a sense of belonging, the retention of a youthful spirit, and independence.

18. Nick Harris and Helen Harris, *A Man in a Hurry: The Extraordinary Life and Times of Edward Payson Weston, the World's Greatest Walker* (London: DeCoubertin Books, 2012).

19. Steve Wulf, "The Gray Wolves, a Senior Hockey Club, Have Found a Frozen Fountain of Youth," ESPN, accessed December 25, 2018, https://www.espn .com/nhl/story/_/id/25478501. Steve Wulf and David Burnett (photographer), "Who You Calling Old?," ESPN (magazine), June 2019, 30–33, featured a photo essay on elderly athletes, including a 59-year-old female skateboarder as well as 95-year-old Marsh Webster's hockey team, in which one of his teammates stated, "You should've seen Marsh when he was 80. He could fly" (32).

20. Ericka N. Goodman-Hughey, "The Splash Sisters Are Still Out Here Crushing the Competition," ESPNW, accessed February 25, 2019, https://www.espn.com /espnw/culture/the-buzz/.

21. Emily McCarthy "At 81, Willie Murphy Is a Competitive Powerlifter," ESPNW, accessed July 9, 2019, http://www.espn.com/espnw/life-style/article/24200181 /at-81-willie-murphy-competitive-powerlifter.

22. Elizabeth C. J. Pike, "Outdoor Adventurous Sport: For All Ages?," in *Sport and Physical Activity across the Lifespan: Critical Perspectives*, ed. Rylee A. Dionigi and Michael Gard, 301–15 (London: Palgrave Macmillan, 2018), 302.

23. Rylee A. Dionigi and Michael Gard, "Sport for All Ages? Weighing the Evidence," in Dionigi and Gard, *Sport and Physical Activity*, 1–20 (quote, 16).

24. Rylee Dionigi, "Competitive Sport as Leisure in Later Life: Negotiations, Discourses, and Aging," *Leisure Sciences* 28, no. 2 (2006), 181–96.

25. Pike, "Outdoor Adventurous Sport," 301.

26. Adam B. Evans, Anne Nistrup, and Gertrud Pfister, "Active Ageing in Denmark: Shifting Institutional Landscapes and the Intersection of National and Local Priorities," *Journal of Aging Studies* 46 (2018), 1–9.

27. Lawrence R. Samuel, *Aging in America: A Cultural History* (Philadelphia: University of Pennsylvania Press, 2017), 161.

28. Sarah Lamb, "Beyond the View of the West: Ageing and Anthropology," in *Routledge Handbook of Cultural Gerontology*, ed. Julia Twigg and Wendy Martin, 37–44 (London: Routledge, 2015).

29. Stephen Katz and Toni Calasanti, "Critical Perspectives on Successful Aging: 'Does It Appeal More Than It Illuminates?'" *Gerontologist* 55, no. 1 (February 2015), 26–33; Tamar Z. Semerjian, "The Role of Gender and Social Class in Physical Activity in Later Life," in *The Palgrave Handbook of Ageing and Physical Activity Promotion*, ed. Samuel R. Nyman, Anna Barker, Terry Haines, Khim Horton, Charles Musselwhite, Geeske Peeters, Christina R, Victor, and Julia Katharina Wolff, 571–88 (London: Palgrave Macmillan, 2018).

30. David Geard, Peter R. J. Reaburn, Amanda L. Rebar, and Rylee A. Dionigi, "Masters Athletes: Exemplars of Successful Aging?," *Journal of Aging and Physical Activity* 25, no. 3 (July 2017), 490–500.

31. Hirofumi Tanaka, "Aging of Competitive Athletes," *Gerontology* 63, no. 5 (2017), 488–94.
32. Bergquist, *Second Wind*, 2.
33. Annemarie Koster, Sari Stenholm, and Jennifer A. Schrack, "The Benefits of Physical Activity for Older People," in Nyman et al., *Palgrave Handbook*, 43–60.
34. Dan Buettner, *Blue Zones: The Science of Living Longer* (Washington DC: National Geographic Society, 2016).
35. Buettner, *Blue Zones*.
36. Buettner, *Blue Zones*, 4.
37. Mike Stobbe, "1 in 3 Adults Eat Fast Food Daily, Federal Study Says," *Chicago Sun-Times*, October 7, 2018, 26.
38. Shari S. Bassuk and JoAnn E. Manson, "Epidemiological Evidence for the Role of Physical Activity in Reducing Type 2 Diabetes and Cardiovascular Disease," *Journal of Applied Physiology* 99, no. 3 (September 2005), 1193–1204; Maureen C. Ashe, William C. Miller, Janice J. Eng, and Luc Noreau, "Older Adults, Chronic Disease and Leisure Time Physical Activity," *Gerontology* 55, no. 1 (June 2009), 64–72.
39. Jinmoo Heo, Robert Stebbins, Junhyoung Kim, and Inheok Lee, "Serious Leisure, Life Satisfaction, and Health of Older Adults," *Leisure Sciences* 35, no. 1 (January 2013), 16–32; Jinmoo Heo and Younghkill Lee, "Serious Leisure, Health Perception, Dispositional Optimism, and Life Satisfaction of Senior Games Participants," *Educational Gerontology* 30, no. 1 (2010), 101–17.
40. Emmanuelle Tulle and Cassandra Phoenix, eds., *Physical Activity and Sport in Later Life* (Basingstoke, UK: Palgrave Macmillan, 2015); M. Rebecca Genoe, "Leisure as Resistance within the Context of Dementia," *Educational Gerontology* 30, no. 1 (2010), 303–20; Cecilie Thogersen-Ntoumani, Anthony Papathomas, Jonathan Foster, Eleanor Quested, and Nikos Ntoumanis, "'Shall We Dance?' Older Adults' Perspectives on the Feasibility of a Dance Intervention for Cognitive Function," *Journal of Aging and Physical Activity* 26, no. 4 (October 2018), 553–60; Malte Nejst Larsen, "Locomotor Activity, Heart Rate Distribution, Enjoyment, and Perceived Exertion from Walking Football for 60+ Women" paper presented at Le FOOTBALL pour et par les Femmes, Twelfth Colloquium on International Football and Research, University of Lyon, Lyon, France, June 20–22, 2019.
41. Cassandra Phoenix and Noreen Orr, "The Multidimensionality of Pleasure in Later Life," in Tulle and Phoenix, *Physical Activity and Sport in Later Life*, 101–12; Barbara L. Marshall, "Anti-Ageing and Identities," in Twigg and Martin, *Routledge Handbook of Cultural Gerontology*, 210–17.
42. Twigg and Martin, *Routledge Handbook of Cultural Gerontology*.

43. Matthew Carroll and Helen Bartlett, "Ageing Well across Cultures," in Twigg and Martin, *Routledge Handbook of Cultural Gerontology*, 289. See Levitin, *Successful Aging*.

44. Ros Jennings, "Popular Music and Ageing;" 77–84; Cathrine Degnan, "Ethnographies of Ageing," 105–12; and Joanna Bornat, "Aging, Nostalgia and Biographical Methods," 113–20, all in Twigg and Martin, *Routledge Handbook of Cultural Gerontology*.

45. Brett Smith, "Narrative Inquiry and Autoethnography," in *The Routledge Handbook of Physical Culture Studies*, ed. M. Silk, D. Andrews, and H. Thorpe, 505–14 (London: Routledge, 2017).

46. Victoria J. Palmer, Emmanuelle Tulle, and James Bowness, "Physical Activity and the Aging Body," in Nyman et al., *Palgrave Handbook*, 531–49.

47. Cathrine Degnan, "Ethnographies of Aging," in Twigg and Martin, *Routledge Handbook of Cultural Gerontology*, 105–12.

48. Smith, "Narrative Inquiry and Autoethnography," 507.

49. Brett Smith, "Disability and Physical Activity," presented at International Society for the History of Physical Education and Sport (ISHPES) Summer School, Paris-Est University, June 24, 2019.

50. Cassandra Phoenix, Brett Smith, and Andrew C. Sparkes, "Narrative Analysis in Aging Studies: A Typology for Consideration," *Journal of Aging Studies* 24 (2010), 1–11 (quote, 1).

51. Arthur Frank, *The Wounded Storyteller* (Chicago: University of Chicago Press, 2013), xii, xvi.

52. Phoenix, Smith, and Sparkes, "Narrative Analysis in Aging Studies" 3, 4.

53. T. Yamagami, M.Oosawa, S. Ito, and H. Yamaguchi, "Effect of Activity Reminiscence Therapy as Brain-Activating Rehabilitation for Elderly People with and without Dementia," Psychogeriatrics 2, no. 7 (June 2007), 69–75; Y. Chang, Y. Nien, C. Tsai, and J. L. Etnier, "Physical Activity and Cognition in Older Adults: The Potential of Tai Chi Chuan," *Journal of Aging and Physical Activity* 18, no. 4 (2010), 451–72; Philippe Cappeliez and Annie Robitaille, "Coping Mediates the Relationships between Reminiscence and Psychological Well-Being among Older Adults," *Aging & Mental Health* 14, no. 7 (September 2010), 807–18.

54. Belinda Wheaton, "Staying 'Stoked': Surfing, Ageing and Post-Youth Identities," *International Review for the Sociology of Sport* 54, no. 4 (June 2019), 387–409; Emmanuelle Tulle, "Life History Research in Sport," presented at International Society for the History of Physical Education and Sport [ISHPES] Summer School, Paris-Est University, June 25, 2019.

1 A History of Aging

GERALD R. GEMS

In prehistoric times there was no concept of aging. Scientists estimate that thirty thousand years ago, one-third of those born did not survive childhood, while those who did rarely lived past the age of 50. Yet old age was not unknown among the ancient Greeks, who even required military service to age 60. We know that the philosopher Socrates, forced to drink poisonous hemlock, died at 70. His pupil, Plato, lived to be 80, and the playwright Sophocles died at 90.[1]

The Greeks, however, provided mixed messages relative to aging. The historian Herodotus, writing late in the fifth century BCE, associated longevity with diet; while Plato, a fourth-century BCE philosopher, perceived old age as a period of disengagement from affairs, "deprived of women, drinking, and fun," a time for greater spirituality. Greeks also believed that wisdom was truly gained after the age of 50 and, in democratic assemblies, citizens beyond that age were allowed to speak first, while more youthful persons waited while their elders disseminated knowledge. Plato's pupil Aristotle noted that "illnesses are the companion of old age."[2]

Galen, a second-century CE physician and philosopher, told the story of another philosopher who maintained that the aging process might be tamed by a judicious diet. He reached the age of 80 but was mocked by youth who despised his pointed nose, twisted ears, and sunken eyes. The

Greeks saw old age as ugly when compared with their idealized concept of beauty displayed in youthful bodies.[3]

Historical sources indicate a long concern with the process of aging. Even the ancient Egyptians recorded cures for wrinkled skin and the necessity of caring for elderly fathers. The Chinese prescribed a balance between the yin and the yang, a regimen of exercise and healthy diet, and respect for the elderly. Other societies in Asia, Africa, Latin America, and the Middle East, and among Native Americans and other indigenous peoples, have emphasized the priority of family life as well as the value of wisdom among the aged. Elder rights laws in both China and India even require children to visit and care for their aging parents or face fines or jail time. The western cultures of Europe and North America, however, have come to value the exuberance of youth over age and experience.[4] Even the word *aging*, defined as "senescent, declining, wearing out, or wilting," carries a negative connotation.[5]

The striving for a youthful appearance was already evident in the sixteenth century, when average life expectancy was only slightly more than 33 years, as noted by author Anna Whitelock in her description of Queen Elizabeth I of England.

> Over the five decades of her rule, Elizabeth changed from being a young vibrant queen with a pale pretty face, golden hair and slender physique, to a wrinkled old woman with rotten teeth, garishly slathered in jewels and cosmetics to distract from her pitted complexion, and wearing a reddish wig to cover her balding head. . . . The Queen's image was fashioned to retain its youthfulness, which necessarily obscured the reality of her physical decline. . . . Such was Elizabeth's desire to preserve the fiction of her youth that she sponsored the search for the "Philosopher's Stone," the elixir of life which would ensure eternal health and immortality.[6]

That quest continues today.

In earlier times lifespans were generally short due to disease, famine, and warfare. If one survived into old age his or her family assumed the responsibility for elder care. As early as the seventeenth century, aging was depicted as a period of decline. In 1601 an Elizabethan poor law provided a measure of community responsibility for the aged and infirm. That stipulation carried over to the English colonies in America, and by 1642 the Pilgrims of the Plymouth Colony in Massachusetts authorized funding for institutionalized elders. The following year the Anglican Church in Williamsburg, Virginia, provided tax relief for the aged poor. They received alms and firewood, but such individuals were required to wear a red or blue letter "P" on their clothes that stigmatized them as paupers, not unlike the scarlet letter "A" of the adulteress in Nathaniel Hawthorne's novel set in the same era. In 1657 Dutch settlers in Rensselaerswyck, New York, established the first almshouse. A year later assistance for the indigent extended to the home care of such individuals. Boston provided home care in 1664, and similar provisions extended to New York, Philadelphia, and Charleston by 1713. The Philadelphia Friends' Almshouse of the Quakers cared for orphans, the mentally ill, the disabled, and the elderly, all labeled as destitute. By 1773 the Baltimore County Almshouse accepted the destitute, the infirm, social deviants, and the elderly, but all were considered "public nuisances."[7]

In colonial times men were judged by their piety, and the elderly were believed to be closer to God due to their impending death. Such a position provided a measure of reverence and authority but also assumed a decline in health and an image of infirmity.[8] Still, few people reached advanced age, and an estimated 10 percent of women died in childbirth. In colonial New England it was not unusual for women to bear as many as eleven children. In 1801 only 8.7 percent of the residents of France surpassed the age of 60. Only 6.7 percent of the British did so, while a meager 4 percent of Americans reached that milestone by 1830. By 1841 life expectancy for the English barely surpassed 40 years.[9] After 1834 the poor and elderly citizens of England were required to compensate for their living quarters in so-called workhouses by their labor. Between the War of 1812 and the Civil War, one-sixth of American almshouse residents were older than 60, and such residency carried the stigma of a public shaming.[10]

Women, less esteemed than men, were valued relative to their reproductive and domestic usefulness. The United States remained a rural culture until 1920, and large families met the needs of farm life. In seventeenth-century colonial America, 36 percent of families included nine or more children, who assumed adult responsibilities by age 7 with little distinction between ages. Complications resulting from childbirth accounted for greater mortality among women until about 1900.[11] Mothers were expected to nurture their children and attend to household chores. In 1864 author Lydia Child documented her annual work as "wrote 235 letters, read 28 books, made 25 needle books for freedwomen, cooked 360 dinners, 365 breakfasts, swept house 350 times, plus innumerable jobs too small to be mentioned."[12]

The Second Great Awakening, a religious revival early in the nineteenth century, prescribed moral norms relative to one's age, and aging still carried a moral connotation relative to proper behavior and etiquette. The ages between 14 and 21 were considered the primary period of character development. Old age might be considered a blessing if one had lived a good life, but sinners might face punishment in the form of disease or poor health. William Alcott, a nineteenth-century educator and prolific author, stated that "the child of future blessed ages would die at 100 years old—if he was a Christian. The wicked, however, would not live out half their days."[13]

European immigrants increasingly traveled to the United States throughout the nineteenth century, bringing alternative religious beliefs. Jews and Catholics formed fraternal organizations dedicated to meeting the needs of the elderly through charity. By midcentury some European governments had initiated economic assistance for the aged. Prussian miners won old-age insurance in 1854. A united Germany (achieved in 1871) provided insurance for invalids and those over the age of 70 in 1889, and Great Britain passed an Old Age Pensions Act in 1908.[14]

Whereas some European governments began to address the needs of their aging citizens, the United States implemented forced retirement. As early as 1861 naval officers below the rank of vice admiral lost their jobs at age 62. Some states and individual companies began to provide pensions in order to retire older workers, but the U.S. government did not similarly cover its elderly citizens until 1935, when the Social Security Act gave full retirement benefits to people aged 65 and older. Life expectancy at that time, however, was only 62, and the legislation was of no help to the indigent or unemployed who had not contributed to the program. Congress increased funding of social services for the elderly in 1952, but it was not until 1965 when President Lyndon Johnson signed the Older Americans Act that adequate housing, income, low-cost transport services, Medicare, and Medicaid gave greater independence to the aged population. Thirty-four countries had preceded the United States in providing such insurance to seniors. Families, however, retained the primary responsibility for elderly care. During the 1960s, managed health care facilities began to provide an alternative, but it was an expensive one unavailable to most. Over the next half century the health care of senior citizens came to be perceived as a drain on the national economy.[15]

At what point in American history did the denigration of the elderly and the elevation of youth become a reality? "In preindustrial Europe and North America much less attention was paid to distinctions between ages. Life was not perceived as a series of distinct, sharply defined stages organized in a certain uniform age-graded sequence.... There was little sense of being 'too young' or 'too old' in a society where most people did not know their own age with any great precision."[16]

In premodern western societies children were treated as adults. In the preindustrial economy, mixed family generations labored on farms, while master craftsmen employed journeymen, apprentices, and helpers from boys to men. An 1866 book, *Athletic Sports for Boys*, offered instruction in activities such as fishing, gymnastics, fencing, horsemanship, and yachting, with no distinction between boys and men. With increasing mechanized industrialization after 1850, many independent craftsmen lost their jobs and the need for youthful apprentices. Factory work engaged children, young women, and adult males in a multiaged labor force. Likewise, children attended ungraded schools with mixed classes that made no distinction based on age. American schools adopted graded schools based on European models only in the middle of the nineteenth century. By 1871 school officials determined that children were ready for schooling at age 5 or 6, with eight grades encompassing children up to 14 years old.[17]

In the field of medicine, nineteenth-century American doctors learned from French physicians how to address the medical needs of children. A children's hospital opened in Paris as early as 1802 to treat youngsters aged 2 to 15. Philadelphia opened the first children's hospital in the United States in 1855, and Boston opened one in 1869. A German doctor who traveled to New York in 1862 founded a clinic to treat children's diseases, and by

1888 the American Pediatric Society was founded, recognizing childhood as a distinct stage of life.[18]

During the same era, recognition of the aged as a distinct stage of life with its own needs became a reality, but with that classification came negative connotations. The terms "gaffer," "fogy," and "geezers" were used to denote elderly men. When physicians, educators, and psychologists began to construct norms applicable to age groups, senility was considered a "continuous, gradually progressive loss" that was normal for the elderly.[19]

In the wake of the American Civil War, older military heroes and statesmen were still held in esteem despite the encroaching negative conceptions of aging. In Asian and Native American cultures, however, the elderly were and are respected and admired for their wisdom. But the United States is a relatively young country. Between 1850 and 1900, life expectancy rose from only 40 years to 49 years. The era was one of unbridled capitalism, which reaped the rewards of the industrial revolution. As such, the value of people came to be measured by their productivity, and wealth superseded piety. Athletic performance too became more quantified and driven by winning results. The young produced more than their older counterparts, and removal from the workplace lessened one's value.[20]

After 1870, as early mortality decreased, "life became more predictable, with longevity a reasonable expectation for everyone . . . and men began to plan their lives around a series of distinct stages from childhood . . . to eventual retirement. Women's lives were planned around marriage and child rearing." Three stages of life became discernible: childhood, adulthood, and old age.[21]

By the late nineteenth century, the growing feminist movement attracted the "new women," young, vivacious, and athletic, who continually transgressed the established gender boundaries and societal norms. Their entry into higher education and the professions previously reserved for men created a crisis of confidence and a threat to the gender order. Men reacted with a greater emphasis on the public display of masculinity. Football surpassed baseball as the major sport on college campuses by the 1890s, and despite the attendant violence that increased deaths and serious injuries, it remains the national sport and a symbol of male privilege.

Among working-class men, physicality had always been important, but the sport of boxing assumed new prominence as a marker of masculine toughness. That public display of masculinity remained a major sport over the next century, and female boxers did not gain entry to the Olympic Games until 2012.

Emphasis on the male physique at the beginning of the twentieth century fostered the media empire of Bernarr Macfadden, publisher of numerous magazines, including *Physical Culture*, a newspaper, and more than one hundred books. Macfadden became a prominent advocate of bodybuilding, healthy diets, and food supplements to achieve a long and healthy life. He featured his own muscular body in publications and promoted beauty contests for both men and women in his search for the most perfectly developed bodies. That emphasis on youth, muscularity, and physical attractiveness continues in current men's and women's magazines. Research shows that physical attraction reaps benefits for the young and beautiful, characteristics no longer available to most elderly adults.[22]

In 1904 G. Stanley Hall, first president of the American Psychological Association and play theorist during the Progressive Era, published a book on adolescence, further promoting the emphasis on youth. By 1912 Lee Walling Squires described the characteristics of old age. "Property gone, friends passed away or removed, relatives become few, ambition collapsed, only a few short years left to live, with death a final and welcome end to it all." His designated age for such decline was 60. Only after World War I did "middle age" gain greater acceptance as a distinct phase of life.[23] In 1922 Hall published another book, *Senescence: The Last Half of Life*. He claimed that decline started after age 40, and old age was marked by increasing isolation. Hall stated that old age had no substance and that it "is now only too commonly a hateful and even ghastly thing" that required greater scientific management.[24]

Hall's 1904 book reflected an ongoing concern with youth as a problematic stage of life, but over the course of the next two decades, youthfulness became extolled as a desirable characteristic. Young women, in particular, rebelled against the simple maternal reproduction functions promoted by eugenicists such as Edward Alsworth Ross and Madison Grant, who preached the necessity of strong white babies to combat the rising tide of alien immigrants to America. Women wanted more out of life, eastern suffragists and pioneers in the western lands had begun campaigning for voting rights by the middle of the nineteenth century. By the latter decades of the century, women employed sport to challenge patriarchy, male hegemony, and prescribed social norms. They began wearing pants to cycle more comfortably, eschewed the customary Victorian chaperones in their social lives, and participated in more active sports such as tennis, baseball, and basketball, while European women engaged in soccer and rugby. Such activity fostered wholesale changes in fashion and personal relations as young women earnestly proceeded toward greater independence, often to the chagrin of parents, psychologists, and governmental authorities. Organizations such as the Boy Scouts, Camp Fire Girls, and adult supervised sports programs were intended to socially control such impulses.[25]

In contrast, magazines, exuberant public dances, and new forms of technology such as moving pictures shown in cheap nickelodeons promoted and solidified a youth culture. By 1910 more than seventy-five hundred movie houses and twenty-five hundred vaudeville theaters in the United States attracted young crowds. Young, beautiful, and handsome movie stars projected vitality and life. One of the progenitors of such a lifestyle, Irene Castle, stated that "dancing is not only a rejuvenator of good health and spirits, but a means of preserving youth, prolonging life, and acquiring grace, elegance, and beauty."[26] Beauty became synonymous with youth, and the unmarried woman became a "despised old maid."[27]

That idyllic quest was interrupted and defiled by the decimation of youth in the horrendous battles of World War I. The devastation of the global conflagration created "a spirit of euphoria when the long, brutal conflict finally ended. Euphoria and disillusionment. These combined with cynicism to foster a spirit of rebellion and carpe diem."[28]

The decade known as the Roaring Twenties extolled youth and its hedonistic pleasures: illicit drinking, dancing, smoking, and sex. The extensive loss of life in the global war and the flu pandemic that began in 1918 encouraged surviving youth to seize the day, as old age was never assured. Advertising became a "proponent of self-indulgence, hedonism, and an abhorrence of tradition" and was a prominent factor in the American economy. The postwar era made a distinct break with the past as new forms of music (jazz), more lively and energetic dances, a growing feminism, and motion pictures and media that glamorized actors, actresses, and athletes as celebrities disrupted the culture and the generational hierarchy.[29]

Women's fashions emphasized a slim, even adolescent figure. Artificial makeup camouflaged perceived inadequacies, as perfume and cosmetic manufacturers nearly doubled between 1901 and 1929. Cosmetics became a necessary means to maintain a youthful appearance. The first facelift occurred in 1901, and cosmetic surgery only increased thereafter, with breast and hip reductions by 1920. Aging males, most notably Harold McCormick, a former tennis star and wealthy heir to the International Harvester Company, sought fertility injections and even submitted to testicular transplants from animals to increase their waning vitality without success.[30]

The advent of gerontology studies after World War I further portrayed aging as a social problem. The devastating economic depression of the 1930s had an even greater effect on the elderly who, unable to secure work when so many younger bodies were available, suffered disproportionately. The federal Social Security Act of 1935, while providing a more stable and welcome retirement for the elderly, also marked them as dependent and reliant on assistance.[31]

The 1930s also marked a resurgence of nutrition studies as part of the scientific management of the aging process. As early as the 1830s Sylvester Graham, a Presbyterian minister, had advocated a vegetarian diet, temperance, and sexual abstinence as a means of gaining piety and better health. He promoted his Graham crackers as nutritional alternatives to spicy foods that might agitate the nervous system. Later in the nineteenth century, Yale University experimented with different diets and training tables to determine the best fuel for its athletes. Bernarr Macfadden also advocated fruits, vegetables, whole grains, and exercise by the dawn of the twentieth century. Nutritional studies of the 1930s advocated a decreased caloric intake as the way to longevity, and similar studies continue today.[32]

A second social revolution after World War II ushered in the rock-and-roll era of the 1950s, much to the chagrin of parents and many older adults. Like the 1920s, the decade revolved around music, dancing, movies, and clothing styles that accentuated youth and delivered its messages daily via the new medium of television. The youthful exuberance, however, was tempered by the political Cold War, which reinforced perceptions of imminent doom in the atomic age.[33]

The turbulent sixties followed with youth, women, and racial groups leading a crusade for civil rights and social change. Young men challenged forced conscription in the Vietnam War, started by old men. A young athlete, Muhammad Ali, became an activist for the poor, the downtrodden, and other disadvantaged people. By the 1970s hippies created a counterculture by eschewing traditional social norms, dropping out of society, and warning other young people not to trust anyone over 30. Sexual activity, previously considered the province of married adults, became commonplace among rebellious youth. Even the American working class erupted in the political and economic upheavals of the decade. In the process the elderly were dismissed and forgotten as largely irrelevant.[34]

The individualistic pursuits of the 1970s also fostered a fitness boom that promoted successful aging through an active lifestyle. The movement spawned greater interest and participation in weightlifting and body building as well as marathon running, but the extremely fit elder athletes who competed in the Masters Games and resisted the dominant ideologies of degenerative aging could also stigmatize those elderly nonparticipants who lacked such interest or abilities as less than ideal citizens.[35]

By 1984 Colorado governor Richard Lamm declared that "sick, old people had an obligation to die and get out of the way." Historian Thomas Cole stated that "growing old is like being penalized for a crime you haven't committed."[36] More recently, journalist Bruce Grierson noted that "old people in the West . . . are so often plunked on an ice floe and shoved out to sea."[37] Some scholars and policy makers have even advocated for decreased medical care for the aged, suggesting they have a duty to die and thus decrease the costs of the federal Medicare program in favor of younger generations.[38]

That condition has begun to be challenged as "older people are urged to think and act young. Rules of good aging, such as retirement at a designated age, that only a short time ago seemed so natural and self-evident are being challenged at every level."[39] The baby boomer generation, born between 1946 and 1964, has come to fruition with an inordinate amount of political and financial influence. The American Association of Retired Persons, established in 1958, advocates for the rights of and better conditions for the aging and elderly. With 38 million members, it has become one of the most successful lobbying groups in the United States. Not long after the organization was founded, the U.S. government began enacting laws against age discrimination. The Older Americans Act, passed in 1965, advocated for the elderly and intended to help them lead relatively independent lives as they aged. It provided for delivery of cooked meals, transport services, support for family caregivers, protection from abuse, and job training. The National Institute on Aging, founded in 1974, became one of the largest research organizations in the world.[40]

Researchers and scholars have proposed various theories and conditions relative to aging, but the negative connotations of the process persist. In the youth-centered cultures of western nations, a youthful appearance, especially for women, is valued. Billions of dollars are spent annually on plastic surgery, acupuncture, and stem cell therapy. "Many otherwise ordinary Americans continued to see aging as a treatable disease, with a host of cures at one's disposal—vitamins, enzymes, B-12 shots, omega-3 oils, herbs, neutraceuticals, and bioflavonoids, or supplements. A fair number of people subscribing to an antiaging regimen were taking dozens of pills per day, some of them adding an extra shot of human growth hormone to the mix." As many as thirty thousand American spend $1,000 per month on the latter despite its illegality.[41] Others preferred "Botox (a brand of botulinum toxin, a neurotoxic protein produced by a bacterium) [which] was fast becoming the cosmetic therapy du jour for its ability to prevent the development of wrinkles by paralyzing facial muscles."[42]

I suggest that the process of aging be reconceptualized.[43] Some have already devised a new etymology, with terms such as *seniors, mature adults, seasoned citizens* (sounds like succulent dinner fare), *wellderly*, and *superadults*.[44] I will leave the labeling to others but propose a paradigm based on the wellness framework of Abraham Maslow, which permits older adults to negotiate and challenge negative conceptions of aging and resist the dominant discourses and power relations that create such stereotypes, as the masters athletes previously presented have done.[45]

Maslow, a psychologist, proposed his hierarchy of physical, emotional, and social needs as early as 1943 and refined it thereafter in a pyramid model. The physiological needs of food, shelter, and clothing form the base of the pyramid, followed by safety, and then emotional needs, such as love. The fourth level is esteem, and the top of the pyramid is self-actualization, or reaching one's full potential in life. Maslow contended that only 6 percent of individuals reached that pinnacle. I contend that the state has an obligation to provide the first two levels, and that family and friends can provide a sense of belonging to a group.[46] Although sport need not be a requirement in any stage, clearly those engaged in the Masters competitions and sport clubs experience a sense of community and camaraderie. Abundant research attests to the value of physical activity in later life, but it need not be of a competitive nature.[47] Physical activity in many forms, from walking to various sports, can and should be pleasurable.

While not all can reach the level of self-actualization (for example, a Nobel Prize winner may have suffered a divorce or be so engrossed in his or her work as to neglect family or physical health), they should be able to reach the level of esteem in which they are valued and respected as they age gracefully.

A 2011 study of fourteen European countries and Israel measured successful aging by such criteria, but researchers determined that only 1.6 percent of Poles and 8.5 percent of all subjects attained the level of esteem. Danes, supposedly the happiest people in the world, led the list with 21.1 percent of successful agers, while the United States can count only 10.5 percent in that category. There is much more to be achieved in that respect as we engage in meaningful research and practice for the future.[48]

Maslow's theory has rightfully been criticized as less than universal in that he concentrated not on the general population but on elite leaders and outstanding students from the United States, groups that generally promote individualism.[49] Communal societies, for instance, value different objectives. Surely there are other exceptions, because not all aspire to the level of self-actualization.[50] That term has also been questioned and might more accurately be "a sense of personal fulfillment," which might be achieved by all.

I believe that any such framework must also consider some class differences based on Pierre Bourdieu's concept of habitus. For the more educated and economically secure upper classes, the upper levels of Maslow's hierarchy are more easily achieved. These groups of people are more likely to engage in sport or some form of physical activity as a necessity for good health.[51] The working class, however, engages in sport to acquire esteem through their physical prowess.

Professional football player George Blanda used sport to gain esteem as well as social and economic capital. He stated, "My father was a coal miner. My first challenge was to get out of that."[52] On his retirement from professional football he remarked that "one thing I learned from George Halas [owner of the Chicago Bears team, for which he played] was that in most cases football should be a steppingstone to greater things, not an end in itself."[53]

I can provide additional examples from my own working-class family. My father was a boxing champion in the U.S. Army. He worked as a plasterer, and in his spare time he coached youth baseball and football teams. Each year he would race the members of his teams, and no one ever beat him until he was 49 years old. The runner who did so was the sectional track champion of the city of Chicago.

A few years later when he was in his midfifties he came down to the local bar where my friends and I congregated. While he was talking with the attendant at the door, a rival group tried to enter the premises and an altercation occurred. My father was about to fight with a young man in his twenties until I jumped between them and assumed the role of protector. A melee ensued, and the police arrived as I was sitting atop the assailant, holding both of his ears in my hands and pounding his head on the concrete sidewalk. The first policeman to arrive on the scene pulled me off the forlorn victim and was about to send me to incarceration when my father ran up and said, "Officer, I'll take care of this one; you've got a lot more to take care of." The policeman unknowingly thanked my father, who then whisked me away from the scene. Dad was, however, greatly upset with me and would not talk to me for an entire week. He reasoned that I had disrespected him by "taking his fight" and by assuming that "he could not take care of himself."

My father was still working at age 65 and was always meticulous about his workmanship. When a younger colleague, perhaps forty years his junior, accused him of being slow, my father challenged him to a race. As coworkers cleared pedestrians from a downtown street, the two contestants agreed to a sprint from one sewer cap to the next, approximately forty yards. My father won and thereby reclaimed his working-class pride and honor.

While his employment may have been mundane and limited as to rewards, his role as a coach enabled him to teach, nurture, and support young men in a medium that was meaningful to them, that is, sport. He served as a surrogate father to those who did not have one, even securing an education for some. Neighborhood youth turned to him for guidance. His life had a purpose as he instilled a love of physical activity in his family and teams. Research indicates that such appreciation for physical activity, as well as values and attitudes, can be generated and maintained across generations in families who value their health.[54]

My mother, always able to turn a tragedy or a mishap into a joke, possesses joie de vivre. At the age of 96 she is raising her third generation of children, for whom she serves as baseball pitcher and football quarterback. She claims that she is the only quarterback who has never been sacked. She did, however, suffer a black eye when her reflexes proved inadequate to catch a line drive off a great-grandchild's bat. Recent research validates the joy and the physical activity involved in the practice of grandparenting.[55] Throughout her life her care has extended to not only the extended family but also neighbors in need.

Despite her advanced age she maintains a quest for knowledge. She reads incessantly and nightly, often into the wee hours of the morning. She remains engaged with the larger society and the political issues of the day.

My mother, like all the athletes mentioned previously, possesses some qualities that greatly enhance the aging process.[56] These people serve as examples for all in leading a dignified and respected life. They are independent yet engaged with the larger culture. They are caring people and cheerful optimists, resilient in times of adversity and hardship. They are resourceful and train the body as well as the mind, and they have found their purpose in life. The chapters that follow provide examples of people who have aged well and offer hope, direction, and guidance for readers.

May we all aspire to such a well-lived existence, respected for our contributions to society, whatever they may be.

NOTES

1. John Withington, *Secrets of the Centenarians: What Is It like to Live for a Century and Which of Us Will Survive to Find Out?* (London: Reaktion Books, 2017), 11–15.
2. A. Diamandopoulos, "The Ideas of Plato, Aristotle, Plutarch, and Galen," *Journal of Gerontology and Geriatrics* 65 (2017), 325–28 (quotes, 326, 327).
3. Diamandopoulos, "Ideas of Plato"; Elizabeth C. J. Pike, "Physical Activity and Narratives of Successful Ageing," in *Physical Activity and Sport in Later Life*, ed. Emmanuelle Tulle and Cassandra Phoenix, 21–31 (Basingstoke, UK: Palgrave Macmillan, 2015).
4. "History of Aging: Confronting Aging, a World in Transition," Confronting Aging, accessed July 10, 2018, https://www.confrontingaging.com/history-of -aging.html; Sarah Lamb, "Beyond the View of the West: Ageing and Anthropology," in *Routledge Handbook of Cultural Gerontology*, ed. Julia Twigg and Wendy Martin, 37–44 (London: Routledge, 2015).
5. Marc McCutcheon, *Roget's Super Thesaurus* (Cincinnati: Writer's Digest Books, 1998), 22.
6. Anna Whitelock, *The Queen's Bed: An Intimate History of Elizabeth's Court* (New York: Picador, 2013), 9.
7. Stephen Lassonde, "Age and Development," in *Encyclopedia of Children and Childhood: In History and Society*, ed. Paula S. Fass, 38–45 (New York: Macmillan Reference, 2004); W. Andrew Achenbaum and L. Christian Carr, "A Brief History of Aging Services in the United States," American Society on Aging, accessed July 10, 2018, www.asaging.org/blog/brief-history-aging-services-united-states, originally printed in *Generations: Journal of the American Society on Aging* 38, no. 2 (Summer 2014), 9–13; Claire Gordon, "Timeline: A History of Elder Care in America," Aljazeera America, February 25, 2014, http://america.aljazeera .com/watch/shows/america-tonight/america-tonight-blog/2014/2/25/history -elderly-care.html; Hyung Wook Park, *Old Age, New Science: Gerontologists and Their Bi-Social Visions, 1900–1960* (Pittsburgh: University of Pittsburgh Press, 2016), 224.
8. Achenbaum and Carr, "Brief History."
9. Withington, *Secrets of the Centenarians*, 18; "History of Aging."
10. Janice I. Farkas, "Grandparents," in *Boyhood in America: An Encyclopedia*, ed. Priscilla Ferguson Clement and Jacqueline S. Reiner, 320–24 (Santa Barbara CA: ABC-CLIO, 2001); "History of Aging"; Achenbaum and Carr, "Brief History."

11. Barnet M. Berin, George J. Stolnitz, and Aaron Tenenbein, "Mortality Trends of Males and Females over the Ages," *Transactions of Society of Actuaries* 41 (1989), 9–27, accessed July 14, 2018, https://www.soa.org/library/reserach/transactions -of-society-of-actuaries/tsa89v414.pdf; Howard P. Chudacoff, *How Old Are You? Age Consciousness in American Culture* (Princeton NJ: Princeton University Press, 1989), 10, 18.

12. Thomas R. Cole, *The Journey of Life: A Cultural History of Aging in America* (New York: Cambridge University Press, 1992), 150.

13. Alcott cited in Cole, *Journey of Life*, 98; Chudacoff, *How Old Are You?*, 18–22.

14. "History of Aging"; Park, *Old Age, New Science*, 11.

15. Achenbaum and Carr, "Brief History"; Chudacoff, *How Old Are You?*, 111–13.

16. John R. Gillis, "Life Course and Transitions to Adulthood," in Fass, *Encyclopedia of Children*, 547–52 (quote, 547–48).

17. *Athletic Sports for Boys: A Repository of Graceful Recreations for Youth* (New York: Dick and Fitzgerald, 1866); Chudacoff, *How Old Are You?*, 9–28, 31–41.

18. Chudacoff, *How Old Are You?*, 43–45.

19. Chudacoff, *How Old Are You?*, 6, 24–25, 57 (quote), 58; Lawrence R. Samuel, *Aging in America: A Cultural History* (Philadelphia: University of Pennsylvania Press, 2017), 2.

20. Cole, *Journey of Life*, 143–73; Samuel, *Aging in America*, 9.

21. Gillis, "Life Course and Transitions to Adulthood," 549.

22. Chris Wienke, "Bodies," in Clement and Reiner, *Boyhood in America*, 88–94.

23. Chudacoff, *How Old Are You?*, 66–71, 106, 110 (Squires quote).

24. Chudacoff, *How Old Are You?*, 109; Cole, *Journey of Life*, xix, 200 (Hall quote); Park, *Old Age, New Science*, 35–36.

25. James A. Mangan and Roberta J. Park, eds., *From "Fair Sex" to Feminism: Sport and the Socialization of Women in the Industrial and Post-Industrial Eras* (London: Frank Cass, 1987); Patricia Vertinsky, *The Eternally Wounded Woman: Women, Exercise, and Doctors in the Late Nineteenth Century* (Manchester, UK: Manchester University Press, 1990); Gerald R. Gems, Linda J. Borish, and Gertrud Pfister, *Sports in American History: From Colonization to Globalization* (Champaign IL: Human Kinetics, 2017), 202–10.

26. Linda Simon, *Lost Girls: The Invention of the Flapper* (London: Reaktion Books, 2017), 108–35, 116 (Castle quote).

27. Simon, *Lost Girls*, 195–96, 200 (quote).

28. Simon, *Lost Girls*, 7.

29. Peter Jennings and Todd Brewster, *In Search of America* (New York: Hyperion, 2002), 127 (quote); Lucy Moore, *Anything Goes: A Biography of the Roaring Twenties* (New York: Overlook Press, 2010); Joshua Zeitz, *Flapper: A Madcap Story of Sex,*

Style, Celebrity, and the Women Who Made Modern America (New York: Crown, 2006); Stanley Coben, *Rebellion against Victorianism: The Impetus for Cultural Change in 1920s America* (New York: Oxford University Press, 1991).

30. Simon, *Lost Girls*, 197–210; Park, *Old Age, New Science*, 37.

31. Samuel, *Aging in America*, 8; Park, *Old Age, New Science*, 63–66.

32. Gems, Borish, and Pfister, *Sports in American History*, 62, 136–37, 178–79.

33. David Halberstam, *The Fifties* (New York: Villard Books, 1993); Howard P. Chudacoff, "Adolescence and Youth," in Fass, *Encyclopedia of Children*, 15–20.

34. Jefferson Cowie, *Stayin' Alive: The 1970s and the Last Days of the Working Class* (New York: New Press, 2010); Samuel, *Aging in America*, 11.

35. Emmanuelle Tulle, "Physical Activity and Sedentary Behavior: A Vital Politics of Old Age," 9–20; Pike, "Physical Activity and Narratives"; Rylee A. Dionigi, "Pathways to Masters Sport: Sharing Stories from Sport 'Continuers,' 'Rekindlers' and 'Late Bloomers,'" 54–68, all in Tulle and Phoenix, *Physical Activity and Sport in Later Life*; Cassandra Phoenix and Meridith Griffen, "Sport, Physical Activity and Ageing," 329–36, in Twigg and Martin, *Routledge Handbook of Cultural Gerontology*.

36. Cole, *Journey of Life*, 169 (Lamm quote), 237.

37. Bruce Grierson, *What Makes Olga Run? The Mystery of the 90-Something Track Star and What She Can Teach Us about Living Longer, Happier Lives* (New York: Henry Holt, 2014), 194.

38. Margaret Morganroth Gullette, "Aged by Culture," in Twigg and Martin, *Routledge Handbook of Cultural Gerontology*, 21–28.

39. Gillis, "Life Course and Transitions to Adulthood," 551.

40. Chudacoff, *How Old Are You?*, 175–80; Park, *Old Age, New Science*, 246; Tamara Lytle, "The Older Americans Act," *AARP Bulletin* 60, no. 3 (April 2019), 6–7.

41. Laura Hurd Clarke and Erica V. Bennett, "Gender, Ageing, and Appearance," in Twigg and Martin, *Routledge Handbook of Cultural Gerontology*, 133–40; Samuel, *Aging in America*, 3, 25, 52–56, 64–70, 88 (quote), 109, 127, 149, 150.

42. Samuel, *Aging in America*, 90.

43. Samuel, *Aging in America*, 2; Cynthia Alford, "Reconceptualizing Aging," *Academic Medicine* 79, no. 7 (July 2004), vii–viii; Jessica Pace, "Reconceptualizing Aging among North American Older Indigenous Peoples," International Network for Critical Gerontology, accessed January 30, 2021, https://criticalgerontology.com.

44. Samuel, *Aging in America*, 2.

45. Rylee A. Dionigi, "Competitive Sport as Leisure in Later Life," *Leisure Sciences* 28, no. 2 (2006), 181–96.

46. Abraham H. Maslow, "A Theory of Human Motivation," *Psychological Review* 50, no. 4 (1943), 370–96.

47. Tulle, "Physical Activity and Sedentary Behavior," 9–20; Cassandra Phoenix and Noreen Orr, "The Multidimensionality of Pleasure in Later Life," 101–12; Gertrud Pfister and Verena Lenneis, "Ageing Women Still Play Games: (Auto) Ethnographic Research in a Fitness Intervention," 149–60, both in Tulle and Phoenix, *Physical Activity and Sport in Later Life*.

48. Matthew Carroll and Helen Bartlett, "Ageing Well across Cultures," in Twigg and Martin, *Routledge Handbook of Cultural Gerontology*, 285–92.

49. Jack Fox, "Maslow's 'Hierarchy of Needs': A Critique," Medium, August 20, 2020, https://medium.com/@lodder77/maslows-hierarchy-of-needs-a-critique -f2669ef9fcc1; Ryan Mutuku, "Major Criticisms of Maslow's Hierarchy of Needs," accessed January 30, 2021, https://www.tuko.co.ke/314803-major-criticisms -maslow-hierarchy-needs.html.

50. Ryan Mutuku, "Major Criticisms of Maslow Hierarchy of Needs," September 17, 2019, https://www.tuko.co.ke/314803-major-criticisms-maslow-hierarchy -needs.html.

51. Tamar Z. Semerjian, "The Role of Gender and Social Class in Physical Activity in Later Life," in *The Palgrave Handbook of Ageing and Physical Activity Promotion*, ed. Samuel R. Nyman, Anna Barker, Terry Haines, Khim Horton, Charles Musselwhite, Geeske Peeters, Christina R, Victor, and Julia Katharina Wolff, 571–88 (London: Palgrave Macmillan, 2018).

52. Hubert Mizell, "Blanda Thrives on Challenges," *Tampa Bay Times*, December 28, 1974, 5.

53. David Condon, "Stabler and Blanda Recall Raider Loss," *Chicago Tribune*, February 13, 1975, 53.

54. Victoria J. Palmer, "Keeping It in the Family: The Generational Transmission of Physical Activity," in Tulle and Phoenix, *Physical Activity and Sport in Later Life*, 69–80; Christine Kenneally, *The Invisible History of the Human Race* (New York: Viking, 2014), 139–58.

55. Sara Arber and Virpi Timonen, "Grandparenting," in Twigg and Martin, *Routledge Handbook of Cultural Gerontology*, 234–42.

56. Amy M. Gayman, Jessica Fraser-Thomas, Rylee Dionigi, Sean Horton, and Joseph Baker, "Is Sport Good for Older Adults? A Systematic Review of Psychosocial Outcomes of Older Adults' Sport Participation," *International Review of Sport and Exercise Psychology* 10, no. 1 (January 2017), 164–85; Joseph Baker, Jessica Fraser-Thomas, Rylee Dionigi, and Sean Horton, "Sport Participation and Positive Development in Older Persons," *European Review of Aging and Physical Activity* 7, no. 3 (2009), 3–12.

2   Life with a Purpose

FRANCES GEMS

My name is Frances Ann Gems, and I was born on a very cold day, February 22, 1925, in Chicago, Illinois. I was told that I weighed barely five pounds at birth and was eager to make my debut. My parents were immigrants from Monreale, a small town in Sicily, in Italy. Though they were from the same town, they did not know each other there but met on the boat that brought them to America. My mother and her family settled in Chicago. My father also settled in Chicago, and since he traveled alone, he was taken in by friends until he could find employment and support himself. The couple eventually married and settled in an area known as Little Sicily, close to St. Philip Benizi Church, where they became parishioners along with other families from Monreale. Much of their social life centered on church activities. An important activity for new immigrants was to attend classes to learn the new language, English, so they could find employment to help support their families. Soon all the families from Monreale were dinner guests at others' homes.

My parents lived in that area for some time and eventually were able to combine their income with the little that my grandparents had and purchase the home I was born in. My father was able to learn the English language well, and that ability helped him to get employment in the building trades. At that time in their lives, my parents and the other Sicilian immigrants in the neighborhood were considered lower class, because many had been peasants with little education and their appearance gave the impression that they were illiterate.

Despite our working-class background, I never experienced any prejudice growing up, not in school nor in employment. We lived in a mixed neighborhood with many other ethnic, working-class groups of immigrant families. In high school I had many friends of different nationalities, and we enjoyed talking about our different cultures with no discomfort or prejudice. In employment I was never overlooked because of my ancestry. I was employed because I was capable of doing the work and was happy to be a part of the working class.

Growing up, I was happy to be a part of our family. I had three older brothers and two sisters (five other siblings were stillborn or died in early childhood). My favorite sibling was my brother Frank, called "Chico" by all who knew him, family and friends. He got the nickname as a youth when his friends misheard my mother calling him "Francisco" in her broken English.

During the summer months our family would meet with relatives and friends, then drive out to a forest preserve picnic area in Wheeling, Illinois (now a northwest suburb of Chicago), to enjoy an all-day picnic with food, music, and games. The men would cook over a large, open grill, while other men played horseshoes and the women entertained the children. There was always someone who played an accordion to entertain us and add to the dancing and laughter. Those picnics would last from early morning to early evening, when everyone decided it was time to go home. Those summer days were very happy ones.

As I grew up, we made our own fun, playing outdoors. There wasn't any extra money in the household budget to spend on so-called fun time. I roller-skated on the street in front of our house, jumped rope with my girlfriends, and drew a hopscotch pattern with chalk on the sidewalk and challenged other kids to compete by jumping through the game without falling. And of course we always played tag. We had to stay close to the house, because in Italian culture the girls are sheltered and my father was very protective, so our social relations beyond the family were limited.

While my childhood was generally a happy one, I also had some sad times in my life, the first when I was only thirteen years old. My oldest brother Sam had been home from the Civilian Conservation Corps (a work program for unemployed young men during the Depression era to build environmental projects in remote areas) only a year when he became very ill, his condition getting worse with each passing week. After many trips to the doctor and many tests, the doctors told my parents he was suffering from a brain tumor without a cure and he was not a candidate for surgery. My brother suffered so much pain, and in the last few weeks of his life he became blind. I felt very sad because I could not help in any way to ease his pain. He passed away on November 2, 1938, at the age of 23, a short time before my eighth-grade graduation. I never had the chance to really get to know him as I grew up, and that sadness stayed with me for some years to come.

My second bout of depression occurred with the unexpected death of my mother at the age of sixty-one. My daughter was born shortly thereafter, but she never got to know my loving mother. My third bout of sadness occurred with the passing of my older sister in 2003. We had been not only sisters but also lifelong friends who lived only a block apart and talked daily. The death of my husband of fifty-nine years only two years later was a huge blow to me and our family. My brother Chico then died in 2017 at the age of 95, another setback but an inevitable culmination of life. He and my husband were known throughout our neighborhood for their charity and help to others in need.

I prefer to remember the good times. We had many fun times, especially holidays. My favorite was Christmas. Our house was the gathering place for at least three or four related families, complete with all the kids coming for dinner and exchanging small gifts. Our day consisted of going to church on Christmas morning, coming home to a small breakfast, waiting for all the relatives to come for dinner, and opening our gifts. The dinner was always prepared by my mother and grandmother. In our Italian culture the sharing of food is a symbol of love, one we continue to share with the extended family today.

Our gifts were minor, sometimes clothing, a new game, or a coloring book and crayons. I enjoyed playing with all my cousins, singing and dancing around the dining room table, until it was time for all the girls to clean up the table and get busy washing dishes. It was really a fun time for all of us.

My older sister Rose and I enjoyed singing together. We put the radio on and sang to all the songs that were popular during that era. My father would tell us to keep the volume down so he could hear his program on the big radio in the front room. On Saturdays after we finished our chores, we could rent a bicycle for twenty-five cents an hour and ride around the neighborhood. We did not own a bicycle, only a wagon that the boys could use to deliver newspapers and make some additional money. There were times on Sundays when my father had a little extra money and we could go to the neighborhood show (or movie theater) called the Easterly for twenty-five cents and for ten cents more get a box of popcorn. For that price we could see a full movie plus two cartoons. Those times remain as fond memories of growing up.

I also have fond memories of my school years. I started kindergarten when I was one month shy of being 5 years old, the usual starting age. My mother took me to Agassiz School on my first day of school and promised me a treat if I was a good girl and didn't cry for her. The teacher took my hand and introduced me to all the other children already there, and I was comfortable in my new surroundings. At noon my mother came to take me home, and I can still remember how excited I was to tell her of all the activity we had that morning. I enjoyed school from that day on.

In that era parents had the choice of kindergarten hours, mornings or afternoons. My mother chose mornings so that I could go to school with my older sister and brother and come home with them at lunchtime. Lunch was always from twelve to one o'clock, so after lunch, children had time to play in the schoolyard before classes resumed again. From grades one to five I was more or less quiet, not volunteering for many activities. I was unable to participate in more organized activities in the schoolyard after school hours due to shyness and parental restraints. From grades six to eight I became more vocal, joining the glee club, library club, and the debating team. I was also the sprint champion in schoolyard races.

Eighth grade brought fond memories. Our graduation program was planned, and I was given a star role, singing a solo. I was thrilled when it was well received by the audience in the auditorium. That was the beginning of my dream to become a professional singer. Upon my graduation, my music teacher, Miss Houlihan, wanted me to go on and take voice lessons, even offering to pay for them. She told me that I was blessed with a gift and should develop it further. My father thanked her but refused her offer, as he wanted me to go to high school and get a good education and, he hoped, a good job. So I continued to sing for my own pleasure and to sing with my sister Rose as we washed dishes. I later got to sing in amateur plays at our church auditorium.

Upon graduating from elementary school, I enrolled at Waller High School, where I enjoyed four years of fun and learning, making new friends and joining the drama club and choir. I did not participate in any sports, as very little was offered to girls at that time, only cheerleading and baton twirling. Sports were dominated by the male students. I can only identify with female athletes in appreciation of their dedication to their skills. As an adult I became much more involved in sports as a supporter and a spectator. My husband coached youth baseball and football teams in his leisure hours, and later the young men of the community formed a semipro football team and prevailed upon him to be their coach. All three of my children, as well as my grandson and great-grandchildren, became athletes. In my childcare duties with the great-grandchildren, I sometimes serve as the pitcher for their baseball games and the quarterback for their football games in my backyard. I remain a loyal and cheering spectator at their local park district and traveling team games.

Today my hobbies and interests are varied. I enjoy music, reading, gardening, meeting people, and travel anywhere, and I always enjoy the company of all my grandchildren when they have time to come for a visit.

Aging can be a difficult process for some. In my culture people are considered elderly when they reach the age of 80. Between the ages of 70 and 80, many people are still healthy and able to participate in exercises and sports. I enjoyed walking and visiting people into my 90s. The government also offers services to assist the elderly such as Medicare (government health insurance), home care for those in need, exercise classes, and in some cases hospice care. As to my own aging body, I find myself curtailed in some ways. I walk more slowly and cannot do as much as I used to do, and I have lost the independence to come and go without restriction that

I enjoyed in earlier years. Now I must wait for a family member to take me to doctor's visits and shopping. I was capable of all that on my own earlier in my life, but now I must rely on family help.

The aging process can, however, be enjoyed with changing habits. Diets can be changed to eat less and healthier, we can use less caffeine and refrain from smoking, and we can continue to enjoy family and an active social life. I have found that a sense of humor can brighten one's day, and I enjoy joking and repartee with family and friends. Physical activity depends on the elderly person's ability to participate in sports such as golf, bowling, yoga, swimming, and daily walking. Much of my activity comes from playing and chasing my great-grandchildren around the house and yard.

As I look back on my life, I am still very proud of a role I assumed many years ago. I was elected the president of the Mothers' Club at St. Alphonsus School, where I also served as the cook for fifteen hundred children. As president of the club, I increased our membership to five hundred mothers, and to my knowledge that number has never been exceeded. Our members had one goal: raising funds to supplement whatever was needed in each classroom. I do have a characteristic of persistence and a commitment to people as a goal in my life. My goal as president of the club was to provide for the children of the school. Under my leadership, all the members put their trust in me, working together to reach our goal. Being able to respect all opinions and to compromise proved to be the key to my success. It was a demanding time in my life but also a fun time. To achieve harmony with five hundred women was a challenge, but it enabled me to become a successful president. To this day I have conversations with some women who still remember me from so long ago in the Mothers' Club.

Such leadership also pushed me to provide charity for other neighborhood residents in need. When a fire destroyed a neighbor's home, I canvassed the neighborhood, collecting food and clothing for them. When another birthed eleven children, virtually one annually, I donated my time to assist her with cooking and household chores. Our neighborhood was a community rather than just a place of residence.

I take pride in my greatest success, being partners with my husband, Gerald. We raised three children (two boys and a girl) to become loving, caring adults who in their own ways have chosen careers that brought them happiness and wise employment. They are now parents with families of their own and show love and respect and involvement in their children's lives.

Yes, "family is everything." To reach that accomplishment, my husband and I took great pride in their schoolwork and in their participation in sports, giving them all our love and encouragement in whatever they wanted to pursue. Their friends were always welcome in our house, and we considered and treated them as extended members of the family.

I remember one occasion when my son, Gerald, wrote an essay about why his mother should be crowned "queen for a day." It was a contest sponsored by a well-known businessman in Chicago. My son's essay told the public about all of the good things I had done and of the love he had for me as his mother. His prize for winning the contest was a family dinner at a famous restaurant, and I received a fur coat. Needless to say, I was thrilled beyond words, and that occasion will be in my memories forever.

During World War II I took pride in writing letters every week to my brother Chico and to all my cousins who were in the military service, telling them what was happening in our families and in our neighborhoods. Letters from home brought comfort to them, being so far away from home. When my brother came home on leave, he thanked me for my letters, telling me that they helped him through some perilous times. Writing cheerful letters was not a hard task compared with what my brother and other veterans lived through.

Besides reminiscing, the particular joys of aging come from seeing your children mature into young adults who define goals for themselves, accept responsibilities, and enjoy long and healthy lives. When the grandchildren come along, aging gives us further blessings. We get to interact with them, answer questions, play games, enjoy all of their antics, attend sporting events they are a part of, and love, spoil, and cherish them for as long as we are here on this earth.

The fears in aging are serious illness, being alone without any social contact, living at a distance away from family, and being alone in an emergency, unable to ask for help. This is so true for many people.

Does age bring greater wisdom? That question has been asked many times over the years, and I would answer that the person making an important decision in their life as to a personal matter, employment, or a financial problem needs to make good choices. I do not think that age alone solves problems, but it helps to give wisdom to people who are struggling. With age comes understanding, compassion, and respect, and these characteristics are what I see as aging being a path to greater wisdom. As a person matures, wisdom should be a goal in life.

The most trying time of my life occurred with the death of my husband. It was not unexpected, as I nursed him through his later years of debility. But still I missed him every day, especially at night, eating dinner alone, not having him close by to speak to about family, sports, and whatever happened at work. I missed going to church with him and seeing him coach young men from the neighborhood in football. Our home was so empty without him. There were times I found myself just looking at his clothes in our closet.

My children were towers of strength and help for me, and I slowly became more involved with my grandchildren, socializing with my friends from my parish church, reminiscing with my brother, Chico, and getting busy with my garden. My children and my brother gave me love, comfort, and total support. They were the pillars of my strength and recovery.

I have been fortunate in that I have never had any serious health problems. One exception is that as I age, I have to contend with glaucoma, but that is being treated with daily eye drops.

Another benefit is my disposition. I consider myself to be an optimist. I wake up each morning to take on each new day, thankful for family and friends. Love has been my life. Love of family and friends and all good things that lead to happiness for other people. Friends have always been important to me. They bring us together in times of joy and in sorrow. I can honestly say that I have enjoyed the friendship of several people from my parish church for fifty years. How many people can say that?

I do engage in nostalgia at times, looking through albums of old photos taken during family vacations and more recent photos of weddings, grandchildren growing up, and family and friends enjoying our fiftieth wedding anniversary festivities. It brings back pleasant memories of my husband.

I have only one regret in my life, that my husband was not able to live long enough to enjoy our great-grandchildren. He would have loved them all, and they in turn would have loved telling him of all their sports activities. He would have told them about his life in the army, when he was a regimental boxing champion and played on a baseball team while stationed in Alaska. Although he never bragged about his accomplishments, as a coach he also served as a mentor to many young men in need of guidance. Our great-grandchildren would have benefited from his counsel.

I would like to be remembered as a loving grandma who not only gave hugs and kisses free with every visit to all her grandchildren and great-grandchildren but also told them all they were my favorites. I want to be remembered for enjoying birthdays and holidays with family, and for cooking special pasta meals for Thanksgiving and Christmas holidays. It wasn't a holiday if we didn't have a platter of pasta, a traditional Italian meal, and of course the threat of using my wooden spoon on anyone involved in any mischief. I also want to be remembered as a grandma who loved each grandchild and great-grandchild for their individual talents, love, and devotion that made my life so happy and so complete, all of them treasured in my heart forever.

As I look to the future, I have several hopes and wishes. I sincerely hope for world peace among future generations. My hope for our nation is that its people come together and remove the divisive hatred that is prevalent in all parts of our country. We should really help the poor people who need more food and better housing, improve education for children who are just getting by, help immigrants to settle in our country, and give love and respect to all people no matter what their ancestry or faith might be.

3 Looking Back

TONY KALETH

I was born shortly after the Second World War, on July 6, 1947. Both of my parents were involved in the war. My father was a trumpeter in the Army Air Corps band stationed in Liverpool, England, where he met my mother. Born and raised mostly in Liverpool, she survived to see the city she knew well reduced to rubble by the German air force. For months at a time, both endured nearly daily bombings, usually together in the underground subway. My father was born in the United States. Both of his parents were Polish immigrants. My mother emigrated from England to the United States immediately after the war. My father joined her in Chicago several months later. They lived with my aunt and uncle in the Albany Park neighborhood, which was, at that time, part of the city's Polish ghetto. While my father did not speak Polish, almost all of his brothers and sisters either spoke it or could understand it.

His family were devout members of the Roman Catholic Church and were active members of the St. Hyacinth parish. I was baptized at that church one week after my birth. My mother, however, was never affiliated with an organized religion. Shortly before my first birthday, my parents divorced. At that time, for reasons never explained to me, I was "placed" by my uncle, who was then a Roman Catholic priest and the de facto head of the Kaleth family, in the home of my father's sister. I remained with her for much of the next twenty years, until I was married in 1969.

I saw my father maybe ten times while I lived with his sister and her husband and their son. I never knew my mother until much, much later in life when we were reunited. I attended St. Andrew School for my elementary education and, later, Gordon Technical High School, both Catholic institutions. We lived mainly in the neighborhood adjacent to Riverview Park, at the time one of the largest amusement parks in the country and probably the world.

During those times, it seemed everyone played outside, and I loved playing whatever game was current. It didn't take long to discover sports. I lived for those summer days when we would play ball from nearly morning to evening. While baseball was my first love, it was actually the first of many. I think that I actually loved football the most. Playing sports gave me more than something to do. It gave me something to be . . . an athlete. From a very early time in my life, I identified myself in this very exclusive manner. I was an athlete. While I also loved music, that was a field that was for all purposes closed to me. My "mom" was well aware of the pitfalls that could befall someone who went into that field. Her father and my own father were both professional musicians. Both suffered, maybe not coincidentally, from alcoholism. As such, I was never encouraged to pursue music beyond listening to it. Music didn't consume me, however, quite like sports did. In high school I was unable to make the basketball team but still played casually throughout the year. I planned on playing football but suffered a season-ending injury while playing a casual pickup game with my college-aged cousin and his friends. Then I saw a poster about trying out for the track team, and the proverbial rest is history. Once I began to train for track, the other sports mostly fell by the wayside. I did enjoy golf during this period and managed to play quite a bit into my forties but did not have a good golfing disposition. So, from 1962 until the present, I have been a runner. I ran in high school and ran when I attended college. After the birth of my son, running became more of a sporadic activity, but I still thought of it as my hobby and identity even though I would not run for months at a time.

I sometimes experienced a bit of discomfort due to my working-class background. I do not think that I experienced any prejudice regarding who I was, but I did feel, in college, that I was a stranger in a strange land. Indeed, on a visit to North Central College in a suburb of Chicago, after my first train ride ever, I remember walking back from the fieldhouse after my visit with the athletic director and the track coach and having an epiphany— "This is where Dick and Jane must have lived!"—as I recalled the long-ago characters from that ubiquitous basic reader series. I knew for certain they didn't live in my neighborhood or anywhere else that I went in Chicago. I don't think that I ever felt comfortable during my college years in the town of Naperville. But that discomfort paled when compared with the turmoil that had been inside me since childhood. My family life had been very unsettling. I suspect that I suffered from depression long before I had a word to describe what I was feeling. And I had what might now be called an anger problem. I have had suicidal thoughts most of my life. I never knew until much later why I didn't "have" a mother and a father. Maybe a more accurate way of saying that was I never knew why I didn't live with them. I have always been grateful for the family that I had, but I can say with a high degree of certainty that I always missed what I didn't have . . . my actual mom and dad. I was never adopted, and no one had actual legal custody of me, but in those days few asked questions. After several years of living with my dad's sister and her husband and son, the husband passed away when I was in second grade. We moved for the third time, and I was placed with my "mom's" sister-in-law and her family for just over two years. I would stay with them for the school week and go home on the weekend. Years later a cousin would share this thought with me. "You cried when you left us and you cried when you left your mom every single week." I have a foggy recollection of those partings. One summer during my tenth year I was exiled to Wisconsin to live with another of my dad's sisters. I have never discovered why this happened, but it wasn't a happy time. I did enjoy school because it gave me something to do during the days, but I lived for after school, to play and to explore. And though I had friends, I always felt lonely. I do not recall ever talking about this problem with anyone as a child or even as an adult for many, many years.

I do recall playing sports at my elementary school and with my friends in the neighborhood. While the school games were well-organized intramural activities like soccer, basketball, football, and softball, the games in my neighborhood were loosely organized. Teams would be picked and we would play, more often than not, in the streets by our homes or at the neighborhood playground. We could play for hours unsupervised. I took great comfort and excitement in these casual competitions. Later, during my high school years, I participated in interscholastic competitions in track and field but still played basketball regularly for fun and relaxation.

I felt very comfortable in my own city neighborhood where I had friends and freedom that only summer brings. I frequented Riverview Park, whose motto became my own: "Forget your cares and laugh your troubles away." I'm fairly certain that I didn't live up to that motto.

A kind assessment of me after completing my college education would be that I was lost. Looking back, I suspect that I was terrified and couldn't find a place in the world. While I never abused alcohol or drugs, I never hesitated to abuse and degrade myself. An abusive internal editor is very hard to live with.

I think that for the longest time my identity was merged with my running—both metaphorically and in reality. I have been a runner since I was 14. My introduction to that sport came in the middle of a Chicago winter, and even the harshness of the elements didn't seem to discourage me. And while I may have had some talent, I never felt that I accomplished what I should have accomplished physically. So, while I might not have been a good runner, I was still a runner. At the time, this status provided me with inclusion in a select group of athletes. It was still rare to come across another runner while my friends and I trotted down to Lincoln Park. And when we did come upon someone else, we always knew who it was. It was quite a comforting feeling that the park seemed to belong to us. Even today, when it's not unusual to see hundreds of runners in a day down there, it's a comforting feeling to recall those days of yore.

It seems I have lived various lives. But in reality, my life can be divided into two parts. The first was before my son was born, and the second was after that moment. I'm not sure what happened, but when I became Anton's dad, my life changed. It is akin to the biblical story of the centurion Saul on the road to Damascus. He sees God, and his life is never the same afterward.

Becoming a dad gave me insight into where I came from and, much to my surprise, where I was going. I was not sure how to be a dad, because I never had one, but even though I was afraid I would fail, I stuck it out. I certainly knew what not having a dad was like, and that was my inspiration. And because of the birth of my son, I had a different identity. I was still a runner, but now I was Anton's dad . . . and I am still Anton's dad today. Once I had an adjunct identity, it seemed that my life took a different direction. I went back to school to earn my teaching credentials. I secured work as a public school teacher. I even managed to get a master's degree and certification as a reading teacher. For the very first time in my life, I managed to have a nearly perfect grade point average. I was motivated beyond anything that I ever recall. And I assumed another identity. I was a teacher. I am now retired, but I still work at a library, trying to help folks enhance their literacy.

While I use the word *demons* cautiously, it seems that I have come to acknowledge them and perhaps put some to rest. Putting these words on paper, letting them seep out of my fingers and onto the keyboard, has been strangely helpful. I'm not sure if this current recollection has helped, but it certainly hasn't hurt. I'm so much calmer and at peace now than I have ever been.

I have several hobbies currently. I collect musical instruments. I love to travel. I actively advocate for literacy. I enjoy sports. I am still a runner, though that is not my exclusive identity anymore. I am a student of the guitar and play regularly. I read daily. I truly love to build objects out of wood. Home repair is a passion of mine. I am a father and a grandfather. I also loved being a teacher, and while it is not my profession any longer, I occasionally revert to that role at the library where I work on a temporary basis when advising parents on their children's literacy development. History is another of my avocations.

As I age, I contemplate the aging process in American culture. I am not trying to be sarcastic, but it has been my experience that the age of 25 or 30 is the dividing line between youth and older folks. In my own experience, I found the dividing line in this manner. I realized early on that the family I grew up in had very defined roles. Most of our family get-togethers took place at a particular aunt and uncle's house. During those gatherings there were three specific locations in which people placed themselves. The kids would be playing in the yard or, when it got dark, playing board or card games in the dining room. The men would sit in the kitchen and talk and generally nurse their beers. The women remained in the living room, talking. Near the end of the evening, everyone would gather in the living room and sing. Afterward we would gather in the dining room for cake and coffee before heading out into the night. I was struck that no adult, male or female, ever ventured into the yard or the dining room to play with us kids. In my observation, it was marriage that demarcated the elderly or those who didn't play anymore. As I've grown older, I realize that I live in a youth-oriented culture that seems to totally embrace youth over everything else.

For most of my life I have been a runner. I view my body, subsequently, as that of an athlete. While I understand some of the factors that have caused my slowness as I age, I do not understand all of them. The fact is that my body cannot perform as it did even five years ago. While ten or twelve years ago, I could have still built a house by myself or with the occasional aid of another, I cannot do that now. As a runner, workouts and competitions that I performed a decade ago are totally impossible. I've grown weaker. But it would be too easy to stop there and understand that this deterioration will continue until I stop breathing one day. While there are restrictions on many things, some things carry no restrictions. I can still create music and still be thrilled listening to it. I can travel more now than ever before. I can become a better husband and friend and dad and granddad. I have more time to read if that is what I choose. In the end, we have to find our own limits and not simply accept what may or may not be accurate. I have never been 72 before . . . what excitement awaits me?

In fairness, some days are harder than others in coping with a body that is aging. Memory is often a difficult companion, especially as an athlete. My workouts were measured and compiled. Clocks don't lie. I can recall specific races and practices. It is this recall that can be so unsettling, as I cannot duplicate those sessions. Sometimes there is a sadness that is hard to bear regarding aging because of the comparisons between the past and the present. But then I realize that if I don't start my watch, the running process is virtually still the same. I can still run fast, and I can, with patience, run far. My body doesn't feel quite the same, but the feeling I now get is close enough to fool me.

I have adopted some coping mechanisms. First and foremost, I think dietary changes have been important to maintain energy levels. Eating intelligently (which I don't always do) is one way to cope. More rest is important. I take naps during the day because I don't sleep soundly for eight hours any longer. I allow more time to complete various tasks because I'm a slower (and way more careful) worker. I arrange for people to help me when I need it in various projects. My balance has never been great, but it's gotten to the point where I don't do any work on the roof. So, when faced with a project that requires climbing above the second story, I get help. In the last few years, I have hired workmen to do projects that I would have taken on myself when I was younger. Even at my temporary library work, I find that my attention drifts after six or seven hours. To improve my general fitness, I have taken to lifting weight to increase the strength of my upper body that had become much weaker than my lower body. I rarely run intensely, as the recovery period is almost astronomical. The risk of injury is high, and the amount of time to heal even a minor setback is substantial. Being mindful of where I am in time and space might sum up my current condition. I am far better at making alterations in a plan than I ever have been. Defining success has changed also. Socially, my wife and I have never been active. When we do engage in something social, it is usually in the daylight hours. Evenings are our less favored time, as fatigue seems to come way too early. In spite of that, I think my wife and I are best friends. I cannot imagine going on this final journey without her. To have someone who supports me and values and embraces the endeavors that I value is priceless.

I can look back with pride on some personal achievements. I don't think anything has given me quite the satisfaction that being a dad to my son has. Because I never really had a dad or a role model for being a dad, I was determined to be my son's father. Fortunately, he let me. Any other successes I may have had along the way flow from being Anton's dad. I have learned to be a good husband, and maybe that success has to do with the third time being a charm. Of all the failures in my life, being an awful husband the first two tries has a lasting sting. I have long wondered if I had a fear of intimacy or a fear of being left. It's quite an academic wonder, as I was not the husband that I've become. Maybe it is because of aging that I've come to appreciate what a wonderful partner I have. I also think my tendency to flee was negated by the realization that many, many years have passed and my wife and I are still together . . . still looking forward and not behind us. I suspect it has more to do with being a dad to my son. Becoming a father terrified me. Once I realized that I can only do my best and will be forgiven for the mistakes I make along the way, I think it was easier to transfer that knowledge to being a spouse.

I also have great pride in the teacher that I became. It was such an inspiration . . . going to school every day and finding myself in the presence of genius. My career was spent with kids who were reputed to be struggling both in school and outside the academic environment. In all honesty, I struggled way more than they did. Their courage and perseverance remain among my most powerful inspirations.

I am grateful to have discovered the guitar later in life. I simply love spending time with it to discover the mystery that is music. Building furniture has given me such satisfaction, too. Running has also been a very special time for me. I was not a very good competitive runner, and because my identity was based on that, I suffered greatly. But the simple and pure act of running has always been so rewarding. The results of competition, less so.

I am not sure that I can identify the qualities that help me to achieve these successes. I think fear played a big role. Certainly reflecting on insight I gleaned as I grew older was beneficial. I also think a certain amount of stubbornness contributed. And I think a willingness to stay in the present was vital to most of my endeavors. Finally, being able to dream and being able to disregard common sense were vital. I don't want to sound righteous, but listening to my heart has been a light in the darkness for me. Keeping hope alive in any way possible is helpful to provide meaning in one's life. Tomorrow is a new day.

One encounters both fears and joys in aging. Even as a little boy, I feared death. In talking with people, I realized that I went to many more funerals by the time I was 10 than anyone else I knew. They left their mark on me for certain. As I approach that time, I'm not quite as frightened. I am also too busy living and doing "stuff" to pay much attention. If anything, death will probably be an inconvenience. I know, however, that death occupies a more prominent place in my psyche these days. My wife and I have talked about it. One of us will know a unique aloneness, and that nearly breaks my heart. Should she pass first, the sadness will be monumental. I will be sad that she is gone. If she's the one left, I will be sad to have caused her such agony. Having said these things about death, it is a real prod to stay in the present.

Some of the joys: I got to see my son mature into a self-sufficient man. I have watched him develop into a wonderful father. I have witnessed my grandson turn 21 and cope with struggles that we've all experienced. I've been inspired by both of them and, by observing them, have come to understand something about my early life and how some of those slings and arrows made me who I am. In regard to wisdom, I'm not sure that I know what that is. I listen to myself more these days than I ever did when I was younger. I try to remember that the present is all we have and to embrace it fully. I am careful of what I say to others. I wear my seatbelt when I drive. I value my friends more than ever.

I think that the setbacks that I faced were invisible at the time but, looking back, I see them more clearly. I think the very first real setback—beyond my athletic failures—was going to college and feeling very, very lost and alone. I was clearly awkward in the company of my fellow students. I was unsure of my ability to survive there intellectually but also emotionally. I also discovered during the first semester that I was considered and marked as poor and underprivileged. The college had regular visitation to a mission they established in Chicago to work with the poor. The problem was that the mission was in my own neighborhood. My father died my sophomore year. We were clearly not close, though I spent more time with him during his last month on earth than ever before. I knew when I left for school that September that I wouldn't see him alive again, but it was still a shock when he was gone. In typical fashion, I would simply store those emotions away. I took sick shortly after his death and had to return home for nearly three weeks of total bed rest. It was impossible to do any schoolwork. The grades that I received that semester were simply gifts. While I eventually graduated from college, I realized, more than ever before, that I was unprepared intellectually for the challenges that college presented. I was subsequently married thrice and even though I knew that I shouldn't have married that first time, I still went through with it. Eventually, I moved away from the only place I knew as home to someplace where I knew no one. I'm not sure of the impetus behind that move, even today.

I cannot count the number of jobs that I've had, and most were unrewarding. I did manage to find a job that was more to my liking at the library in Denver and have remained connected to that job (and subsequent ones within that organization) to this day. I also became a teacher, which was one of the very best experiences that I've ever had. It was, looking back, a true vocation.

Depression has been a constant companion. I have felt suicidal at times. While I have never acted overtly to end my life, I have put myself in very dangerous situations where I might be accidentally killed. I do not know that I have ever coped with many of these setbacks and subsequent swings of emotions. I compartmentalize much of the uncomfortable memories that I have. Oddly, I think running may have helped . . . it was a tool to engender fatigue. I have always listened to music to soothe my soul and to lift my spirits. Reading has helped. I have sought out professionals for help, both doctors and psychologists. I've also let myself be consumed by various projects. For instance, when I did resign from that teaching position, I was distraught and totally lost. But I also happened to commence painting my house. It was a big house and hadn't been painted for at least a quarter of a century. Conservatively, I would think, that summer I spent at least ten hours a day prepping and painting. Fortunately, I was also married to my third wife, who was a good listener, among other things. The look of pain that I recall on her face that summer has never left me. Clearly, these were things that I did to alleviate the sadness or the fear that I was feeling, but at the time, I just wanted to get through the day.

By most measures, I would think that the term *optimist* fits me more than *pessimist*. Outwardly, most people would agree with that emphatically.

On the inside, it is more of a battle. Having said that, however, I do look forward to tomorrow and the next day and the next. At 72 years of age, I know that resiliency is a necessity because of the challenges life gives us. I do engage in nostalgia. It is like a brother to me. Yet I would wholly endorse the classic definition that includes the pain of looking back. But I have always seen time accumulation. While an event may seem in the past, it is part of the present . . . if that makes any sense. I know it makes sense to me, but I'm not trying to proselytize anyone else.

Friendship and love have surely helped to heal wounds. Without a single whisper of doubt, I know that without love I would not still be in this world. It is the alpha and omega of my life. It is the one thing that keeps us tethered to life on this planet. Without friendships and, more important, love, what is the point of hanging around?

I have some regrets, most notably the pain that I've caused in the lives of others, particularly my ex-wives and those with whom I've had conflicts during various employments. I have wasted inordinate amounts of time and squandered valuable opportunities. The list goes on. In the words of one of my favorite poems, "It was a summer of limitless bites . . . or hungers quickly felt and quickly forgotten." Having said that, to my own amazement, it seems like some of the behaviors that haunt me most were necessary to get me to the present. I very much look forward to the next day and the surprises that might await me. I am happy to have gotten to know my son and my grandson and appreciate the inspiration that they've given me. I cannot imagine life without my dear wife. About death, it would be inconvenient if it showed up tomorrow. I actually like the feeling I have now about where I am and how I got here. I am not sure if that's fulfillment, but I'll take it regardless of the word.

I have not thought about my legacy. I want my son and my grandson and my wife to know that I will love them forever just because of who they are, not because of something they've done. When I taught school, I wanted the kids to know that I cared about them and that they were way smarter than they felt. I guess, in a way, I have thought about my legacy and it is this: he was someone who gave hope and tried to make his world a happier one.

I only really look toward the future in a few instances. When will the snow melt so I can finish various projects? If it's snowing, where will I run my workout? After having spent much of my life in the past or in the future, I've been attempting to be in the present in whatever I am doing . . . even if it's petting the cat. We do plan vacations and stuff like that, which is always something to look forward to. What's left for me? I'm not sure, but I'm eager to see what happens this afternoon or tomorrow. The best table that I've ever built might be sitting out in the garage . . . a bunch of rough maple boards just waiting to be shaped into a beautiful table, or a song that I've not been able to arrange might fall into place, or this afternoon's run in the snow might be a transcendent experience.

4 It Was Not Easy!

MAHA EBEID

I am an Egyptian woman working as a professor in the Faculty of Physical Education for girls at Alexandria University in Egypt. You probably wonder about the title of this chapter, but let me explain it. I thought, when I was asked to write about my life experience, it would be a piece of cake, but that is not so. I found it difficult to talk about myself because I never had done so before, not even in my dreams! But here I am, doing it with the hope to inspire readers of this book and help them realize that they can change their lives whenever they want.

I am a second child, who came after a spoiled sister and before the only brother, who took all the attention. I was the quiet one, which made my mother forget about me most of the time. Years passed quickly, but I remember hearing myself cry for the first time when we moved from Cairo to Alexandria without my mother. Later I learned the meaning of *divorce*. I became closer to my father, who was a police officer and seemed always to be away from home because of his work. He was very kind, however, and loved us more than enough. Because of that love, he gave my mother a divorce on one condition: that we children live with him! Before we got used to a new city and a new school, we moved again, this time to a busy house full of children and a woman who made me realize the meaning of a second new word in my life: *stepmother*! She was a widow with three daughters close in age to my siblings and me. Together we became a big family. A few years later we had two new sisters, one from my stepmother and, coincidentally, another from my birth mother, whose husband, a military officer, made as a rule for their marriage that she must never see or meet us again.

I was about 12 years old, however, when I reunited with my mother, after six years. Her husband had died two years previously, and since that reunion my siblings and I would spend a few weeks at a time in her home in Cairo. For me that was a happy ending.

In Egypt you don't have much choice in your college career; it is largely determined by your grades during your last year of secondary school. I wanted to study art, but my grades in that area were insufficient. Luckily, I took a qualification exam for the Faculty of Tourism and I passed. I was so happy, but when I told my father, he refused to allow my enrollment there because that school was in Cairo, where my mother lived. At the same time, my stepmother convinced my father that I should join the Faculty of Physical Education, where she was working. She believed that I would be successful in such studies because I was a swimmer. They insisted I pursue that route through the faculty qualified exams, and of course I passed. I was not happy with the proposed curriculum, which required that I retake many of the same courses of my last year of secondary school, but my father found out I had been accepted when he received a letter from the school with my name on it. It was obvious to me, however, that I had chosen an undesirable education career!

Success

I seems as though I did not stop crying during my first year of college, and I didn't pay much attention to my studies. But when I joined the theater group in the faculty, I was happy during play rehearsals every day after school. On the day of the play's opening, someone asked to see me after the performance. He was a famous film and theater director in Egypt, and he asked me if I would agree to join his play production and become a professional actress! I agreed, even before telling my father, who also agreed after I begged him. He used to take me to the theater for rehearsals every night from 11 p.m. until 2 a.m. One day the dean of the faculty sent for me and made it clear that I had to choose between being an actress and becoming a staff member after graduation. I left the theater life. I was surprised to find that even after paying little attention to my studies, I ranked third among all the other first-year students and had a very high grade! If it was that easy for me, what could I achieve if I worked hard? With more focus, I became the first-ranked student in the second year. I graduated and became a staff member in a career that I didn't choose.

Getting Married

In March 1976 my older sister got engaged, and there was a big party at the house. There I met Khaled, a friend of my sister's groom. At the end of the same month, Khaled invited us all to his family's home to attend his sister's engagement party, and when his family met me, they approved! Yes, in Egypt all children live in their parents' home throughout their lives even if they are male, unlike traditions in other cultures. Another custom is for parents to approve who their children marry. By coincidence, Khaled was in the same career I had chosen to study, but he was older than me by seven years. He had just obtained his master's degree and was a handball player on the Egyptian national team. He has a strong personality, is full of confidence, and loves me very much. It wasn't long before we were engaged, when I was 18 years old, soon after my second year of studies at the faculty. When I finished my last year of undergraduate education, we got married on August 8, 1980. I was pregnant while I finished my master's degree and became a mother to a beautiful girl, Lobna. I was 25 when Khaled, Lobna, and I left Egypt for the Sultanate of Oman, where Khaled assumed a new job as a coach of the Oman national handball team. I returned to Alexandria to finish my PhD before earning a leave of absence. I was not sad about spending approximately six years away from the faculty; I was still not emotionally attached to it.

Different Careers

Living in the Sultanate of Oman was among the best times of my life because my mother was living there. She had been working in an institute of education for girls, where she was successful and had a good relationship with the dean of the institution. She persuaded me to work with her, but after I had been accepted there, I had to submit my file to the ministry of education in Oman. There I had a loud argument with an administrator who disrespected me. Despite an apology from the manager, I decided not to take that job. I was not sad about losing it.

Many of the women I knew in Oman were working in various embassies. One day I applied to work at the Sultan Qaboos University, but when I learned I would be expected to work from 4 p.m. until 7 p.m., I decided that position was not suitable for me. The next day one of my acquaintances told me that the Saudi embassy was looking for an ambassador's secretary. I went for the interview with nothing but my PhD certificate and no hair cover! The councilor who interviewed me was surprised; maybe I, as a university graduate with an outgoing personality, was different from the other applicants. Our meeting ended up with "we shall call you." I left feeling sure they never would. Two days later, at three o'clock in the afternoon, I received a phone call from the Saudi councilor asking me to go immediately to the embassy. I replied that it was not acceptable to call me at lunchtime and expect me to come over; besides, I was busy. Instead of the reply that I expected, he apologized and said, "You are right." I hung up after telling him I would come tomorrow. I started my new job after meeting the ambassador, a very nice, civilized, well-educated man. I worked for six years as a successful secretary; even the ambassador's wife became a friend of mine.

After my family and I moved back to Alexandria, I still had two years of leave before I had to return to the faculty. I decided to try another line of work. Through one of the family friends, I got a position at American Express. Most of the time I worked in Cairo, which was difficult for me and my family, especially now that we had two daughters. That is why I left that work, but I did not give up on finding an alternative to the Faculty of Physical Education.

Another friend provided me with work as a fashion designer at one of the fashion companies in Alexandria. I spent about a year and a half in that new experience, and I made a huge financial profit for the company. The clock was ticking, however, and my free time was up. I had to return to work in the faculty, and I finally did, in 1991.

Back to the Faculty

I had been away from the faculty since 1982 and didn't know what happened during that period, not only in the faculty but in the whole country. When I left Egypt, my female colleagues had nice hair and clothes, but on my return, I saw only long dresses and hair coverings everywhere! I looked very different from them and refused demands to cover my hair. It is a free country! They gave up on trying to change me and accepted me because I had always looked different. I have always relished my independence. I resolved to keep myself busy and to earn an academic promotion. I engaged in hard work day and night until I got my final promotion as a professor doctor. I was the youngest professor in the faculty.

IAPESGW and a New Path

Lucky me! We had a most powerful dean of the faculty who was and still is my role model. Professor Nabila was one of those women who dare to have a different vision, one that I admired and respected. I was starting to lose my passion for work, as I felt bored when repeating the same lectures and doing the same routines. Then my dean asked me whether I was planning to attend an upcoming international conference. I told her I could not afford it, but she surprised me by saying that having a paper accepted for any conference meant that the university would cover all the expenses of attendance. I did not sleep that night until I googled the conference information and decided to attend the meeting of the International Society for the History of Physical Education and Sport (ISHPES) in Bulgaria, where I first met Gertrud Pfister, who was the ISHPES president at that time and remains one of my friends. I had a new goal to keep me going at work, and I worked hard to finish my accepted scientific research. The trip to Bulgaria was my first experience with an unfamiliar culture and people, but I had no problem in dealing with them. I was afraid of being alone, however, but by keeping myself busy with all the events at the conference, I succeeded in that experience, which pushed me to attend more international conferences. When I came back home and went to work, I met my dean to tell her what happened in Bulgaria. She told me that she had decided to host the biggest international conference of the International Association of Physical Education and Sports for Girls and Women (IAPESGW).

Most of the faculty members on the staff could not understand or speak English, though I could. That ability was the main reason my dean picked me to be a member of the organizing committee for that conference, which involved technology and emails that even she could not understand. I remember how surprised she was when I connected her with Margaret Talbot, the president of the IAPESGW, in a live chat through the computer. I started to feel attached to the faculty and found myself going every day because of the conference. We managed to acquire a donation of 25,000 LE (Egyptian pounds) for the conference. The opening ceremony was scheduled for September 11, 2001, the same date as the Twin Towers attack in the United States. We were about to cancel the conference, as I started to receive many emails from registrants who said they would not attend. But with two strong women, Professors Nabila and Talbot, we did not. Of the original 350 potential attendees from all over the world, thirty came. Still we managed to have a powerful and perfect open ceremony. I was engaged in the multiple tasks of reworking the program offerings and events daily, a tiresome duty, but I was so happy to break up my usual work routine with such a big event. My hard work was not only noticed but appreciated, as the IAPESGW president accepted me as a member of the executive board of the association. With that, I started a new chapter in my life.

In 2000 I joined a Greek project named Be a Champion in Life, which became an international teacher's resource book by the Foundation of Olympic and Sport Education in Athens. In 2001 I was chosen by the British Council in Alexandria to be part of its project named Dreams and Teams, which developed young citizens through sport and international educational links with the British Council in London. In 2004 I became a member of another project named Equal Opportunity in Mediterranean Sporting Activities, through Thé Association (Femmes, Sport, Culture, Mediterranean) in Nice, France.

Leaving My Country

I started to pull myself out from the faculty and have a wider target. I travelled the world to attend international conferences, be a part of meetings of the IAPESGW, or accept invitations to be a keynote speaker. I broadened my international network with friends and colleagues. But I was still doing the same routine at the faculty. I needed something new, something to add to my academic experience, which had reached the top at my institution. I had a feeling of confidence through all my travelling, and I needed a new challenge. I applied for work at two universities, one in New York and another in Washington and waited for their replies.

A week later I received a reply from the New York State University in Cortland (SUNY Cortland). The institution required, in addition to a telephone interview, some documents, and because of my wide international network I sent them three recommendation letters, one from my dean and the others from individuals in the United Kingdom and the United States. They also asked for proof of a research project in the field of physical education pedagogy. Finally, they asked me for a face-to-face interview in New York. My husband was totally understanding of the challenge I was undertaking, and he supported me. A week later I went to the unknown. I was not afraid because I had been there before for a visit and the people I met were like many others I had met before. I was afraid only of failing, but I never did. A long day of interviews went from 7 a.m. until 6 p.m. It seemed as though I went through the activities they had organized for the interview with one breath: meeting the search committee, giving a twenty-minute lecture to students, meeting the head of the department, meeting the dean, making another presentation to staff members about one of my scientific research projects, meeting the university president, and finally meeting again with the search committee. I left the next morning for New York City to wait for my flight back home in two days, but before leaving the city, I received a phone call that changed my life. "Hello, Maha? I would like to tell you that you won the job and will be one of our staff members soon." Now I took my second breath quietly and happily. I was moving to the United States to work. What a victory! I did it!

I left home and my family and went alone to Cortland for another target in my career. I was determined to succeed in my mission. I intended to stay for only two years and not renew the agreement with SUNY Cortland, and thus I was more focused in my work there than I otherwise would have been. It was not easy to be part of the American system concerning work. I know very well how to teach, but I had to follow the university's system, which meant attending all my colleagues' classes for the three modules I was assigned to observe their method. But they were very nice to me and understanding about the transition in my life. Later it became easy for me to follow the system, but my biggest problem was the students themselves. I felt that I was walking among them with a big heavy question mark over my head! One day, however, a student came into my office and said, "I logged into the country you came from, and I didn't find anything but the pyramids and a camel. Who are you?"

It was a Friday when she told me that, and I didn't sleep that night. I wrote to Margaret Talbot in England, whom I considered to be my mentor. She answered back, "Maha, be yourself and act as the real Maha I know, and never be afraid; they are just students. Let them understand who you really are, let the beauty you are hiding reveal itself in your address." I realized that I started my first class with only my name as an Egyptian and the statement that I would be their teacher, then went directly to the course description. It was not enough for them. I realized they were not convinced that an Arab woman could teach and help them learn. I kept talking to myself and remembered my first encounter with an American taxi driver, who wondered whether I was Italian or Mexican. But when he found out that I was Egyptian he asked me very fast, "Where is your hat?" Now I believe that my students had the same stereotypical thoughts as the taxi driver had.

I spent my weekend in front of my computer making a Power Point presentation with a lot of pictures about Egypt, from its ancient beginnings to the modern era, and some pictures of my family with a hope that the students would understand that Egyptians are people like them. After the first class on Monday morning, I hadn't taught my students any of the course material, but they did learn about Egypt and who I am. I had invited my colleagues to attend the presentation too. All were silent with open mouths! After I finished, for the first time I heard students asking me about myself. Did you get your education in the United Kingdom? Did you take off your hat (hair covering, or hijab) before coming? Do men kill women who play sports in Egypt?! I was shocked by the number of questions, but I answered them quietly and with a smile. After that day my relationships with students and staff members changed. It became traditional for me to do the same presentation with every class each semester.

Another challenge during my work in the United States was having a student assistant while teaching the practical swimming class, because I thought that I had to have CPR training and a lifeguard license to be on my own while teaching. I could not accept the perception that I was an incompletely certified teacher, so I decided to sign up for the lifesaving class to get that license. When I told the head of the department about that, he said, "You are not young enough for that high-intensity course and I doubt you can make it." I did not listen to him and became a student in that class and a teacher in the next. There is no need to tell you how difficult it was to swim every day for an hour, then go to the gym after work, but I was determined to succeed and I did it.

I rented a two-bedroom flat with a nice terrace and furnished the place. I used to go to work on a bicycle one of my colleagues gave me, but winter in Cortland had an atmosphere I had never experienced before. It became clear that I would need a car to move around. I decided to get an American driving license, but the driver services office did not recognize my Egyptian or Omani driving license and I was told I would have to go through the entire American process. But first I asked to go through the written driving test just to know what it looked like even if I believed I would fail. The officer gave me a small book to study, then told me to come back for another written test. I spent the weekend studying and returned for the written test, which I passed, as I did the driving test, on the first trial.

It was a huge day when my daughters came to visit, and I took them to a volleyball match in my department. All my students were there and quickly started to talk with my daughters. The students were surprised at my daughters' English skills and their comprehension, and in no time they made friends. I was happy when one of my daughters invited one of the American friends to visit us in Alexandria, Egypt, and stay in our home. I found that visit a great opportunity to present an authentic experience in all that I had shown my students in presentations about my homeland. I had to convince the young woman's parents that she would be safe and would return to them. Susan came to Egypt and never wanted to go back home! I laughed when she told me, "What are you doing in Cortland while you have such a beautiful life and country?" I told her my two reasons: first, I needed a new objective to advance in my career, and second, there was no better place than the United States to learn or to promote my career. I reached my target with an A-plus and will never go back to Cortland. Susan did not know that before she traveled to Egypt, I had finished my appointment agreement with Cortland and refused the offers they made for me to stay. My mission and target were done, and I had accomplished my goals in the United States.

New Target

Until I had a new goal in mind, my work in Egypt was the same as it had been, though I did change my ways of teaching and assessment according to what I had learned in Cortland. Quality assurance had come to Egypt, and education accreditation became a must for all faculties and schools. One day I received a phone call from the ministry of higher education asking me to be a member of the Egyptian committee that would create the physical education standards for the entire sports faculties sector. The project was titled National Standards for Undergraduate Students in Physical Education in Egypt and was under the auspices of the National Authority for Quality Assurance. The new assignment was very promising, and I agreed to be a part of it. Working hard for about two years to come up with the standards document was not easy, but I did it with the committee. Another mission had been accomplished. What was next?

I thank Margaret Talbot for helping me set a new national and international target. I joined a project with Cambridge University in the United Kingdom to develop a new curriculum model and teaching guide for physical education in Egyptian schools. As part of the project, Cambridge chose me to tutor Egyptian physical education teachers in how to use the curriculum guide and apply it in schools. As part of the Cambridge International Examination Nile Egyptian School Project—Retrain Teachers, I spent about five years giving face-to-face lectures and teaching online courses.

It was a normal working day in 2010 when the faculty dean sent for me and said, "Maha, you will be the head of your department [Sports Training and Movement Analysis]." I never thought I had to be so attached to my work. I still had the same ambivalence about my career path, but now I would have to follow my first academic goal and get more involved with the faculty itself. I accepted the challenge despite my own misgivings. As head of the department, I was to set new goals for all the staff members. I had to develop the department program and its modules, as well as descriptions for accreditation. With the help of others, I worked day and night until the peer reviewers came to make their decision about our program and modules description. They passed. I did it.

I suddenly asked myself, "Why I am not a peer reviewer?" That was my next close target, and I joined the nine modules in Cairo and became a peer reviewer for accreditation.

In the summer of the same year, the dean again sent for me and this time said, "Maha, I chose you to be vice dean of graduate study and research." She added, "You used to work in the dark; it is time to let the light show how hard and creatively you are working." Should I have been happy to become even more involved in a career I did not choose? To tell you the truth, I was glad for the first time! Finally, I came out into the daylight in my new role and decided to set another big goal for myself.

Vice Dean

I had a big office, which I reorganized, searching the files to set priorities and review the numbers of graduate students we had. Finding that we had only two international students as well as an unfinished file for the credit hours system, I realized I would have to address these two major issues. I worked with all the departments in the faculty until the system for credit hours was approved by the higher education ministry, and my first target was completed successfully. I pushed announcements for our new study system, conducted a lot of meetings, uploaded the web page of the faculty with all the programs we had for graduate studies, and highlighted the possibility of earning a master's and a PhD in two years. The plan started to work as the first fourteen international students signed up for our programs. I paid a lot of attention to the students, and that is why the number rose in the next semester. Through five years as vice dean, the fees income for the university reached 22 million LE, an accomplishment of which I was very proud.

My third target was to issue an international scientific journal besides the Arabic one, and I worked for two hard years until the *International Sports Science Alexandria Journal* made its debut. I also created a website for it. All my three major targets were accomplished successfully. I can say that I enjoyed the work in the faculty, maybe because I made a difference in every responsibility I accepted but also because of the feelings I had before my interest started to fade. I needed more.

Surprise Election

In Egyptian universities, choosing a new dean of any faculty was done through the current dean. He or she offered a name to the university president, who usually approved that choice. In my case it was different.

What happened in Egypt on January 25, 2010, changed every system. When the Muslim Brotherhood took control of the country, it was a big shock for most people. At that time the hiring for every position at work changed to an election system just when I was thinking about applying for the dean position, which was the biggest and last goal in my career. I was disappointed with the new system because I am not one of those who can win through elections; most of my colleagues at work, who were not comforted by the fact that I was different, were not my friends. I paid attention only to work and to whoever wanted to be part of that success. I started to rethink applying and stayed quiet doing my tenure as vice dean.

Everything changed again with the accession of our country's current president, Abdel Fattah al-Sisi, who changed the rules for choosing the dean from the election system to one in which the best in quality of work and personality was the goal. I knew at that moment I could win.

Dean of Faculty

I spent about a month preparing my portfolio with all original documents to apply for the position of dean of the faculty. Another four colleagues were doing the same; it was a competition I relished.

Some of the members of the search committee I knew; others I didn't know. The group consisted of seven professors, including the vice president of graduate study and research for Alexandria University and a former university president. I had to give a twenty-minute presentation about my vision to promote my faculty. I saw my portfolio in front of everyone when I started my presentation, which took less than twenty minutes as I was well prepared. They asked me lots of questions. I was firm and answered straight to the point; then I left.

In November 2014 I received the letter of my appointment, signed by President al-Sisi, to be dean of the faculty for three years. What a victory; I did it!

Last Academic Mission

I had a vision for my faculty, but would I be able to fulfill it? That was a question only for myself, and to achieve that goal I promised myself not to be attached to negative colleagues. Their negative energy might catch me! I will always look and move forward.

In my first meeting with faculty staff members and administrators, I tried to break the ice between us by stating that I was looking not for their love but for their respect and I would roll with the punches that came my way. And I did that.

After I went through the files, I noticed that the infrastructure for the faculty was about to fall down. After one week as the dean, I traveled to Cairo, where I met the minister of youth and sports, and asked for his help to turn all the green-grass playgrounds into artificial green ground. Why? Because it cost the faculty 23,000 LE every year to renew the grass even though it lasted for only two months. I convinced the minister of the rightness of this proposal by explaining the community service we offer in allowing neighborhood children to use those fields for sports. I was clever, and he agreed. Target one was accomplished.

For the infrastructure, I got a donation to renovate one of the administrative offices, which cost 20,000 LE. When I received a letter of thanks from the staff there, I felt so happy. With another donation, I renovated the locker room and bought ninety new lockers for students. I changed the system of recording morning attendance for the administrators. Instead of having teachers record attendance by hand, I got a machine to do the job. I succeeded in acquiring 3 million LE from the university to construct a new building for graduate students, whose enrollment had increased to about three hundred. I renovated one of the main conference halls that had remained the same since 1980. I built another two classrooms for students and furnished them. I built two new table tennis facilities, indoors and outdoors. I updated the gym and its locker room. I created a new area filled with seats for the students' break. I rebuilt the indoor swimming pool and changed its heating system. In the middle of all that, the new artificial green courts were finished and we had a big ceremony for their opening that was attended by the minister himself, the university president and his three vice presidents, and all the staff members and students. That was a day I felt proud, and I think I deserved it.

For my students and young researchers, I provided grants. Two of the young researchers travelled to Greece for one month each, and another two went to Austria to finish their PhDs with their foreign supervisors. Another one traveled to Germany for a semester to study for a master's course. My vision was to let students have experiences that might change their lives as happened with me. I made their dreams come true. I also persuaded the university and engineering faculty to partner with Magdeburg University in Germany in starting a master's program in sports engineering, which would be the first such program ever in Egypt. The engineering dean and I traveled to Germany twice to facilitate that program.

Academically, in 2015, I held the international symposium for the Union of Arab Universities in my faculty with the attendance of the former higher education minister, the university president and his vice presidents, and all staff members and graduate students. In 2016, my faculty and other peer faculties in Cairo and Tanta in Egypt, Magdeburg University in Germany, and Sfax University in Tunisia cooperated to organize an international conference in Tunisia, and many of the Egyptian staff members attended the conference.

In 2017 the faculty held the biggest conference of the International Society for the History of Physical Education and Sport (ISHPES). This eighteenth ISHPES congress was titled The Transformation of Sport and Physical Activity through Time: Journeys in History. I had followed the ISHPES for three years of conferences in Qatar, Croatia, and then France, where I gave a presentation and some handouts and won the hosting rights for my university. I was so happy but knew how much hard work I would face and was determined to succeed. On April 3 the opening ceremony in the big hall of the Alexandria Library was attended by more than two thousand persons, of whom about fifty came from outside Egypt. The ISHPES members and the president, Annette Hofmann, were very supportive, and I felt I did not fail them with this conference. And finally, I increased the income of the community services department from 1 million LE to 2.5 million LE.

I had a vision about what to do to renew the accreditation of my faculty that had occurred two years before the previous dean left. I knew it was my chance to leave a gift for my faculty and the university. The reviewers came after I left my position, and just as I had hoped, the faculty was officially accepted and got its second accreditation, which made me so happy and proud.

I left my position as a dean, but I am still a professor, teaching graduate students, supervising their research, and still helping the sports engineering program to become a reality. With all that, I did not forget about what I really love to do, and away from work I paint and have finished my first novel. As I meet my goals in life, I continue to challenge myself with new interests.

Many of my colleagues and friends used to ask me, "When are you going to grow older?" I always laughed and gave them some advice for staying young or at least youthful: eat healthy, sleep well, and exercise. Because I did not have enough time to go to the gym, I bought a treadmill that I use every day before sleeping. But early in the morning before work, I do some stretching with yoga videos on YouTube. I never eat between meals, and I always keep my food plate colorful. The more salad colors you consume, the healthier you are, and I don't eat red meat and only occasionally eat chicken. My big secret for keeping my skin soft is to have a spoonful of olive oil every morning. Try it; it's like watering your plants. I never eat fried food; bake it or grill it. And always drink water with slices of lemon. Stay healthy and you will look and feel younger.

The truth is that I would not have been able to accomplish any of what I have been through without my husband's support and understanding, maybe because he reached the position of dean of faculty before I did and knew what it took to attain the job and do it well. He continued his successful career as the president of the Egyptian Handball Federation and a member of the Egyptian Olympic committee. It was my good destiny to have a husband in the same career and with the same vision. I have tried to be a role model, and my daughters are proud of me. My younger daughter is now pursuing her master's degree in fine art history, and she used to tell me, "I want to be like you." My happiest time now is spent with my two grandchildren, a girl and a boy named Rola and Adel.

My personal motivation, my career, and my international travel have helped me to realize that we should not judge our destiny but can change it for the better if we believe in ourselves. It will bring the best out of you.

I did it, so you can too.

5 My Life of Physical Activity and Fitness

JAMES R. COATES JR.

I'm a 72-year-old African American man who stands five feet six inches tall and weighs 185 pounds. No, I'm not fat. In fact, I consider myself quite the opposite. Sports, fitness, and physical activity are and always have been a major part of my life. My hobbies and interests include participating in sporting activities, such as softball, jogging, pitching horseshoes, disc golf, and above all else body shaping via weightlifting activities. I also enjoy watching and attending sporting activities. I was born in Annapolis, Maryland, on February 5, 1950. I'm the first-born male of my family's six children. All of us, with one exception, were born at a home on Spa Road in the city of Annapolis. Our brother was born at a home on Greenfield Street in Annapolis. There are four girls and two boys. Our oldest sibling is eight years older than I am. The next oldest is seven years older. The next oldest is three years older. I'm next in the order of children, and then we have our youngest sister, who was one year younger than I am. She passed away from cancer just before her sixty-fifth birthday. Our brother, who is the youngest of the six, is eight years younger than I am. Including my mother and father, that was the total membership of our immediate family.

We were raised in the beliefs of the United Methodist faith, practicing at Asbury United Methodist Church in Annapolis, Maryland. In 1976 my wife and I were married in that church. And, in 1979, our son was baptized there as well. The extended family in which my siblings and I were raised, however, consisted of grandparents, aunts, uncles, cousins, and other distant relatives. Our neighborhood was pretty much one massive family. At times many of us lived together or stayed at one another's homes. I would estimate that at least 75 percent of the homes in our neighborhood were inhabited by one of our relatives. In my opinion, this was by far the greatest community and neighborhood environment that anyone could ever possibly obtain.

The neighborhood we lived in was extremely poor, but the larger community contained African American families from upper, middle, and lower socioeconomic classes. During my developmental years, the city's Black living areas were named. Our community was called Spa Road. The others were In-Town, O'Berry Court, Larkin Street, Down Town, East Port, Parole, and Annapolis Neck, and all of them marked racial boundaries. When integration began in the city and gentrification of neighborhoods resulted, the city began development of other Black communities such as Annapolis Gardens, Newtown Nineteen, Newtown Twenty, and Robin Wood, but the one truly upper-class socioeconomic Black community was named Highland Beach. It was founded and developed by Frederick Douglass, the great African American abolitionist. While the name Spa Road is one of the streets in the city, when spoken of by African Americans, most often it refers to the community of the Black neighborhoods located thereon, as location signified race.

Annapolis, in Anne Arundel County in Maryland, was also the location of Wiley H. Bates Junior-Senior High School, the only middle and high school for Blacks in the entire county before integration. That school was in the Spa Road community. Ironically, the major white public high school for the city and parts of the county was also in this same community. The road to the white high school, Greenfield Street, had a fence and gate across it to divide the white high school from the Black community. That fence also had barbed wire atop portions of it. At night the gate was pulled across the road and locked. The image of this fence is fresh in my mind because the front door of the house that I grew up in was no more than seventy-five yards from the front door of the white high school. That gate and fence were no more than forty feet from the front door of our house.

The head custodian of the white high school was an African American, Travis Jackson. He and his family lived in a house provided by that school system right on the school's property. Our families were pretty good friends. Although they had kids my age (a daughter was even in my class), I rarely interacted with the family unless asked to do something by my parents or Mr. Jackson. We knew when the gate would be closed for the day because Mr. Jackson was the one responsible for it, and he would inform someone in the community if there was going to be a time change in the process. Black lives were thereby regulated.

The location of these two schools was no small matter. The county, which then was the third largest in the state, sent to our community every Black student who was to be educated. Some students traveled for over an hour to get to school in the morning and the same length of time to get back home. Drives of over thirty miles to attend school were not uncommon for some of these Black students. Just like the city, these Black communities within the county also had names to identify their members, which included Brown's Wood, Mulberry Hill, Pumphrey, Brooklyn Park, Lothian, Mayo, Edgewater, and Shady Side. Regardless of where the students came from, Black or white, if they were going to attend a football game for either school, they went to the same football field, which was owned by the city. The two schools played one another only twice in their histories. Those two games came during the last two years that Bates was open as a public high school. Within the depth of this provided scenario, you will find the development for the basis of my intrigue with sports, fitness, and physical activity.

Beginning Endeavors in Physical Activity

Growing up in a house that was just over five hundred square feet, with four sisters, most of them older than me, and a much younger brother, I was limited as to the type of activities I could participate in, especially on rainy, stormy, or snowbound days. On most such days, we engaged in board games of all types but also played card games, jacks, paddle and ball, hopscotch, and jump rope. When other kids in the community came together to play, we participated in the activities just mentioned but added others, including sporting activities, such as tag, hide-and-seek, tin can in the alley, horseshoes, sprint footraces, football, basketball, baseball, and fighting. Fighting was not a game, but on many occasions the sporting games resulted in such altercations.

The board games and card games were something we normally did when night fell on the neighborhood, when we were ill, when the weather was foul, or when we were being punished by our parents. Not being allowed to go outside for play was the softer side of such punishment. The main board games were Monopoly and Scrabble. The card games were war, gin rummy, tunk, spades, and Pokeno.

The game of jacks was played on the linoleum floor, outside on the concrete sidewalk, or inside on the table, which we had been warned not to do. All of these games and activities were done not just with immediate family but also the larger community.

At any level of schooling, sporting activities included people from each of the Black communities. While participating in school recess, physical education classes, play days, and team sports, I came to understand that running fast, jumping long and high, moving quickly, being stronger, catching, and throwing long, hard, and straight were the abilities that helped an individual or a team win competitions or contests set up by teachers, or by students themselves. I was always one of the smallest boys, if not the smallest, in all of these activities. But I was always one of the first persons selected by the various captains to be on their teams if I was not a captain myself. Even though I was smaller, I possessed enough speed and strength to be successful in physical activities. Why did I have these skills? Well, not knowing the actual components of fitness at that age, I just gave credit to great eye-hand coordination from playing jacks and paddle bat and ball with my sisters; body control and coordination from jumping rope and playing hopscotch; quickness and running fast from always playing with the older boys and having to try to keep up with them to play; and a sense of toughness from having to fight often or play rough.

Many of these skills were useful to us kids in other ways besides sports and recess activities. To get to one of the elementary schools we attended (Adams Park Elementary School), we had to walk a few miles. That walk included having to travel through at least one white community. On more than a few days each week, many of these white families would have their pet dogs out. Of course, this era was before leash laws were enforced, if they existed. The loose dogs always chased us, making us run. Another option for getting to school, even though our parents and law enforcement authorities warned us against doing it, was to jump onto a moving freight train going in the direction of the elementary school. We all made a pact not to tell our parents to avoid getting into trouble with them. Those running, jumping, strength, and coordination skills proved useful in this situation. In all the years of kids doing this that I can remember, there was only one major injury.

Youth League Sports

Sometime during my late elementary school years or in junior high school, it dawned on me that very few of the boys from my community who were in my age group participated in any organized league sporting activities such as football, basketball, baseball, track and field, lacrosse, wrestling, gymnastics, boxing, and sailing. The reasons for their lack of participation varied, but I continued and enjoyed being a part of these activities. The guys from the community always wanted to play against those of us who did play in these leagues to prove that although they didn't play in these leagues, they were just as good or even better at athletics than those of us who did participate. Naturally this rivalry raised not only the competitiveness in the games but also the number of physical altercations.

Participating in organized leagues gave me access to coaches who reinforced the things that physical education teachers were teaching us. We did the normal stretching, pushups, jumping jacks, leg kicks, pull-ups, and more. The coaches were always telling me, being smaller, "Get some size on you, Coates." I did eat a great deal. I also participated in a great number of activities at school, at home, and in youth league games. This activity kept me burning a lot of calories. Keeping my body slim was what I thought made me fast and quick compared with other boys I played with and against.

When I got to junior high school, the coaches were always talking about lifting weights. I saw the high school athletes in this combined junior-senior high school and thought that they were just born that way. After the coaches had me start lifting and I saw the difference that it was making in my body, I was hooked. By that time, my parents allowed me to work out at the United States Naval Academy, where my father worked. He worked at the academy for fifty years, first in the mess hall as a head supervisor and later in the facilities management division when the academy contracted out its food service division. During my many routine trips to those grounds, I worked on a lot of gymnastic equipment, since I had been taught routines in physical education classes at the junior-senior high school. I could see that these gymnastics workouts were also shaping my body in a way I liked. Others might not have noticed my development as much, since I was still very slim. But I certainly noticed it. My friends who participated in youth league sport and I took part in other sporting endeavors on the Naval Academy grounds, where we played at tennis, basketball, track, football, handball, indoor baseball, sailing, and lacrosse.

My older cousins and other boys in the community were then playing at Wiley H. Bates Junior-Senior High School, and they always took the time to play games with us younger boys in the neighborhood and teach us how to be better athletes as well.

All of my youth league sporting activities took place during the early years of the integration periods of the 1960s. On one occasion, when I was 12 years old, I was told, not so very politely or professionally, to get my "N——a A——" off the field, because I would never play for this white team. Recently my high school graduation class held its fiftieth anniversary. One of the white alumni who had been a high school athlete with me and went on to play professional lacrosse noted to me and a group of other classmates that he remembered meeting me for the first time. We were 12 years old. He had been on the youth league tryout fields when I and another Black guy from our neighborhood tried out for those teams. He said that he and the other boys there were shocked at how we had been treated by the coach. They had heard from members of the younger youth league teams that I was a good player and were looking forward to seeing me play or getting to play with me. Because of the adult white coaches and their racial perspectives, I was not afforded that opportunity with that team. By the way, the coach who said derogatory things and denied me that opportunity was one of the most prominent names in Annapolis City and in the sports history of the state of Maryland.

During the summer months that we were not in school, one of my cousins and I would take our dogs and go to play in the swamps early in the mornings. We were both members of Boy Scout troop 268, organized at the Black junior-senior high school and were always doing things to get merit badges. The swamp hunts helped us get our nature merit badges. For the rest of the day, we would join the other youth, male and female, in playing some type of sporting endeavor. Many times, a parent had to send another kid to come get us all to come home.

On one of our early morning swamp trips with our dogs, we came upon a very big man putting down sod grass on the new football field for the white high school. A new semipro football team, called the Annapolis Sailors, was going to play on this field, and they had contributed funds to upgrade the new field and stadium at the white high school. The Black high school was to continue using the city field. We asked the man if he needed any help. He said yes. So we spent the next two weeks working with him to place that sod on the field. We learned that the man's name was Al Larrimore, and he was the assistant football coach at the white high school. Of course, he asked our names as well. We told him but figured just like anyone else, he wouldn't remember us.

High School Sports

During the school year beginning in 1964, the political forces in Anne Arundel County finally decided to follow the 1954 U.S. Supreme Court ruling on *Brown v. Board of Education of Topeka* and fully integrate the public schools. The countywide all-Black high school would eventually no longer serve as a segregated high school. Black students from miles outside the city would now attend the school closest to their homes. My three older sisters, however, would graduate from Bates, the Black high school. The youngest of those three sisters graduated in 1965, and the last graduation class from Bates as a high school would be in 1966. Knowing that my youngest sister and I would not be able to graduate from Bates, our parents moved us to the formerly all-white high school in 1965. This move was good and bad for us. The good part was that we had to walk only about seventy-five yards to get to school. The bad part was also that we were only seventy-five yards from school. Getting to school was easy, but skipping classes or staying home from school was not good because you couldn't go outside without being seen by truant officers. This circumstance didn't bother me, though, because I attended the third grade through the twelfth grade without missing a day of school. Yes, I was one of those nerds who even went to classes on "senior hook day," when seniors were expected to skip all classes. I was not alone in not skipping classes that day, but many of the senior class teachers, who were expecting a "free period" from teaching, were not pleased to see a few students showing up for class.

My first year at Annapolis High School was a big transition. In most of my upper-level classes there were only two or three Black students. Our white teachers on many occasions would get us confused with one another. Grading periods were awful times if more than one Black student with the same last name was in a class. I experienced this type of error so often in my biology and zoology classes, with the same teacher, that it wasn't funny.

By this time, however, I had developed a pretty good reputation as an athlete. I was still extremely small, but with skill development, I had learned how to play a great number of sports with athleticism. I went out for the football team, thinking that as a sophomore I would make the junior varsity (JV) that year. When the team tryouts were held, I was one of only about five male students from the all-Black school who showed up. Other Blacks came out, but they were either just moving into the area or had gone to other white schools on experimental bases. There were 250 or more people trying out for the ninety-five positions on the varsity and JV teams combined. As usual, I was the smallest person trying out. How was I going to get attention from coaches with all these bigger guys around?

Using skills and techniques that I had learned from neighborhood games and youth league coaches, I was able to stand out not only for my small size but also for my performance. I was surprised to learn that the assistant coach I had helped lay sod a few years earlier was now the head coach, and he remembered my name. I did not know much about this man except his name and that at least in my eyes, he was huge, standing six feet three inches tall and weighing 350 pounds. During the two-week tryout period, I tried to be impressive in all the drills. I was among the fastest runners and demonstrated a lot of quickness and agility. But I was still small, weighing just over 100 pounds at that point. The time came to pass out equipment. I got all the equipment everyone else received, except there was no helmet for me. That meant I would have to sit out all the hitting drills. I got mad about that after one day. The next day I started going out on the field and hitting without a helmet. Larrimore, the head coach, stopped the drills, and I thought I was in trouble. Instead, he walked over to an assistant coach and screamed, "Get that kid a damn helmet." The next hurdle was cut-down day, when the less skilled players would be dismissed from the team.

On cut-down day each of the boys trying out for the teams would report to the school's locker room doors, where two lists of names were posted. If your name was on either list, you were to continue practicing with the team. I was elated to find my name on the JV list. All of the advice from previous coaches and other athletes, even those from the Naval Academy, about working out and being in shape when preparing for a sport had seemingly paid off, that is, until I found out that the JV coach was the man who hadn't given me a helmet during tryout sessions. I was doing well in practices and feeling good about myself, knowing that I was among only three Blacks who had made the squad. Then the fact that many white teachers and coaches don't know one Black kid from another took hold again. One of the other Black kids who tried out for the team but didn't make it got into some trouble in the school. The JV coach thought it was me. I was in this coach's physical education class as well. He told me that I could no longer be on the team. I tried to explain that it was not me who committed the infraction but rather a young man name Kirby. The coach didn't want to hear it. If any of the kids in my family ever got into trouble in school, that kid would have hell to pay for that poor behavior. It took me about three weeks before I was no longer embarrassed about being removed from the team for something I had no part in. I continued to work out with a few other athletes and stay in shape by doing gymnastic routines with another of the assistant varsity coaches, who taught a lot of such concepts in his classes.

What I didn't know, however, was that the head varsity coach, Larrimore, who actually controlled both varsity and junior varsity programs, didn't know that I had been removed from the team. After school one Friday, when the JV team had a game, I decided to leave the gymnastic activities and go watch the game instead. On the way from the gym to the field I heard someone calling my name. I turned to see the varsity coach, Larrimore, coming in my direction. He started asking me questions. The first one was "Don't the JV have a game now"? I answered, "Yes, sir." He then asked, "Are you injured? No one told me about your injury." I said, "No, sir, I'm no longer on the team." He said, "Why? Did you quit, son?" I then said that the coach put me off the team. He responded with "What? Come with me." We walked back to the football locker room, where he immediately confronted the JV coach. He told the coach that this was his program, and when he put a player on either varsity or JV, they are on it until he removes them. He turned and walked away, saying to me, "If you have any more trouble, you come to see me." From that day on, the JV coach never had a good thought about me.

I took that experience and worked exceptionally hard in preparing for my junior-year athletic season. With the Black school now officially closed, players from that school were trying out for the integrated team at Annapolis Senior High School. Of the extremely large number of guys trying out, eleven Blacks made the team. Three, including me, were from my neighborhood. I had gained twenty pounds but was right at 120, still small for a football player. The star player from the Black school was one of my childhood friends in our neighborhood. He was a fast, powerful, and tough running back. When the hitting started, he became everything he was rumored to be. By having played with and against him in our community, I was able to tackle not only him but also the other bigger running backs. The coaches noticed my play, and I made the team.

Not having played on the senior varsity level before, I had no idea what to expect for the first game. While we had two or three scrimmages (practice games) against schools that were not in our league, those practice games were nothing like playing in front of the large crowds that turned out for our home games. When I did not play during the first half of that first game, I was disappointed because I was coming from leagues where

I was accustomed to playing. Then I realized that I was playing behind a two-year starter on the varsity who was also the star player, Dave Hart. Not only was he starting at cornerback, the position I played, but he was also the starting quarterback on offense. In fact, he was selected as the best quarterback for the entire county two years in a row. His father was the head men's basketball coach at the United States Naval Academy. Dave was also the starting point guard on our basketball team. Upon graduation he went to the University of Alabama to play basketball. (During the era of Bobby Bowden, the famed football coach at Florida State, Dave was the athletic director there.) At halftime of my first varsity game, because Dave was slightly injured, the coach told me I would be starting the second half of the game at the cornerback position. I started every game at that corner-back position the rest of the season. During the ten games we played, our defense allowed only three teams to score on us. Two of those teams scored six points each, and during the final game of the season, our rival, Severna Park High School, scored twelve points. We were undefeated that season.

At the end of the season, the coaches gave each player a goal to meet before the next season. They told me to gain some weight. Everyone on the team giggled when the coach stated my weight aloud. Living only seventy-five yards from the school building, I never missed a session when the coaches conducted their summer weightlifting and workout program. I did experience pain in my back during some of the training sessions. A coach had me go to see doctors in the city. Each of the first four doctors I visited told me I had deterioration in the thoracic section of my vertebrae and that I should not play football anymore. I visited a fifth doctor, who said the deterioration was an old injury, and he saw no reason why I shouldn't play football. I decided to play. Participating in the summer training program, I gained five or six pounds. But what was more noticeable was my muscularity. I now weighed 126 pounds, still small by any standard. But I was pleased with how my body looked. The rewards of physical activity were beginning to take hold for me, both physically and mentally. I was hooked on lifting weights and working out.

At the beginning of my senior year in high school, I looked forward enthusiastically to the football season. At the time, no one on our team had any idea that one of our JV team members was to become one of the greatest football coaches in National Football League history. He was an offensive lineman whose father was the head lacrosse coach at the Naval Academy. That player became the current New England Patriots head coach, Bill Belichick. He was elevated to the varsity at the end of the JV season, which was always a couple of games shorter than the varsity season. After the success of our previous season, our schedule was loaded with teams that had great reputations as powerful football programs. As usual we started the season playing well and easily won the opening game. But unfortunately for me, I was injured in that game. My knee was damaged. I missed the next game against one of the best backs in the state at Cambridge High School. While not being able to play in the game, I was, however, able to go into the radio booth and comment on our game for a local station that also carried the games of the Naval Academy. I truly enjoyed that aspect of sports, and I continued in broadcasting later in my professional career. That game was special for several other reasons as well. First, we were playing in Cambridge, Maryland, the same city that not one month before was the site of one of the most noted racial riots of the civil rights movement, led by activist H. Rap Brown. Tensions were extremely high, to say the least. Second, the Cambridge running back, an African American who was highly touted as among the best in the state, was injured during the game and could not return. Our team demolished Cambridge after his injury, but we did not escape the wrath of the local whites in that city.

Cambridge is on what is known as the Eastern Shore of the state of Maryland. That section of the state, at that time, was reputedly among the most racist parts of the entire country. After our victory, we hurriedly boarded the team bus and left the city but not before racial epithets and physical objects were hurled our way. When we stopped in the nearest city, about fifteen minutes away from Cambridge, we encountered some racial animus as well. One of the perpetrators was the star tight end on that city's high school team. The following week, I returned to playing. My knee hurt, but a doctor told me that if I kept the leg muscles around the knee strong, I would be okay. The coach moved me from the starting cornerback position over to play safety. I played extremely well the rest of the season and made the all-county team, a selection of the best players at each position for the entire county made by the coaches and newspaper sportswriters. To this day, I'm still the smallest player, weightwise, ever to make that team.

I completed my senior year by playing on the baseball team, which had been a desire of mine since playing in Little League and then meeting one of my middle school teachers who was also a former professional minor league player. When the Black junior-senior high school closed, he transferred to the school where I had damaged my knee during football season. He was now the baseball coach there, and he played in the local fast-pitch softball league. Being an older man who still played extremely well with much younger men, he impressed me and served as a role model. I wanted to stay fit like he had. What I did not realize was that my knee injury was much worse than I had been told.

College Activity

By the time I went to college that autumn, there was very little stability in my knee. The college I selected to attend, thinking that I could still play football, had an enrollment of about fifteen hundred students that semester. During my college career, however, by the time the spring semester arrived each year, the school could have as few as 750 students. I tried to play in college that first term, but I was much too far from recovering to even think about playing. I did associate with the freshmen team members and had most of them in my classes, since I was majoring in physical education. To my surprise, also attending the historically Black Maryland State Teachers College (the name was later changed to the University of Maryland Eastern Shore) was the star running back from Cambridge High School who had been hurt while playing against my high school team the previous season. His knee was injured to the extent that he too could no longer play football beyond a light-contact level. Most of the players on the football team were some of the biggest human beings I'd ever seen in my life. In the 1960s many of these men went on to play in the National Football League.

Our physical education activity classes at this undergraduate school were competitive sessions. Most of the male students in our classes were current or former athletes. The size and athleticism of some of these guys was amazing. But my background in various activities had prepared me well for such an environment. In fact, when it came to participating in gymnastics, wrestling, archery, and field hockey, the professors relied on me a great deal because many of the other students had very little if any knowledge about or experience in these activities. Sometimes even the professors themselves had very little knowledge about or experience in directing or participating in them.

Putting away youthful activities was hard for me, at least partly because one of my undergraduate professors, Dr. Howard Davis, had always emphasized the idea of lifelong fitness, retiring from work, and enjoying what he called the good life. Dr. Davis was also the chairman of the Health, Physical Education, and Recreation Department at the university. As the president of the physical education majors club, I traveled with Dr. Davis to professional conferences on more than a few occasions. His constant conversation was about perseverance as a Black professional physical educator, not just a "gym" teacher, and about committing to lifelong fitness. I had been voted the most promising physical educator and most outstanding physical education major in the program at the University of Maryland Eastern Shore my junior and senior years. Dr. Davis would say to me, "Coates, we don't worry about you, but you have got to help get some of the other majors interested in doing things besides coaching." To me it seemed as if the faculty and other members of the physical education majors club were pushing or encouraging me to go farther in the professional world.

After College and Beyond

On leaving college and entering the professional world of teacher education, life changes increased for me. By that time, I had gained weight and was up to 150 pounds. I was leaving the predominantly Black culture of the college and community in which I lived and was heading for the larger-majority culture of mainstream society. I had been substitute teaching since my first year of undergraduate school, and I felt well prepared when I received my first full-time position in 1972 at Corkran Junior High School. This was a life-altering beginning for me. At that school I was to meet Frances Bain, a white art teacher, whom I began dating, and four years later she became

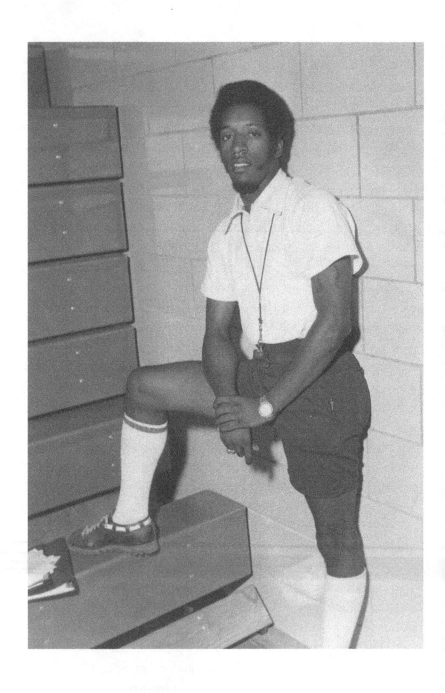

Aged 22, at Corkran Junior High School. Courtesy of James R. Coates.

my wife. I also had the privilege of working with my first two students who later went on to obtain national and international acclaim. One was a young lady who later became an alternate on the U.S. Olympic Team as a high jumper. The other was Toni Braxton, who became an internationally renowned pop singer and entertainer. My soon-to-be wife, Frances, taught Toni, her three sisters, and her brother during their junior high school years at Corkran Junior High School.

The notion of participating in youthful activities was still a very large part of my favorite hobbies, so I continued playing baseball, basketball, and flag football in adult recreational leagues, and turned to fitness training for myself. The fitness training was not just to improve my performance in the athletic endeavors that I was undertaking but also to fulfill the lifelong fitness pledges I had made to Dr. Davis during undergraduate school.

The main issue for me, however, was that by the time I was leaving my undergraduate school, I had come to understand that my knee was pretty much destroyed. I learned that I had torn my anterior cruciate ligament, my medial collateral ligament, and my lateral collateral ligament in the same knee. I had to undergo total knee reconstruction. Keeping my leg muscles strong would help me to continue doing some activities as long as I wore a brace on that knee. So, I continued to participate. I even formed a weightlifting program for the junior high school kids and faculty at the school where I was teaching. My wife was a part of that program, even after I left the school, and she won a recognition award from the students for her work in the program. I was just as proud of that award as I was of any special recognition that had been given to me.

My wife and life partner, Frances, was also fully into fitness. She in fact was a member of her college synchronized swimming team. We would go to the YMCA every day for exercise. Frances would swim nonstop for over an hour. I would swim one lap, get out of the pool, and go into the weight room, which was right next to the pool, separated from it by only a glass wall. When we had our kids, we continued the same routine. Our son began swimming lessons when he was 6 months old. Our daughter, whom we adopted at age 5, also went to the Y every day for family exercise time. While my family worked on swimming, I was primarily in the weight room.

Keeping my knee stable with weightlifting lasted for about five years before surgery was truly necessary. While the entire process from surgery to getting back to participating in sporting activities took about a year, I was back to engaging in all my physical-fitness activities. The surgery was scary, however, because the doctors told me at the time that if I damaged the knee again, the only thing that they could do was to fuse the knee together. That was something that I did not want, but my desire to participate in sporting endeavors overrode my fear of injury at that time. In other words, I probably wasn't using common sense.

While working on my PhD as a graduate assistant at the University of Maryland, College Park, I regularly participated in the intramural sports program and the faculty noontime basketball activity. It was during this basketball activity that I was to destroy my knee again, ten years after I last had it repaired. I was scared to see the doctors again, but I had no choice. I had decided to undergo fusion of my knee and thus end my athletic participation days. On arriving at the doctor's office and telling the doctor which position I wanted the knee fused, I was relieved by his reply. He told me to relax and said that due to new techniques and procedures, my knee no longer had to be fused in a stationary position. The second surgery went well, and the lessons I had learned after previous procedures served me well in the rehabilitation of this one. My desire for fitness also fostered my recovery efforts. The surgical procedure involved freeze-dried muscle fascia from a cadaver, Gore-Tex material, and realignment of my leg muscles to repair my knee. Less than nine months after this surgery, I went on a two-week backpacking trip in the Grand Canyon. I also continued to participate in weightlifting competitions in the intramural program. My success there compelled me to participate outside the university in amateur competitions at various fitness clubs.

As I got older, my perceptions about my aging body began to change the way I thought about physical activity. No longer did I have a desire to compete. I turned my attention to body shaping and toning. I moved from doing a great deal of fast-twitch muscle activities to participating in short-distance endeavors, like 5K races. My regular workout routine came to include runs of one to five miles and then an hour or so of light

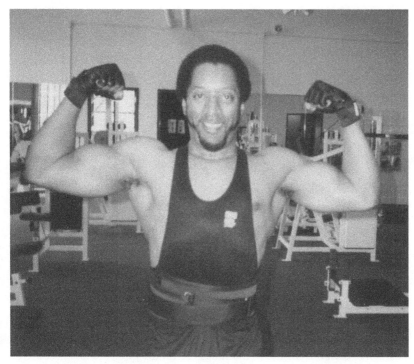

Aged 46, North Carolina A&T State University. Courtesy of James R. Coates.

weightlifting. Now that I'm 72, my runs are more of a one-to-two-mile jog. The weight workouts, however, are still a large part of my workout routine.

The coping strategy that I apply to the aging process is consistency. I continue to exercise four or five days a week. I listen to my body, however, and take a few days off from workouts when I feel the need for such a break. Also, every three or four months, I take at least one week away from all planned workouts. I continue to do a great deal of yard work. And because my wife is a wildflower artist, we hike in the Shenandoah National Forest to look for certain flowers. Despite all my fitness activities, I'm still a junk food junky. My wife keeps me on the right track, however, making sure that my diet is balanced. That regimen includes my intake of water. I estimate that I've had more water in the past five years than in the previous sixty-seven years combined.

Because my life is multicultural and multiracial, being considered elderly

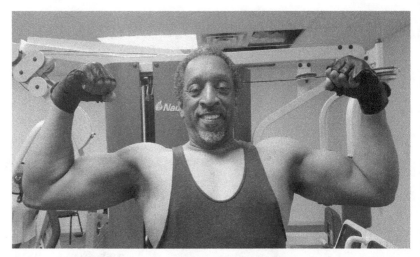

Retired, aged 69, at the gym at home in Virginia. Courtesy of James R. Coates.

encompasses different connotations in each segment. In my wife's white culture, being elderly is noted by the government as someone over 66 years of age. In the culture of the Black community in which we associate, being elderly is noted by the activities that one is physically still able to do. In other words, one's physical mobility is crucial. My mother, for instance, will be 95 years old on her next birthday. She is on the go and more active than I could ever keep up with each night of the week.

The services offered by the government to the elderly in my cultures vary. In my Black culture, the city of Annapolis offers social activities to the elderly with trips to museums, theatres, book readings, social conversations, tax preparations, affordable housing, and more. In my white rural community, few services for social activities are provided. Individuals are expected to provide for their own health and cultural needs and desires.

As for my social life, it is strong. My wife and I travel occasionally. We go to Washington DC; Annapolis, Maryland; and Arlington, Virginia, on a regular basis for museums, baseball games, theatres, dinner, and social visits. We are active in our local community. I even serve on our community association board of directors. We have over 960 homes in our gated, mountain lake community. I just recently persuaded the community to spend thousands of dollars to upgrade our community fitness room, which is only a small part of the fitness and social activities provided here. Some of the other amenities include a 240-acre lake with three beaches, picnic areas, swimming, and fishing tournaments; two playgrounds, a volleyball court, basketball courts, tennis courts, an eighteen-hole disc golf course, a bocce ball court, and horseshoe pits; hiking, biking, and walking trails; a dog park; community social dinners; major holiday celebrations; and a large number of social clubs for quilting, card playing, yoga, astrology, gardening, and more. A major project that the community is currently dealing with is the golf course. It has not been operational for several years, but some residents still play a hole or two of the course, regardless of its condition.

With all these social activities to choose from, I find myself participating in programs that are for the larger community. I'm the legal redress chairman of the Winchester, Virginia, branch of the NAACP (National Association for the Advancement of Colored People). I'm a member of the Lake Holiday Country Club Estates board of directors. I serve on the board of directors of the Virginia Tri-County OIC, a local Head Start program for underprivileged families using federal and local grants. I serve on the Frederick County, Virginia, Public Schools Equity Task Force, and on the Winchester, Virginia, Public Schools Equity Committee. As a retired university professor, I present public lectures at the Handley Library in Winchester, Virginia, and I continue to read, write, and study American sport history.

While I grew up in a lower socioeconomic environment, mainly due to a blatantly racist society, my family environment was rich and strong. Regardless of the activity I wanted to try or the organization I wanted to join, my family was always extremely encouraging and supportive. Above all else, education was a strict requirement in our family. As I progressed and met those who had little or no educational skills, it became exceptionally clear just how academic skills, when applied, assisted with societal inclusion and advancement. I feel an extraordinary sense of pride and good fortune in my past. From my parents, sisters, brother, brother in-law, extended family and friends, and our religious faith, my self-esteem was formulated and enriched. I was also fortunate to have some excellent teachers at the segregated schools I attended in Annapolis. They helped to educate but also to instill pride, perseverance, uplift, and self-esteem in each of their students' individual makeup. I stated above that at least one undergraduate professor had greatly influenced my educational and fitness beliefs. But it was after undergraduate school that another sense of pride, influence, and growth took shape. I met my wife to be, Frances, and we started our life together, including the birth of our son, James, and the adoption of our daughter, Almeda. Through the good, the bad, the rough, and the smooth, they have been there with and for me. My pride and self-esteem have been greatly enhanced by my supportive family.

Along our path, I taught school at the junior high and high school level. I coached young people in the sports of football, basketball, baseball, softball, track and field, and my first assigned coaching position when I was fresh out of undergraduate school, the pompon team. I then received the opportunity to teach and coach on the college level. I was the head men's basketball coach and, one year, an assistant coach of baseball at Chesapeake College. Teaching and coaching at that level was trying but also enlightening. At the same time, when I went to the University of Maryland to work on my PhD, first as a graduate assistant and later as an instructor, I met many white people with characteristics I thought existed only in the one I had married. Their ability to relate to, accept, educate, and confide in me changed me as an individual. Four of those individuals truly changed my life. Two of them were professors, Dr. Nancy Struna and Dr. Joan Hult. The other two were colleagues, Jerry Gems and Guy Hays. All four of them had profound impacts on my professional development after graduate school.

My first opportunity in higher education after receiving my PhD was at Shenandoah University, where I served as associate dean of students. There, I was the only African American with faculty rank. The only other African American employee was a recruiter in the admissions office who also was an assistant basketball coach. I was able to teach a class or two as well as serve in that administrative role. While working at Shenandoah, I also taught U.S. history at nearby Lord Fairfax Community College on weekends. At the same time, my community service, especially with the local branch of the NAACP, led me to more than one encounter with the Ku Klux Klan. After those encounters, my name and that of the president of the local branch of the NAACP were placed on a Klan enemy list that came out of Guilford County, North Carolina. It's ironic that during the same year, 1992, I moved with my family to that county, specifically the city of Greensboro, where I took a full-time teaching position at North Carolina A&T State University, a historically Black school. Through grants that I helped to obtain for community service, I developed a friendship with a white middle and high school parent whose older brother married a Black woman and younger sister was dating a Black man. I found out later that their parents were responsible for the Klan publication in Guilford County. Whatever racist, hateful propaganda they had been taught, it did not take hold with any of these individuals in adulthood. That parent also got me into some of the weightlifting and bodybuilding competitions at one of the local gyms in Greensboro. Such relationships indicate that racism can be alleviated with greater acquaintance and an open mind.

From Greensboro, I went to Green Bay, Wisconsin, where I spent the last sixteen years of my professional teaching career at the University of Wisconsin, Green Bay. For most of those years, I was the only African American faculty member, although there were several African American nonfaculty staff members. My personal community service led me to working with area and regional school districts on issues of racial and cultural diversity. In 2002 the then Brown County executive (Green Bay is in Brown County) authorized the formation of a diversity committee that was to investigate and review all complaints from citizens. In 2004 I served as the chairman of that committee. The pushback from political leaders and their media supporters who opposed such an oversight committee was strong. When I became the chairman, a local conservative radio talk show host, who truly thought of himself as equal to the national talk radio superstars, was relentless in his attacks on me and the committee. I saved many of his recordings and still have them.

In 2010 the then mayor of Green Bay, Jim Schmidt, appointed me to the five-member Citizens Police and Fire Commissioners Board. The board oversaw all aspects of the police and fire departments in the city, including the hiring process, bill-payment approval, and the discipline and removal process.

Another of my combined community and work-related responsibilities in Green Bay led me to the Green Bay Packers of the National Football League. Working with the directors of player development for the Packers, I helped create a program for current players and staff members to complete undergraduate degrees they had begun at other institutions or to obtain graduate degrees at the University of Wisconsin, Green Bay.

The life I have led, especially my growth and development, gives me a prideful feeling. While I have felt this pride in my past, I am now also experiencing the joys of getting older, which include an eye on retirement and longer periods of leisure. I have also experienced fears about getting older, including greater concern about my health and a decrease in neuromuscular coordination (the lessening of balance, power, speed, agility, reaction time, and kinesthetic sense). Aging also provided me with some powerful reflective thoughts, not thoughts of wisdom but rather questions like "How in the world did I make it through those experiences?" Those experiences, however, allow me to share a great deal of reflective advice with those who seek such information or guidance.

As I reflect on fitness and health issues throughout my life, I feel extremely blessed and fortunate. I've had many injuries but my reflections on them bring sadness and disappointments, not depression. I always believed that despite my diminutive size, I was a tough guy who would and could fight through anything. I know this attitude is not realistic, but in dealing with my injuries, that mindset worked. I accidentally chopped off my left index finger with a meat clever when I was 10 years old. I had my kidney bruised while playing football when I was 12. I was also shot in the eye with a homemade arrow (a soda bottle cap being the head of the arrow) while playing cowboys and Indians at age 12. I tore the ligaments in my left knee at 17, and I had my front teeth damaged while playing football at 19. At least twice I suffered a broken nose. My three major knee surgeries have already been mentioned, but in addition I experienced a torn Achilles tendon at age 46, groin hernia surgery at age 52, navel hernia surgery at age 55, and torn rotator cuff and labrum at age 67.

Through all my life experiences I have considered myself a fortunate individual with outstanding family and associates. I've leaned on their experiences, good or bad, to blaze my own path. So I would consider myself optimistic and resilient. And as a reflective thinker, I can't help but engage in some nostalgia. The only thing I truly long for from my youth is the soul music of the late fifties, the sixties, and the early seventies. I guess anyone can guess what my musical collection consists of.

Just like most people, I suspect, I wish I could have done a few things differently. I would like to have done more for those I love and who have loved me through all my trials and tribulations. I wish I could have done more for my mom and dad. My father passed away twenty-one years ago. I am still trying to get my wife her own small art gallery to display her work. Although she tells me that she doesn't need such a place, my pride in her work makes me want to share it with others.

With all that I've experienced in my life, I've never really contemplated a personal legacy. I've never seen myself as great at anything. But I will try, try, and try again to succeed at what I undertake. No, I've not always been successful. But I did seek to obtain. At this stage of my life, I now seek, with my wife, to share what we can describe as the good life. To us, that is enjoying retirement, sharing our time together, and traveling to visit sites and artifacts we desire to see. To me the good things in life include being with family and participating in fitness activities at levels that are appropriate for me and my health. Lifelong fitness! Okay, maybe I could stand to lose a pound or two, but I'm still not fat, at least not yet! But I do love to eat.

6 Aging, Antiaging, and Infinite Youth in Taiwan

CHIA-JU YEN

The greatest Chinese educator, Confucius, kept his own account of his gradual progress and attainments. The Master said, "At fifteen, I had my mind bent on learning; at thirty, I stood firm; at forty, I had no doubts; at fifty, I knew the decrees of heaven; at sixty, my ear was an obedient organ for the reception of truth; at seventy, I could follow what my heart desired, without transgressing against what was right."[1] I have tried very hard to imitate his discipline to experience well-being at an advanced age. As I approach 60, however, it is still hard to abide by his goal for 40—to have no doubts. There are still many puzzles in my daily life.

My father, born in 1934, and my mother, born in 1937, sprang from peasant families in the southern part of Taiwan. When World War II was over, the political environment in China got worse and civil war broke out. It was then that the KMT (Chiang Kai-Shek's Nationalist Peoples' Party) government moved to Taiwan. At that time of general poverty, it was hard for young people to receive a good education. After completing his elementary education, my father, only a teenager, had to go to Taipei to earn money to support his parents and family. My mother had less education than my father did because her father prohibited her from attending school, fearing she might be bombed on her way there during the war. In addition, her health was so poor that she couldn't do farm work. So she became an apprentice to a tailor at around the age of 12. My relatives told me that my mother always dressed well and had long, beautiful black hair. It was unusual to dress up like a lady in the countryside. Because of my mother's interest in personal appearance, she wanted me to wear my hair long like hers. I was not allowed to cut it short until I attended junior high school, when I had to comply with school regulations. She was very sad to see my short hair. Maybe my long hair had reminded her of the happiness she experienced with hers during her youth.

Taipei is a modern and economically flourishing city, with more opportunities to get jobs than in the countryside. When my father first moved there, he worked in a wholesale grocery store in the most prosperous and famous business district—Dihua Street (迪化街) in Taipei. It is well known by foreign visitors and overflows with tourists during the Chinese Lunar New Year Festival. My parents got married in their twenties and settled down in Taipei. I, their eldest child, was born in 1960. When I was in grade 3 of elementary school, my father owned his own grocery store in Sanchong City, a suburb of Taipei. After school, my two sisters, brother, and I had to help in the grocery store. As a student, I had no summer or winter vacation like my friends and classmates did. I disliked the holidays because I had to work at the store. The work was not only hard but boring, and we had only one day off each year—the first day of the Chinese Lunar New Year. Moreover, working hours were from 7 a.m. to 11 p.m. I believe my parents were overworked, as my mother died at 44 and my father at 50. They both led short lives, whereas my grandparents, who lived in the country, led natural, happy long lives and died in their 90s. My great-grandmother died the day after her 100th birthday.

The story of my life begins in Taipei, where I completed my studies. From kindergarten to university, I lived with my parents and siblings. After school was finished each day, I went directly home to help my parents. Because our store was in a market, the whole day was busy, especially in the evening, when vendors supplied grocers in preparation for the next day of business.

But, thanks to my desire for knowledge and despite a stressful schedule during my school days, I always had good grades and could attend a high-quality high school and, later, university. I graduated from the Fu-Jen Catholic University with a bachelor's degree in library science in 1982. I then entered the Academia Sinica as a librarian in the Institute of Mathematics and Information Science, where I worked for ten years. During my school days and the first several years of my working as a librarian, I didn't have much time to exercise. I did, however, join an aerobic dance group that met for one hour twice a week for three years. I didn't like sports in general, because being sweaty was uncomfortable.

In May 1992 I took a job at the National Taiwan Sport University (NTSU), where I worked again as a librarian. This change turned out to be a great turning point for me, as I gradually began to like sports. In the beginning, I tried to play table tennis. I bought formal sport outfits, shoes, and quality paddles, since one of my office colleagues told me that before you learn to excel in a sport, you should have professional sport clothing and facilities. Regretfully, I gave up playing table tennis when a coach told me that my posture when playing was like that of a patient with pediatric paralysis.

Then I discovered what was to become my hobby: badminton. This time, luckily, I had an encouraging coach, who always cheered me up, whether I played well or not. I still remember his voice at the court during that time: "Very good!" "You got an A+++. You are soooo excellent as an athlete!" All these cheerful words inspired my passion for badminton, which lasted for more than ten years. I joined a morning badminton club that met at a junior high school near my home, played with my university colleagues at lunchtime, and then, after work, attended an evening badminton club. I was also a member of the university staff team but not the key person, because we had many retired athletes. In interuniversity competition, I was always the one who stood near the net to hit low shots. My partner was a retired badminton athlete who could last the whole game. Once she told me that she felt like she had three enemies on the court. Anyway, I did my best in the competitions.

I have two sons, both of whom like sports very much. When they were little, they learned to swim at the university during summer vacation. Both are good swimmers. My elder son taught me to swim the backstroke. I still recall his sweet voice when he was age 7. "Mami, you must relax, as if you completed all your housework, then you can float up!" So, my first swimming style was backstroke. People said that it is not easy for a newbie to learn the backstroke in their first swimming class.

My sons play sports regularly. Both play basketball in their leisure time. My younger son is a member of an amateur baseball team; he has a full set of baseball equipment. Now, he is a travel guide. Sea activities are his favorite, so he likes to go to Pattaya Beach in Thailand, and to Hawaii and Guam, to surf with travelers.

Continuing My Studies

In August of 1996 I switched from the catalog section of the library to the reference section. As a librarian at NTSU, I certainly expanded my knowledge of sports. Moreover, I had much more contact with readers. My job was not only to assist them in finding books or research information but also to help them to translate academic papers. That work gave me a chance to know more about sports-related science.

At this time, I decided to end my unhappy marriage. It was quite a hard time for me. I consulted a psychologist several times and read some relevant books to strengthen my mental power. Although I thought that I had prepared myself well, the divorce proceedings set off a neurotic disorder. Six times in one year, I had to go to the hospital emergency unit for vertigo, vomiting, or diarrhea. Thanks to my close friends and officemates, I was able to get through that time of suffering. Of course, sport played an important role in my recovery, for it helped me relax, feel happy, and sleep well.

After my divorce, I decided to continue my studies at NTSU. I prepared for the master's exam, reading many books and notes; I also attended many junior referee lessons or coaching classes to increase my sports credits. I was very lucky to pass the entrance exam in 2001. Before the new semester began, I took my sons and my younger sister to the American West, visiting such places as Los Angeles, San Francisco, Las Vegas, the Grand Canyon, Yosemite National Park, and other places of interest. When I first saw the Grand Canyon, I was astonished by its uncanny structure—a wonder of creation.

Adventure education was the most impressive and interesting course for me. I participated in many outdoor activities, such as sky wooden bridge, sky rope, and rock climbing. All these activities were very stimulating. I believe that activities can strengthen my mind. For me, participating in these activities can be considered a rite of passage in gaining confidence. And the teacher of outdoor activities, Chih-Mou Shieh, became the faculty adviser for my thesis. The term "serious leisure" attracted me very much. Why must leisure be serious? After one year of work, my master's thesis was born. The title was "A Study of Serious Leisure Participation and Relational Factors, Taking Taipei Municipal Library's Teacher, Lin, Telling Stories as an Example." The master's courses gave me a chance to make friends with more people; almost all my classmates came from the sport world. I found them to be open, enthusiastic, and passionate; it was easy to get along with them.

I had insatiable hunger for learning and began my PhD studies in 2005. It was a hard but colorful time for me. PhD students are supposed to master courses at other universities, so I selected Gender and Sex and Field Study at National Tsing Hua University. It took me one and a half hours to get there, but I enjoyed the courses very much and was obsessed with anthropology. Regretfully, the professor of anthropology I studied under, and who inspired me most, died of cancer a few years ago at the age of 54.

There is a Chinese saying: "Reading helps us learn so much about beauty and truth that we can live a better life in our own ways." For me, reading lets me figuratively travel the world. But because I was eligible to attend international conferences to increase my academic credits, I could literally travel to many countries. I had never dreamed before that I might have the precious chance to study in Germany for almost one year. That turned out to be an amazing experience. One day in 2008, I found that the Physical Education Institute website posted sponsorship information from the DAAD (German Academic Exchange Service). I immediately began to prepare for it by studying the German language. Pronunciation and grammar were challenging for a long time. I followed the requirements step by step to complete the application and was the first person at my university to apply for sponsorship by the DAAD and the National Science Council. As a result of my efforts, my dream came true. I remember that in the summer of 2009, before I went to Germany, my reading club played Time Capsule. We were supposed to write down our dreams for the centennial of the Republic of China, which would occur in 2011. We put all the time capsules in an exquisite box, which we buried in the front yard of a member's house. After ten months of studying in Germany, I flew back to Taiwan on New Year's Day 2011. At the first meeting of the reading club in 2011, we opened the time capsules. I was the only one who had made his or her dream come true.

My stay in Germany was unforgettable. I told my friends and my family that it was like a dream and that the value of those ten months was the equivalent of ten years in Taiwan. I, as an Asian person in a western culture, gathered a lot of new and special experiences during that period. I went through the lowest temperature of my life—minus 17 degrees Celsius. My academic adviser, Annette Hofmann, taught me how to ski. Although it was a very short lesson, it was very exciting for me. In 2010 I enjoyed the FIFA World Cup broadcast with students from Taiwan and a bunch of local people in a historic beer brewery. We drank beer and sang songs loudly together to celebrate the victory of the German team. I also played—for the only time in my life—in a soccer game in Muenster with professors and the staff of the Institute of Sport Science. Before the game, I told them that I am a librarian, not an athlete, and that I can't play soccer. A dance teacher told me that she couldn't play soccer either. She persuaded me not to worry too much. Actually, she played much, much better than I expected. I didn't know how to play it at all. The only strategy for me was to run after the ball. I once forced an opponent off the field successfully. I heard his partner scolding him, and he put the blame on me. At that time, I was so proud of myself. But then, with the ball right at my foot, I unfortunately headed toward a bunch of people who turned out to be my opponents. At that moment, I drew a blank—"What can I do, now?" An intermission whistle from the referee saved me from finding an answer. After the game, I was tired out and my body ached all over. What a great soccer game that was!

I liked the cheerful song of the 2011 FIFA World Cup, "Waving the Flag," so I saved the video on my laptop. In Germany, whenever I was discouraged, I watched the video and sang with it to cheer myself up. One day, I visited my neighbor, an architect from Taiwan. His two cute daughters danced to another song of the 2011 FIFA World Cup in front of reflective

French windows. At the beginning, I stood aside and my body swung just a little with the rhythm, but when they pulled me to dance with them, I yelled, "No! No! No! I can't dance!" The younger sister said, with pop-eyes, "How come? Someone can't dance?" My answer was, "Yes, it is curious that some people can't dance." The truth was that I was shy to dance in front of them. My shyness sometimes blocked me from the world. There were times, however, when I was forced to be brave. For example, when the two-month-long portion of the German course in Bonn was about to end, there was a farewell gathering. After dinner, my classmates and I descended the stairway to the dancing saloon in the basement. I felt sleepy and bored, though, and the room was too noisy. But a girl pulled me by the hand to the dance hall. She and other girls gathered in a circle and pushed me to the center to do a solo dance. I ran back out three times but was pushed to the center again and again. "Here goes nothing," I thought and danced some sort of belly dance, causing my classmates to scream. Finally, I showed how brave I could be.

Muenster is the bike capital of Germany. It occurred to me that the bike was a third leg of its inhabitants. My landlord lent me her husband's bike and taught me how to ride it. I remembered that she supported me when we first practiced, and unfortunately, I pushed her down into the bushes and almost hurt her. Because the bike was too high for me, my feet couldn't touch the ground, and I felt unsafe. But I did manage to have a bike adventure. My academic adviser, Annette, invited me to her home for breakfast and said that it was only a thirty-minute bike ride from the campus, where I lived, to her home. Suspecting that with her biking experience she could travel much faster than I could, I thought that riding my "grandfather's" bike would take double the time. I left home at seven o'clock and thought I would arrive at her home at eight punctually. Even though her home was not on my city bus map, I followed the bus route smoothly at first. Unfortunately, the route was detoured due to construction. I tried to find my way but wandered and finally got lost. I panicked because I had missed the appointed time and had no idea where I was. I stopped at a convenience store and asked the clerk to help me contact Annette. She came, and I followed her car to her home. Because the road was hilly, I spent all my energy following her car, although she drove at a very low speed. It took me over three hours to get to her home! When I arrived at almost 11 a.m., I was deadly thirsty and drank three big cups of water. The meal we had together ended up being lunch, not breakfast. Nevertheless, on the ride back, I enjoyed the beautiful scenery and saw horses grazing leisurely in a pasture. People in a beer cart with pedals were singing songs and drinking. What a tough trip for me! I felt as if I were like "Hänsel und Gretel," lost in the woods. After taking a bath, I ate two sandwiches and then took a long nap. That was the longest bike trip I ever took in my life.

As a librarian, I like to do research. But perhaps the stress of completing my work while also overseeing the construction of a new university library led to colon cancer in the summer of 2015 after I returned from the conference of the International Society for the History of Physical Education and Sport held in Croatia. An operation and chemotherapy left me so weak and tired that I needed to rest after a meal or a bath. After a stay in the hospital, I recuperated at my elder cousin's home and was kindly cared for by his family. When I came home, I still needed to recuperate for two months, so I went to a nearby park to exercise with the Infinite Youth Qigong club as much as my body would allow. It was hard to follow the club's tempo, but gradually I became stronger and stronger. I liked the members of the club; I felt as though they were my family. When I was sick at home, they prepared food for me and came to see me often. I am grateful for their help and would do the same for any of them if they need it. Now I practice Qigong almost every day. My strength and fitness have returned. There is still one thing to adjust to, however—the need for a reduced workload. It is still hard for me to say no to others, but I try to remember to say yes to myself; then I can have an easier life in the future.

Aged People in Taiwan

After the government of the Republic of China moved to Taiwan in 1949, a series of political, institutional, and economic reforms were carried out there from the 1950s onward. Those changes brought Taiwan from poverty to prosperity. The country's economic growth, as measured by the gross domestic product (GDP), averaged 7.91 percent between 1960 and 1990.

Between 2010 and 2016, however, the highest rate of growth was about 5.05 percent, with the average being 2.90 percent. In 2016 it was only 2.17 percent. In 2017 the growth in GDP for the entire country was 3.31 percent, equal to $590.780 million, or $25,080 per person, in U.S. dollars.[2] In 2018 the growth rate was only 2.96 percent.[3] These figures show clearly the decline of Taiwan's economic growth. China's economy, on the contrary, is growing very fast and has absorbed much of Taiwan's capital; its cheap labor force is attractive to other countries as well.[4] Many factors have weakened Taiwan's economy, as reflected in young people's low income and reduced pensions. Conditions have become worse in recent years.

Young people with lower incomes hesitate to get married. Poor income leads to delay in marriage and childbearing age, and thus a low birth rate. The average fertility rate in Taiwan is 1.06 percent. And immigration is declining year by year. Furthermore, life expectancy has reached an all-time high of 80.4 years. Taiwan is becoming an aging society and is approaching the status of a superaged society. In 2025 the elderly over 65 years old will account for one-fifth of the total population, approaching 5 million.[5] To deal with this rapidly aging population, the Taiwanese government has executed some plans for caring for the elderly, such as the Long-Term Care Plan 2.0, which covers the years 2017 to 2026. It offers person-centered, community-based, continual care and has four goals, the first being to establish an accessible, affordable, and universal long-term care service system of high quality. The second is "aging in place," or remaining in one's home and community as aging progresses, as a policy goal. The third is upstream prevention to delay disability. And the last is downstream preparedness to provide a discharge plan for home-based medical care.[6]

I learned that reduced pensions for former government officers forced some of them to move out of a quality private nursing home. One of my former colleagues, who had retired in her fifties, had a disabled husband and was very angry about the annuity reform, which makes it harder for her and her husband to stay alive. She has had to adjust to a life without regular payments. In the summer of 2018, I went to my parents' hometown to visit my uncles and aunts, all of whom were in their eighties. When my mother's younger sister-in-law fell and her husband tried to help her, both were seriously injured. Their children all live and work far away from them. The community care unit manages their lunches and dinners. And I witnessed an aide coming to my aunt and uncle's home to help my aunt to take a bath. The couple was satisfied with the service and cost. I also heard about respite care service, which can give a break to those who have to care for seriously disabled elder family members. This service resembles a kindergarten in that older people are transported to the center and can participate in various activities offered there. Most elderly people like to attend this "school," where they can talk with their peers and play together. I believe that such a program benefits both the older people and their family members who care for them regularly.

Research Resources

My research resources involved interviewees, observation of persons close to me, published articles, and media and web reports. The major part of my research consisted of personal interviews and completed questionnaires. The study did not go as smoothly as I expected. For example, my younger sister refused to participate for fear of an invasion of her privacy; others were afraid of stirring up unhappy memories. From the interviews, however, I did learn more about my friends' lives. I appreciated their honesty and generosity in sharing their experiences with me and helping me to complete my research. I noticed that if someone has a happy married life, he or she likes being interviewed and expresses contentment with his or her life. But most people skip the dark sides of their lives, although some confessed to having physical problems, such as diseases.

More complete information would enrich my research, so I interviewed people from various parts of my life, such as my officemates, former classmates, neighbors, a lady in charge of a breakfast, a hairdresser, members of a conference, members of a Qigong exercise group, members of my church, and more. There were thirty-three women and thirty-seven men, aged 50 to 86; only twelve of them were retired, eight were housewives, and eight were currently single. The types of income of the retired interviewees were pensions, bank deposits, investments, rental income, and support from their children. Housewives' financial support came from their husbands or their children. Only one person stated that he lives alone; the others said they stayed with family members, including children and even grandchildren. Most of the men said they felt ten years younger than their age. Two of them reported feeling older than their age: one said he was disabled, and the other had just recovered from a serious illness. Women were more confident than men about their appearance. Among them, one felt younger than 41–45, six felt like 40, four felt younger than 35–40, and one told me that her son thought she looked as young as 18. My interviewees tended to eat light meals without too much oil, salt, and sugar. Only one man and one woman were smokers.

My interviewees' hobbies and activities included gardening, flower arrangement, painting, travel, reading, cooking, singing, playing cards, going to movies, watching TV, photography, playing with grandchildren, meditation, chanting, going to hot springs, playing basketball, playing golf, playing table tennis, walking, hiking, swimming, mountaineering, biking, gymnastics, practicing Qigong, and volunteering to help needy people. There was one man, aged 56, who rode a large, heavy motorcycle, an adventurous sport. My adviser retired last year at age 65, and he planned to follow all nine routes of the Camino de Santiago religious pilgrimage in Spain, already having completed the eight-hundred-kilometer Camino Frances (from St-Jean-Pied-de-Port to Santiago de Compostela) and the thousand-kilometer Vía da la Plata (from Seville to Santiago de Compostela). He shared his experience through speaking engagements and thus attracted people to join him on the journey, making it a fad in Taiwan. My junior colleague joined a group called Happy Run, starting with 5K runs and proceeding to 54K ones, and participated many times in marathons (even a supermarathon) to improve his stamina. A coach told me that she attends a group whose members are a retired handball team; their average age is 54. They practice regularly and go abroad to participate in games with foreign teams. My interviewees generally were not enthusiastic about joining clubs—only eight men and six women had done so. Some of them belong to religious groups and flower arrangement clubs, and others participate in exercise groups for yoga, hiking, tennis, softball, Qigong, and other activities. The men were more optimistic than the women and were more satisfied with their marital status. A lady told me that her divorce made her feel regret for her sons, for she could not offer them a "complete" family. And another lady, aged 54, regretted having no boyfriend after her divorce. Most interviewees paid great attention to their families, hoping that their children would grow up well and follow a smooth life trajectory. Furthermore, two interviewees stated that they regretted having been unable to spend much time with their aged parents before they died.

Two Taiwanese elders are exceptional. One, whom I call Senior Rambo, at age 85 had teeth strong enough to chew hard fried peanuts and sugar cane, and even to open a beer bottle. He took up jogging at 60, and between the ages of 62 and 77, he participated in triathlons. He ran the national road marathon of 113 kilometers in seven hours and two minutes. He proudly said that President Yingjiu Ma ran along with him. He learned to ride a unicycle after falling many times. He claimed that people should try to stay healthy, not mind their age, and do whatever they want to do. Another exception is Jet-grandma, aged 81. I learned about her from media, which proclaimed her a legend. She introduced herself with complete self-confidence. "I am a jet grandma; my granddaughter said that I am a hyperactive grandma!" She runs seven kilometers a day, but even more admirable is that at age 79 she successfully climbed the highest peak in Africa, Mount Kilimanjaro, setting the record for Taiwan's oldest person to reach the summit. She has often represented Taiwan in the International Evergreen Athletics Competition, winning medals and breaking records almost every time.[7]

A professor told me that he helps care for a community, Garlic Mayuan Community (蒜香麻園社區), which is near the university he works at in Yunlin County, an agricultural area. He brought his students there to entertain the aged and organized some activities to cheer them up.[8] Some social organizations and the government have designed projects to help aged people in their daily routine and tend to their medical needs. I was already aware of the Huashan Social Welfare Foundation (華山基金會), whose purpose is to serve the elderly and whose slogan is "To protect the elderly is to protect your future." The Huashan Foundation, formally established in 1999, is a free at-home service for the elderly who are disabled, are homeless, or suffer from dementia. It provides 387 community halfway stations to offer local and regional services. Such organizations are important to help aged people enjoy well-being in later life.[9] Another excellent welfare group, Hondao Senior Citizen's Welfare Foundation, established in 1995, has lasted for twenty-four years. It has three goals—dreams never get old, filial piety, and community care—and offers care and services for senior citizens, including an award for families representing three generations residing together to encourage respect and appreciation for the parents and grandparents. Nationwide Volunteer Stations and Volunteer Services offer forty-six stations with a total of 1,514 volunteers providing free services to the homes of senior citizens. Time Dollar–Mutual Support coupons create the Volunteer Hours Bank through the volunteer hours exchange service, in which volunteers can store their service hours and "withdraw" the hours when they need assistance. Hot Meal Services and Community Care Checkpoints allow senior citizens to live in familiar surroundings while enjoying care and support from their neighbors. Domestic Care Service provides help with household chores, a regular caregiving service, and body care service. Senior Citizen Day Care Service performs case management, daily care, rehabilitation, bodily revitalization training, basic nursing care, and leisurely activities. Halfway House–Short Stay provides shelter for seniors who need temporary housing or rehabilitative care. Senior Citizen Leisure Activities and Senior Citizen Welfare Service Consultation communicate with seniors, their family members, and the general public regarding social welfare information relevant to seniors.[10]

The government has collaborated with several nongovernmental organizations to provide necessary services to the aging population. Some organizations, such as the Infinite Youth Qigong Association, which I was involved with in 2011, are independent, however, and have no sponsorship from the government. They encourage people to practice Qigong and provide support systems to cancer patients in recovery.

Conclusion

According to United Nations statistics, life expectancy is rising. In 2050 the proportion of the global population over 65 will reach one-sixth, and an initial estimate of that population is more than 1.5 billion. This demographic change will have an impact on every nation's social welfare system, especially in Asia and Africa.[11] Managing the growing aging population will be a challenge for the entire world. What's worse is that since 2015, there has been a growing trend of abuse of parents and other elders over the age of 65. Wei-Yan Lin, director of the Department of Protection of the Ministry of Health and Welfare in Taiwan, estimated that this trend may be related to more long-term care and dementia among Taiwan's aging society. Nowadays, families are smaller and pressure to take care of the elderly is growing. When family support is insufficient, family relationships become fragile and prone to crisis.[12]

Growing older comes with fears of becoming disabled or afflicted by dementia. When my surgery required a stay in the hospital for ten days, I felt like a prisoner in my bed. All my care was managed at my bedside. Three nurses bathed me while their tutor stood aside and instructed them in how to do it. The first time for me was awkward. I didn't know whether to keep my eyes closed or open. I was naked as a newborn and had to watch and listen as they cared for and discussed how to handle my body. Moreover, I was astonished to find that when I got up for the first time after seven days in bed, I couldn't stand firmly or move by myself. I needed my son to lead me to the toilet. I was shocked that my body was so feeble. I had always thought of myself as strong and independent. I remembered that I had handled all staff requirements and did every precheck before the operation by myself, whereas, after it, I became a "real patient." This lesson reinforced my desire to stay healthy and not become a burden to my family late in my life.

How to age successfully is an important subject, not only for the aged themselves but also for their families and even the whole country. People say that if you have money, good friends, and a sound body, then you can have a good quality of life in old age. While average life expectancy in Taiwan is eighty years, the average number of healthy years in a lifetime is only 71.2. To avoid nine years of poor health, it is important to learn how to make them good years.[13] Luckily, weakness is reversible. The key points in preventing disability are eating well, exercising a lot, and making new friends. Jin-Chuan Ye, a former director of the Department of Health, Executive Yuan, said, on his Facebook page, that exercise fights disability.[14]

From my research, I discovered the following results:

1. *Live long and live better; community is a basic unit for antiaging.* We all know that exercise is very important for health, but it is hard to get in the habit without any partners. Community is the basic unit for antiaging. I, for example, exercise with Qigong in the park near my home from five thirty to seven every morning. I do it not only for physical health but also for psychological health. The group is like my alternative family. Members often go to breakfast or on holiday excursions together. Sometimes I have a chance to enjoy someone's homemade cuisine. And some of the group members are on medical staffs and thus can act as health consultants for other members. I appreciate the importance of that group and its members to me; without them, my life would be boring. There are still some exercise groups in the park such as healthy gymnastics, tai chi, yoga, and table tennis.

I did research on walking groups in the Nangang district of Taipei in 2017. I interviewed some volunteer leaders of the walking groups. They told me that walking not only improved their health and gave them joy but also enhanced community cohesion. One of the leaders, in his sixties, said that he enjoyed caring for two ladies in their eighties every evening; it made him feel valuable and important. The director of the community very often invited experts to teach members about health and to show them how to walk correctly. Most of them gained confidence from walking together, and they also felt younger than their age. A leader, aged 70, told me that he overcame depression following an occupational injury (one eye blinded in a chemical accident) by walking in a group. He paid much attention to the group and devoted himself to maintaining the walking paths. As a Chinese saying goes, "a far-off relative is less helpful than a near neighbor."

It is easy to consider demographic characteristics in providing community resources for the old. Community programmers must recognize and accommodate cultural diversity and remove the social and cultural barriers to service accessibility.[15] For example, there is a historic temple near which many older people often sit. The government grasps the chance to organize medical staff to speak to these elderly people about health and medicine and national policies, and to even do some minor physical checks like testing blood pressure and blood sugar. This service not only improves health but also protects the elderly from being cheated by unscrupulous vendors selling fake medicine. And the host of the temple often organizes travel groups for a low fee (for it receives many donations) or holds festivals on God's birthday as well as traditional festivals. People of the community play and eat together, thus entertaining not only the old people but everyone. It seems that the temple has become a congregational meal site.

Many local agencies on aging have worked to develop partnerships with the private sector to meet the needs of older adults in their communities.[16] In my community, near the famous Chang-Gung Hospital, there are many nursing homes. On sunny days you can see a lot of elders in wheelchairs accompanied by their helpers. The proximity between the hospital and the nursing facilities makes it convenient for old people to get medical services. Research has shown that it is vital to invest in the humanitarian and social capacity of leaders and volunteers, in the maintenance of partnerships within the community, in the connection to social welfare organizations, and in the improvement of community capacity in various aspects of day-care units.

Introducing young people to the aged world is also a good way to reconcile the gap between young and old. Once, in a church meeting, we discussed the relationships that young people had with older people, such as grandparents. Most of the female members did not have good relationships with older people; some of them even were mistreated by them due to cultural patriarchy (discrimination against girls). Luckily, I had a wonderful relationship with my grandparents and the other seniors in my family. When I was a little child, aged 8, only a junior elementary school student, I was responsible for taking my grandparents to other relatives' homes or to outdoor traditional dramas whenever they came to Taipei. Of course, my grandparents thanked me for my considerations by giving me extra pocket money. Sometimes I acted as a bridge between them and my parents. I was, for example, able to be a spokesperson for my mother to my grandparents. In the early years of Taiwan, in agricultural society, a daughter-in-law had few rights to express her opinions in front of her parents-in-law.

Some researchers showed that the aims of the intergenerational programs developed since the 1980s in countries overseas were to develop positive attitudes of the young toward their elders and to mutually share the experiences of different generations through curricular plans. A community curriculum in the elementary schools in Taiwan is the proper way to set up an intergenerational program because it emphasizes the importance of community resources and cultural heritage. The study took the second-grade students at an elementary school in Pingtung County, the southernmost county in Taiwan, as a research object. And it showed that most of the participants gave the curriculum positive feedback, approved the values of the curriculum, and said they would like to participate in it again.[17] Generally, nursing students have a negative attitude toward elder people, so research done with nursing students incorporated music therapy into a practical geriatric nursing course at a nursing home to see whether it could cultivate positive attitudes toward elder adults. The result concluded that music can be integrated into a gerontological nursing course to enhance students' motivation to learn, empathize, and approach elder adults.[18] Moreover, young people pay attention to the seniors' needs for clothing that can be worn in a variety of ways and is convenient for them to wear.[19]

Therefore, letting the young and old get to know each other will create a harmonious society. And becoming older is the future of young people.

2. *Keep on working.* During the second month of my chemotherapy (such therapy is six months long), my doctor told me that I could go back to work, for I am a restless person. He said that work is good for my recovery. How could that be true? I felt so weak at the time. Actually, going back to work did help me regain my energy quickly. For older people, I thought, maybe doing nothing is not beneficial. One of my interviewees, Senior Rambo, opened a mechanical company in mainland China at 65. He sent a reliable Taiwanese overseer there and still visits his company a few times a year, managing it by reviewing digital reports every day. He said that he is half-retired.

Accordingly, a Japanese professor named Noda said that in the past ten years, the walking speed of people aged 75 to 79 was equal to that of people eleven years younger. They walked normally and healthily and could expect to live for twenty years. It was wasteful and dangerous for them if they could not work.[20] In Japan, the definition of "old" is blurry. In addition to health, the financial situation must be considered. The latest recession and reduced pensions have made things harder and harder. Nowadays, in Taiwan, the number of gray-haired workers is growing. And some aged people care for their grandchildren to help their children out, perhaps earning money for that work. Maybe we should change our stereotypical way of thinking that aged people need to work only for financial reasons.

3. *Activate the third act.* Edward Kelly stated that normally, after retirement, people will have twenty or thirty more years to live. He called these years "the third act." "In the first and second acts there is always someone to blame, family, business; in the third act there is no one left to blame." Longevity is a new phenomenon, according to Kelly. He suggested the following: What we should do is to sense that longevity unavoidably changes the vision of our life. We should insist on growing, evolving, and go back to the depth of the heart to be a real human being, quieter, more intelligent, and kinder and dare to love.[21] I also admire my former classmate Xiang-Ru. Her parents enjoyed a long life, but she was struck with cancer in her forties. She told me that nothing is permanent in life, so seize the day and enjoy it.

Bronnie Ware, in her book *The Top Five Regrets of the Dying*, stated the five most common regrets she heard: "(1) I wish I'd had the courage to live a life true to myself, not the life others expected of me; (2) I wish I didn't work so hard; (3) I wish I'd had the courage to express my feelings; (4) I wish I'd stayed in touch with my friends; and (5) I wish that I had let myself be happier."[22] All the five regrets hit me seriously! It is time for me to ponder my own retirement. How can I manage my third act well?

Relative to the third act, I admired a person, Dan Huang, who is my writing teacher's husband. At the age of 65, he was the deputy general manager of an information science company in America. After he retired, he not only became "Clown Egg Yolk," giving charity performances all over Taiwan in nursing homes; he also used the "three, three, three" allocation method—taking care of the body, challenging oneself to learn, and being a volunteer to give back to society. I thought that this is a perfect arrangement for retirement. People intend to pay attention to the first two parts but neglect the last one. For the second part, I noticed many aged people want to make records or break records. For my retirement, however, being a clown is a good choice for me. I like to make people laugh, and I can gain happiness from them. I remembered that the founder of the Hershey Chocolate Company, Milton S. Hershey, once said, "One is only happy in proportion as he makes others feel happy."

NOTES

1. Ze Hou Li, *Analects of Confucius: Current Interpretation* (Taipei: Asian Culture, 2000), 51–53.

2. Hui Ling Lin, "Opportunities and Challenges for Taiwan's Economic Growth," [in Chinese,] accessed May 15, 2019, http://www.tri.org.tw/trinews/doc/1061214 _3.pdf.

3. National Statistics, R.O.C. [Taiwan], https://www.stat.gov.tw/ct.asp?xltem= 37407&CtNode=3564&mp=4.

4. Wanyu Wu, Jingyi Chen, "Taiwan's Economy Has Been Declining: What Happened in These 20 Years? *Academia Sinica* Report Revealed," [in Chinese,] *Commonwealth* 636 (November 20, 2017), accessed May 15, 2019, https://www .cw.com.tw/article/article.action?id=5086269.

5. Taiwan Ministry of Interior, Department of Statistics, "The Rank of Life Expectancy at Birth by Country, 2017," [in Chinese,] accessed May 15, 2019, https:// www.moi.gov.tw/stat/news_detail.aspx?sn=13742. According to the World Health Organization, if the proportion of the population over 65 years old is 7 percent or more, a society is called "aging"; if 14 percent or more, it is called "aged"; and if 20 percent, it is called "super-aged."

6. Pau-Ching Lu, "Long-Term Care 2.0 in Taiwan: Respond to an Aging Society," accessed May 24, 2019, https://goo.gl/bqi65T.

7. SET News Web, "Admirable! 81-Year-Old 'Jet Grandma' Runs 7 Kilometers a Day and Climbs to the Highest Peak in Africa," [in Chinese,] accessed June 1, 2019, https://www.setn.com/News.aspx?NewsID=352422.

8. Garlic Mayuan Community Building Association (蒜香麻園社區營造協會), "Lifestyles of Health and Sustainability," [in Chinese,] Facebook, May 12, 2019, https://www.facebook.com/ssmayuan.

9. Huashan Social Welfare Foundation, "Our Services," accessed June 1, 2019, https://elder.org.tw/.

10. Hondao Senior Citizen's Welfare Foundation, "Current Services," [in Chinese,] accessed June 1, 2019, http://www.hondao.org.tw/.

11. People.cn, "The Global Population Will Reach 9.8 Billion in 2050: Aging Is Increasing, Ecological Threats Are Increasing," [in Chinese,] accessed June 5,

2019, http://industry.people.com.cn/BIG5/n1/2018/0713/c413883-30144434.html.

12. Wanyu Qin, "On Average, Domestic Violence Occurs Every 5 Minutes: The Number of People Who Have Been Abused Is 3.8 Times What It Was 10 Years Ago," [in Chinese,] accessed June 5, 2019, https://www.cmmedia.com.tw/home/articles/11670.

13. Zishan Peng and Chen Jie, "Hope We Can All Be Aging Slow and Smart," *Commonwealth* 674 (June 2019): 70–94.

14. Peng and Jie, "Hope We Can All Be Aging Slow and Smart," 54–66.

15. Robbyn R. Wacker and Karen A. Roberto, *Community Resources for Older Adults: Programs and Services in an Era of Change* (London: Sage, 2014), 8.

16. Wacker and Roberto, *Community Resources for Older Adults*, 19.

17. Mei-Ju Chen and Fin-Land Cheng, "The Effects of an Intergenerational Program on Elementary School Students' Attitudes toward Elders," *NTTU Educational Research Journal* 18, no. 2 (December 2007), 67–103.

18. Hui-Chuan Lin and Ping-Yi Lin, "The Effects of Group Music Therapy Activities Integrated into a Gerontological Nursing Course on Students' Attitudes and Willingness to Work with Older Adults," [in Chinese,] *Changhua Nursing* 23, no. 2 (June 2016), 28–36.

19. Ching-Hui Lin and Pin-An Su, "The Study of Clothing Design for Wearing in a Variety of Ways by Senior Citizens," [in Chinese,] *Journal of the Hwa Gang Textile* 24, no. 7 (September 2017), 391–96.

20. Zishan Peng and Chen Jie, "Hope We Can All Be Aging Slow and Smart," *Commonwealth* 674 (June 2019), 54–66.

21. Zhang-Han Zhong, "The Third Act," *Commonwealth* 666 (January 2019), 92–100.

22. Ware cited in Ann Kaiser Stearns, *Redefining Aging* (Baltimore: Johns Hopkins University Press, 2017).

7   A Matter of Perspective

SAMUEL O. REGALADO

Not long ago on a rainy night, as I sat in my car outside a small tavern on the outskirts of San Francisco, I decided to hit the pause button for a quick review of my life. I thought to myself, "Here I am in my midsixties and I just played on a stage in a sweaty room with a rock band." Bands at our level, to be sure, have no roadies, layers of loyal fans, high-tech sound systems, or someone to pack up our gear. It's the bush leagues of music, and I love it. But other aspects of my life I equally love. For instance, only a few days earlier, I gave an interview to a writer for *New York Magazine* who sought my thoughts on the Donald Trump administration's policy regarding Cuban baseball players entering the United States. And I saw in a Wikipedia post a citation of my research on Muhammad Ali's celebrated Supreme Court case. In a matter of a few weeks, all three experiences spoke to my life as a whole. In short, I took satisfaction in the versatility of my personal goals. Being a jack-of-all-trades, in a manner of speaking, kept me grounded for most of my adult life and, as I grew older, gave me perspective. Personal enrichment, for instance, always took a backseat to personal satisfaction. And I was good with that. "Work like you don't need the money. Love like you've never been hurt. And dance like nobody's watching," said the legendary baseball player Satchel Paige. And through all the bumps and bruises, these were the traits that, in one manner or another, guided me through life, one that had its start in Glendale, California.

Family Background

I came along on March 22, 1953, to Salvador and Eva Regalado. Dad was an "LA" guy, born near the downtown center in 1925. His parents, of Mexican ancestry, had migrated from El Paso, Texas, to Los Angeles sometime in the early 1920s. My paternal grandfather, Manuel, was a common weekday laborer both in El Paso and in Los Angeles. But, on weekends, baseball consumed his attention. In his heyday, he both played and managed ball teams. In fact, letters he wrote in the 1920s suggest that among the many players he coached was a member of the infamous 1919 Black Sox squad who played for grandpa under an assumed name. My uncle Rudy, also born in Los Angeles, played for the Cleveland Indians, even making a World Series appearance in 1954.

My mom was born in 1927 in the Mexican state of Sonora. The eldest girl in a family of seven, she grew up in the Mexican wasteland where poverty was the norm. To help the family, she left her village at age 15 and by herself immigrated to the United States in 1944 through the entry center at Douglas, Arizona. She worked as a cook and nanny for an Arizona legislator's family before moving to Los Angeles where, in 1950, she met my father, then a navy veteran of World War II. Between the two, my biological mix is of Mexican, Yaquis Indian, and Italian roots, the last of which is indicated by my maternal grandmother's name, Bercini.

Early Years

Unlike my parents, whose upbringing came during the Great Depression, a horrific world war, and, in my mom's case, migration to a different country, I was brought up with three meals a day in comfortable homes. Thanks to the GI Bill, my first home was part of a housing project that sat near the Los Angeles River, adjacent to Glendale. My dad was a truck driver, and mom worked at a tile company alongside my grandfather. After my younger sister was born, the family moved to the suburbs in the San Fernando Valley, which lies northwest of downtown Los Angeles.

It was there that my more conscious self and formal education began. From 1955 to 1972, I did my K-12 schooling in "the valley," played competitive sports, was introduced to romance, and learned to play musical instruments. I was a baby boomer, and much of what occurred in that era helped shape my identity. Little things, like advancements in television, such as the transition from black-and-white broadcasts to color, made huge impressions on me as the pictures on the screen suddenly became more real. Years later, while filming a segment of the documentary *Viva Baseball*, the producer and I sat in the stands at AT&T Park in San Francisco, chatting. He asked me what I most recalled about the first time I attended a major league baseball game. Thinking back to August of 1962 when my grandparents took me to Dodger Stadium, I told him that what astounded me most was the green grass, the color of the uniforms, and the red brick of the infield. He pointed out that up to then, I had seen baseball games only in black and white. A little more than a year after my first in-person game, the stark image of an American flag draped over the coffin of an assassinated president at Arlington National Cemetery brought into focus the fact that, for many baby boomers, the age of innocence was now past.

Little Sun Valley, the neighborhood where I grew up, was like other middle-class suburban neighborhoods in the San Fernando Valley. Communities were ethnically diverse and, as such, aside from family gatherings, food, and related holidays, I initially did not identify with my Mexican heritage. My parents largely spoke English in the household, and my friends who were Mexican Americans came together not to discuss our ethnic similarities but to play ball and such. Not until my closing years as a college undergraduate did my ethnic identity start to surface.

I attended public school from kindergarten through grade four. But that changed in 1963 when my mother enrolled my sister and me into our Catholic parish parochial school. I remained in Catholic school through high school; those years, 1963 to 1971, were a most eventful time. Two months into my first term at Our Lady of the Holy Rosary School, President John F. Kennedy was assassinated. Two months before my high school graduation, the U.S. Supreme Court held for Muhammad Ali in a case called *Clay v. United States*, by which his conviction for having refused induction in the armed services was overturned. In between, civil rights, the counterculture, Vietnam, and an array of movements became the new norm, as were the

Beatles, rock and roll, Motown, flower power, Woodstock, long hair, and bell-bottom pants. But sports, particularly baseball, also were part of my new norm.

Baseball

Growing up in a family that included two uncles who played professional baseball and a paternal grandfather who had roots in many levels of the game over thirty years before I came along laid the groundwork for my familiarity with the national pastime before I even tossed a baseball for the first time. My uncle Greg played in the Yankees organization, and my uncle Rudy, as stated above, made it to the big time. My grandfather, for his part, ambitiously took the lead when it came to indoctrinating his grandkids in the game. My indoctrination hit a high point early on with that August 1962 trip to my first game at Dodger Stadium, a twenty-minute drive from my San Fernando Valley home.

To say that I enjoyed myself is understating my experience. From the moment I, at the age of 10, stepped onto the vast stadium parking lot and reached our seats in the inexpensive left field pavilion was nothing short of Nirvana. From the organ music to the starting pitchers bouncing out of the dugouts to warm up as if simultaneously choreographed to do so, everything was festive. Taskmaster that he was, my grandpa also taught me how to keep score. When all was said and done, the home team Dodgers defeated the St. Louis Cardinals and, more important, at least to me, the game added a happy new disciple to its roster. Now, some fifty years later, my affinity to the game and my reverence for its history remain strong. And, as long as I am in the park, I still don't care where I sit.

Not surprising, I started Little League the following year and continued in competitive baseball through pony-colt, junior varsity, and varsity high school baseball. I learned quickly, however, that my uncles' hitting genes abandoned me. But I had a good arm and pitched at each of those levels. My romanticized fondness for baseball did not, however, exempt me from frustration and heartache that came at the competitive level. While I experienced many moments of joy wearing the uniform, at other times the outcomes were not so joyful. For every moment that I walked off the mound having struck out the other side, my competitive spirit also brought out my anger when I was relegated to the bench. And those instances did not always bring out my best side. In the social Darwinist conventions of the day, open expression of emotion, short of crying, in the athletic arena was considered a sign of strength. But strength did not always equate to wisdom. As such, for whatever skills I brought to my respective teams, my diplomatic shortcomings too often undermined my merits, particularly when dealing with coaches. Such were the trappings of a boy in need of guidance and maturity.

Still, my personal temperament on the field did not deter my overall love for the game. In fact, by the time I reached St. Genevieve High School, my reading about the game's history, such as Jackie Robinson's story, inspired me. While the great Robinson ended his career before the Dodgers moved from Brooklyn to Los Angeles, his legacy was strong and became a bullet point as the impact of the Civil Rights Movement and that of other groups who sought social justice grew on me. As early as 1963, thanks to the wisdom of my parochial-school teachers, students like me read books like *To Kill a Mockingbird*, learned about Dr. Martin Luther King Jr. and Cesar Chavez, and started to see the merit of a pluralistic and tolerant America. Of course, I conflated my growing sensitivities to civil rights with my passion for baseball. Jackie Robinson's story led me to learn more the legendary Black leagues, which in turn brought me back to tales of racial discrimination. In high school I knew as much about Black stars such as Cool Papa Bell, Josh Gibson, and Satchel Paige, who came before my time, as I did about Maury Wills, Willie Davis, and Willie Mays, who were the players during my upbringing. While I learned about the Black leagues, I also wanted to better understand the reasons such leagues existed to begin with and the racial trauma the ballplayers lived with daily.

Thus, history itself captivated my interest in the ensuing years and became the centerpiece of my intellectual curiosity. By the time I completed high school, the groundwork for my cultural, ideological, and professional identity had been laid. And the game's presence in my upbringing was an instrumental component of that foundation. Of course, at 18 years of age, I still had ahead of me more years to lace up my cleats. And I did.

My competitive appetite continued to be strong, and while I experienced frustration as a high school athlete, there also was an upside. I played on championship teams in both baseball and football. As a sophomore, I was a starting pitcher on a junior varsity team that took the league crown. And at the varsity level as a bullpen pitcher, I was part of a club that came one out away from capturing the California Southern Section state title. I also played JV and varsity football. And in my senior year, when I was a three-year letterman and a wide receiver on the varsity squad, we won the 1970 state title with a 12-0 record, a high school record, I am proud to say, that stands today. Thus, following my high school years, it never crossed my mind to abandon my participation in competitive sports, especially baseball.

After High School

In such an unsettled world, the familiar landscape of a ball field with fellow players was familiar and stabilizing. As Satchel Paige once said after stepping for the first time on a major league mound in 1948, "The mound and home plate were in the same place that they were in the Negro Leagues." After high school, I played on a variety of teams at different levels of competition: municipal city leagues, Mexican American leagues, and semipro collegiate level. And playing ball took me to different places in southern California, the southwestern United States, and even Mexico. That said, by age 20, I gave up thoughts of pursuing a professional career and turned my attention to academics.

History and Intellectual Curiosity

Following high school, I opted to enter junior college (as it's called in California) because, as opposed to a university, it was financially free. And, upon reflection, it was a good decision. I was determined to free my parents of the burden to finance my education, which they had already so generously done by putting me through parochial school, and the high cost of a university education made little sense when I still hadn't figured out what my career goals were. I went into junior college with the hope that I might get a fix on my future. Truth be told, I was not the most serious student on campus. After a regimented life in the religious confines of a Catholic school with fewer than five hundred students, I was one of several thousand students at junior college and had few constraints. As such, I landed in academic probation not just once but twice as I struggled to reach some modicum of maturity. But from the rock pile came a nugget: I loved my freshman-level U.S. history class. Though I had enjoyed my high school history classes, the professors at the JC took me to a new level. Such was the value, I discovered, of lower-division general education classes whereby students are required to take courses in a variety of disciplines. Doing so not only exposed me to classes in areas I might not have previously explored, like science and the humanities but also helped give me much-needed direction. While I took few things in life seriously, my history courses were among those few things. Learning about the past helped to bring some sense to the troubling dynamics outside the classroom, like the Vietnam War. And it brought into focus the one and only public issue that had moved me since my youth: racial discrimination. In short, my political ideologies started to take shape in my time at Los Angeles Valley College. However primitive my knowledge about the issues was at the time, I had nonetheless discovered my sense of purpose.

While I did not become a good student overnight, I did start to pay more attention to the events around me, and not a minute too soon. Less than a month after I picked up my high school diploma in June 1971, President Richard Nixon certified the Twenty-Sixth Amendment to the United States Constitution, which lowered the voting age to 18. Such timing made me eligible to vote in the 1972 presidential election, and I couldn't wait to hold my ballot. Rebellion, after all, was in the air, even in the world of sports. On June 28, 1971, the U.S. Supreme Court, in a case called *Clay v. United States*, unanimously held in favor of Muhammad Ali, then the former heavyweight boxing champion, in a case that stemmed from his refusal to report for induction into the military draft based on his position as a conscientious objector to the Vietnam War. And in other arenas, norms were challenged and overcome. Basketball's Spencer Haywood, who took on the National Basketball Association's rule that prevented a player from joining its ranks until four years after his high school graduation, successfully employed the Sherman Antitrust Act to make his 1971 case that he should be able to play with the Seattle Supersonics. And baseball, too, underwent similar challenges. To end the game's "reserve clause," which denied free agency to players, the St. Louis Cardinals' outfielder Curt Flood in 1969 challenged his trade to the Philadelphia Phillies. Though the challenge proved unsuccessful, he triggered a string of events that ultimately led to the end of the reserve clause in 1975.

My immediate concern was the draft, for which I was eligible in February 1972. With the Vietnam War still being waged, the months leading up to the so-called lottery day were akin to waiting for an execution. Given that I was not a person of means nor even remotely qualified to be a conscientious objector, I could only hope that my number, based on my birthdate, would be among the last of the 365 ping pong balls plucked from the large glass jar at the Department of Defense. As it happened, Lady Luck smiled on me as my March 22 birthdate was the 343rd overall pick, meaning that the chance of my being drafted was remote. And, as it happened, in December of that year, secretary of state Henry Kissinger announced in Paris that "peace was at hand"; in January 1973 the war thankfully ended. Richard Nixon, not with my help, was reelected in November 1972 in a landslide over my favored candidate, Senator George McGovern, a war hero with a PhD—in history, I might add. By the mid-1970s, my career direction had become clearer.

Music

The 1970s also saw my development as a musician. Prior to that decade, my early forays into music were a disaster. At age 12 I tackled the violin and trombone. But neither won me over, and at that stage of my life, attempting to learn such instruments bored me. Seven years later, amid the sixties rock scene, my sister, Suzanna, a gifted musician and singer, generously took the time to teach me to how play the piano and the guitar. By age 17, I was ready to take the plunge into music again.

At 18, through friends at St. Genevieve, I found other like-minded musicians and entered the local San Fernando Valley band scene. Like most boys my age with no formal training in music, most bands I joined had one or two players with advanced skills and other members with more enthusiasm than proficiency. I was usually in the latter category. Still, most bands hung on to me, and through baptism by fire, I learned the finer points of music at the performance level. And my singing was a little better than most of my bandmates'. I dabbled in songwriting, too, and most bands I joined included my songs on their playlists. In time I landed in some good bands, some of which opened for name groups like We Five and Iron Butterfly. I also played in a band that shared the bill with Sam the Sham and the Pharaohs.

While my music activities were a far cry from my baseball appetites and developing career as a historian, I saw them as a way to create balance in my life. And my interest in developing my stripes as a songwriter rivaled that of my professional academic goals. I welcomed the diversity and felt I could practice history and create music at the professional level. By my midtwenties, my compositions led to some small opportunities in the music industry. I had joined the music rights organization BMI in 1980, and through its representative, some of my songs were channeled to various established performers. Also, I did some freelance writing for Warner Chappell Music and DeWalden Music (an affiliate of EMI, a multinational music publishing company). Ultimately, apart from a few nibbles, my brush with fame never materialized. But, of course, establishing my musical identity was only one of my goals. By the early 1980s, I took a major step in pursuing the other.

Balance

While bouncing around in the music world had its merit, my interests in academics increased. By the late 1970s, I had become a serious student of history. In 1976 I entered the history program at California State University, Northridge. With an initial goal of earning a teaching credential, I soon scuttled those plans and decided, instead, to think in terms of a possible advanced degree. Also, I grew intrigued with the idea of entering a program outside southern California. Rarely had I spent much time outside the Los Angeles basin and started to realize that to develop personal growth my world needed to expand geographically. Dr. John Broesamle, my mentor at CSU Northridge, encouraged me to ambitiously explore history graduate programs throughout the nation. Eventually, after having raised my grade point average by taking extra courses at the postbaccalaureate level, I made myself academically competitive for grad school. But acceptance was not automatic. Some schools rejected me, though I was hardly deterred. After all, I was a musician and, thus, rejection was not unfamiliar. I was confident that at some point, I'd get my shot. And I did. In the fall of 1980, a letter from Pullman, Washington, invited me to enter the graduate program in the Department of History at Washington State University. Euphoric as I was to be accepted into a graduate program, I was also leaving home.

In January of 1981, I left Los Angeles forever and pointed my pickup truck northward toward Pullman. In doing so, I also left my family, friends, a good job in a hospitable pharmacy, a working and profitable band, and a region with which I was familiar. I was also then engaged to be married. My fiancé accompanied me to Vancouver, Washington, where she had family and from where she flew back to Los Angeles. As if the aforementioned factors were not already traumatic enough, as I made my way across the state toward Pullman, the weather got considerably colder. It was, after all, January, and I had never before lived in temperatures below thirty degrees. When I arrived in eastern Washington armed with only a high school letter-men's jacket and tennis shoes, the region greeted me with subzero-degree weather. Indeed, the term *windchill* was quickly added to my lexicon. Such a drastic change proved to be extremely trying. Between February and June of that year, homesickness caught up with me and proved to be the biggest challenge I had ever faced. My artistic creative fervor evaporated as did my engagement, my trusty guitar sat unused, and only California license plates appeared to keep me in touch with my roots. Adding insult to injury, my arrival in Pullman came as white supremacists, who had gathered just north of town, sought recruits on campus. Apparently I did not go unnoticed, as I was, one morning, greeted with a flyer left on the windshield of my truck that announced, "Open Hunting Season on All Mexicans."

Such challenges notwithstanding, I remained curious as to my capabilities. In short, throughout the entire trip, I asked myself, "Could I cut it as a graduate student?" On my arrival in the department, the graduate adviser took me to meet my mentor, Dr. LeRoy Ashby. I was familiar with Dr. Ashby's name because my mentor at Northridge spoke highly of him and recommended that I consider studying under Ashby. Broesamle's advice was sound. Ashby was warm and friendly. More important, he was key to my transition.

Graduate School

As I settled into Pullman and the graduate program, some important dynamics in the history discipline would benefit me in a major way. In the early 1970s, U.S. historians began to dispense with top-down perspectives of the American past and were introducing bottom-up ones. This new school of thought, referred to as the New Social History, emphasized the roles played by ethnic minorities, the working class, women, and other groups long ignored in previous studies. It was within this realm that sport gained traction as a viable area of serious and studious review. In 1972 an interdisciplinary group of scholars formed the North American Society for Sport History (NASSH) to both provide a forum and advance scholarly works about the impact sport had made on the American and international historical stage. The society's chief conduit to a larger audience was the *Journal of Sport History*, which introduced scholars across the academic spectrum to new ways that historians could digest and introduce their own areas of specialization. By the end of the 1970s, departments of kinesiology at prestigious schools such as Penn State University, the University of Maryland, and the Ohio State University took the lead in introducing programs in sport history studies at the graduate level. By 1980 notable scholars like Allen Guttmann and Ronald Smith, both of whom had academic training in history, literature, and kinesiology, produced highly acclaimed monographs that advanced the legitimacy of sport as a scholarly research area. By 1982, the organizations' tenth year, NASSH had come into its own and the work produced by those in its circles gained respected visibility in the discipline of history.

I did not pursue graduate school with the intention of writing sport history. But neither did I lose my affinity for sport. I participated in intramural sports, held season tickets to Cougars games, and, when environmental conditions were right, managed to get a radio signal from my hometown that allowed, even for a few moments, my "friend" Vin Scully to keep me company and bring to me my beloved Dodgers games. Still, the study of sport in the history discipline was not then entirely embraced by my elders and graduate peers. Thus, it never occurred to me that, short of a brief term paper, I could write extensively on a topic related to sport. Nor did I ever see any assigned or suggested reading lists that included topics on athletics. As such, by 1982, I had settled on exploring the relationship between social Darwinism and positivism in the U.S. and Mexico. But "Fernandomania" changed all of that.

A year earlier a Mexican rookie southpaw named Fernando Valenzuela took the baseball world by storm while pitching for my hometown team, the Los Angeles Dodgers. Dubbed Fernandomania by journalists, his fame, which triggered a renaissance of Mexican pride that enraptured my mother, caught the attention of some of my professors at Washington State University who themselves were baseball fans. One of them, Dr. Richard Hume, suggested that it might be worth my while to see if any scholarly studies of Latino baseball players in the major leagues had ever surfaced. It didn't take me long to learn that the topic as a historical study was yet unexplored. And with that, sport reentered my life, this time as an area of study. With Dr. Ashby's blessing, I entered a whole new phase that included what became a basis not only for my professional identity but for my personal and cultural identity as well.

In 1982 a research grant allowed me travel to New York City to interview Hall of Famer Monte Irvin, who then worked at the Major League Baseball Commissioner's Office, to discuss his career in relationship to Latino players. Not only was the famed Black outfielder informative, but he also gave me several contacts that proved helpful. Things moved quickly after that. During the summer I used my limited funds to establish some oral histories and engaged in archival work. Later that year, a graduate peer of mine came across a "call for papers" announcement by NASSH. And with the blessing of my mentor, I put together a research paper from my master's thesis, about Latino players since 1945, which NASSH coordinators accepted for presentation in the spring of 1983 at Mont Alto, Pennsylvania. Within days after having earned my master's degree, for the first time I presented a research paper at a professional academic conference. Personally, I was in awe of NASSH and its participants. I was in the company of scholars from a variety of disciplines, graduate peers from other universities, many who became lifelong colleagues and friends. Plus, the program presentation topics expanded my horizons in a way I could scarcely have believed. My first meeting of NASSH, in short, completely inspired me to pursue sport as a chief topic of my academic mission. By then I had been admitted into the doctoral program at WSU and was determined to lay the foundation for a definitive study of the Latino experience in the major leagues since the late nineteenth century.

Professionalism

Under no circumstances could I, years earlier, have envisioned seeking a PhD in history, let alone doing so by writing on the topic of baseball. But timing was my friend. By 1984, sport history had made important inroads in academia. My association with NASSH kept me in touch with all of the new developments in the field. Moreover, the *Journal of Sport History* had increased in stature. A few years later the American Historical Association ranked it among the top ten most cited academic journals. More important was that NASSH drew both established historians and recognized publishers like Oxford University Press and the University of Illinois Press, among others, seeking sport history topics. Thus, the incentive to complete my dissertation and join the professional ranks was a great one. In 1987 the PhD was mine.

Of course, history departments were not inclined to hire faculty strictly on their sport history gravitas. In the late 1980s, hiring committees remained largely in the province of historians still on the fence about the acceptability of sport as a research area. As such, and with sound guidance from my advisers, I tailored my doctorate to fit into the academic trends in my discipline, paying attention to the Pacific Rim region and, secondarily, Latin America and East Asia. So, in a competitive hiring environment that averaged 100 to 150 candidates responding to each job announcement, my diverse areas of study in growing fields won the day. By responding to trends in history, I had opened the door to return to the story of Latino players once I settled into my new job back in California.

Return to California

California State University (CSU), Stanislaus, sat in the middle of the state's San Joaquin valley, approximately ninety miles east of San Francisco, in the small town of Turlock. Moreover, it was among the smallest of the twenty-plus CSU campuses, with a student population of six thousand. In need of an instructor to cover their Asian history classes, as their specialist was on a one-year sabbatical, and to be resourceful, the history department at Stanislaus found that my diverse academic fields best suited their needs. For my part, in need of a job and ecstatic at the prospect of being back in California and only a four-hour drive from my parents, I took the gig.

As it turned out, what started as a one-year replacement position turned into a thirty-year-long rewarding career at CSU Stanislaus. Of course, the transition from grad student to professional instructor had its bumps. Affirmative action being among the leading issues of the day, it hung like an albatross on me during my transition from graduate school, where some of my peers made clear their opinion that my presence among them was in part due to the policy, to my hiring at CSU for the same reason. I had much to prove.

But I was young and had ambition and incentive. In my first decade at Stanislaus, I presented at several major conferences, loaded my curriculum vitae with published essays and reviews, and for two terms chaired the publications board of the prestigious *Journal of Sport History*. Four years into my time at CSU, I earned tenure and promotion and was named a Smithsonian fellow. By the mid-1990s, I signed a contract with the University of Illinois Press for my manuscript on Latino baseball players, and in 1998, at long last, *Viva Baseball! Latin Major Leaguers and Their Special Hunger* appeared on bookshelves and was heralded by the *San Francisco Chronicle* as among its top five most recommended books for that year. And, as had been the case throughout my career, I was also the benefactor of good timing, as my book's appearance came amid the fabled home run race between Mark McGwire and Sammy Sosa. Sosa won over the American public with his charming demeanor and good sportsmanship. Indeed, so good were my book sales that only a year later, Illinois Press had me throw together a second edition that included the McGwire-Sosa 1998 season. In 1998 the University of San Francisco awarded me its own Davies fellowship. But while my notoriety, much of which was highlighted by my appearances in several documentaries on Latino players, came as a result of *Viva Baseball*'s success, I did not want to be typecast as a historian who wrote about Latino players only because of my own heritage. My appetite for stories had grown beyond those that had made my scholarly reputation.

After 2000 I became increasingly engaged in Japanese American baseball and legal history, the latter of which I drew from my lifelong commitment to social justice. Having grown up in culturally mixed neighborhoods that included families of Japanese heritage, I used some of my college years to explore my interest in incarceration of Japanese American citizens during World War II. As my career came together in the late 1990s, that history struck me as a story that required attention. To that end, my interest was expressed through journal articles and keynote addresses I delivered. By 2010, and following the third edition of *Viva Baseball*, I set all aside to concentrate on the Nikkei story. And by 2013, following several years of intriguing oral interviews and research, *Nikkei Baseball: Japanese American Players from Immigration and Internment to the Major Leagues* landed on bookshelves. Prior to the book's release, the Japanese American National Museum bestowed on me a place on their scholarly advisory board. In 2013, *Sport and the Law: Historical and Cultural Intersections*, an anthology of landmark decisions and legal cases involving sports and sports figures that had been edited by Sarah K. Fields and me was published by the University of Arkansas Press. And with a coauthored textbook titled *Latinos in Sport* (Human Kinetics Press), an award-winning anthology, *Mexican Americans and Sport* (University of Arkansas Press), and an accumulation of forty-plus published articles and reviews, the goals I had set for myself years earlier were more than realized. Outside the academic world, my activism grew as I participated in a variety of rallies for social justice causes and even served a term as vice president of the American Civil Liberties Union's Modesto chapter.

So, too, did I see dividends from my musical ambitions. Like an artist who continues to draw sketches even when not professionally active,

I continued to create songs at home if for no other reason than to keep myself musically sharp. New technologies in the nineties afforded me the opportunity to own a small four-track recorder, and with it I wrote and recorded songs. Ten years into my academic career, I got back into the band business, returned to playing gigs, and delighted in the camaraderie with other musicians. And it was invigorating. By 2010, with the growth of the indie music industry and advancements in the internet, independent artists like myself no longer needed to turn to the large music labels to have their compositions heard. Armed with more financial resources, I recorded several songs and established a modest profile of my creative works that I, like thousands of others, posted online. Between 2009 and 2019, I toured annually and, having purchased a condo in beautiful Monterey, found and joined an artistic community that, on my 2015 retirement from the university, proved to be rewarding for a vital part of an identity predating my professional academic career.

Sport in Later Life

Along with my musical endeavors, I continued to play competitive baseball into my forties and fifties. When I was 39 and believed my playing days had ended long ago, an adult baseball league was formed in Turlock. While I had played a little softball, it lacked the level of competitiveness that always drew me to baseball, and the new league afforded me the opportunity to return to the game I loved. As a thirty-and-over league, it signed up former college, semipro, and professional players (including two former big-league players still in their thirties). For the next seventeen years, I spent the lion's share of my summer Sundays on the ball diamond and in the company of players who, like myself, were transitioning from our prime years into retirement. Not a beer league, it held many games in minor league parks and at major league spring training sites during tournaments. Aches and pains eventually caught up to me, and I left baseball when I turned 58. But the league had dividends for me that were not insignificant. Sunday ball gave me incentive to stay in shape, helped me establish lifelong friendships with teammates and competitors, and provided, at times, needed sanctuary from the stress that often accompanies an academic career. And it was fun, a virtue, when kept in perspective, not unimportant during the aging process.

Summary

On reflection, who I am now, in my midsixties, and the success that has smiled upon me are largely the result of luck. Luck in that I was the benefactor of having had good parents, siblings, teachers, and friends, all of whom provided me with guidance, inspiration, and assistance. It really did take a village. The importance of perspective, the art of seeing the bigger picture that my parents and sister taught me, segued into my academic and musical interests. Such perspective, in time, helped me develop a realistic sense of strengths and shortcomings. And, as such, irrespective of my limitations, I played to my strengths. Perspective, for instance, made clear to me that if I couldn't hit, I could still pitch. If I couldn't master lead guitar, I could still sing and play rhythm guitar and keyboards. My limitations at throwing a football didn't preclude my ability to catch it. And just because I did not graduate summa cum laude did not mean I couldn't still be a good historian. The principles of such perspective came to me early. My parents were especially good at making the most of what they had. Dinners were almost always a combination of leftovers from previous evenings. My dad, each year, always used leftover paint to beautify our little vacation trailer. Used equipment, in our household, was still good equipment. And we did not have to sit behind home plate to enjoy a ball game. The cheap seats were good seats because we were just happy to be there. For fifty cents—children's admission in the sixties—in the left field pavilion, I sat only twenty feet away from some of the greatest players in the history of the game. One did not have to be financially wealthy to be rich. And it was this important tool, perspective, that kept me grounded during some of the toughest moments in life.

Of course, it wasn't just luck and perspective that brought me to my goals. Hard work, incentive, and determination were necessary to survive the pitfalls along the way. Having always been a bit of a loner, I realized that earning my keep in life meant freedom from having to answer to anyone and freedom to determine, for myself, my own direction. As such, I worked throughout my college years and paid my own tuition. And when CSU Northridge handed me my degree, I successfully left my undergraduate institution without a dime of debt. Six years later, when I left Washington State University with a master's and a PhD, my debt was a paltry $2,500, which I paid off after my first semester of employment. In fact, I was good at making the most of what I had. My ability to make money from music, in short, tempered and all but eliminated what might have otherwise been high costs for my schooling.

My education also triggered my sense of cultural identity. Courses in Mexican American history and those related to it brought me in touch with my heritage. I had never been unaware or unappreciative of my Mexican heritage, but my college education and graduate school gave it more meaning, particularly as a conduit to my social justice leanings. Fernando Valenzuela's celebrated 1981 season afforded me the opportunity to include sports, in this case baseball, into my research. And research let me develop a relationship to the larger historical story of Latinos and immigration in the United States, all of which fed into my incentive to tell their story.

I retired from the university in 2015 and became a professor of history emeritus, having accomplished much of what I set out to do. And aside from the normal physical ailments that accompany the passing years, I reached my midsixties free of any major illnesses, due in part to a lack of destructive habits and sheer good luck. Never throughout my life did I ever smoke. I kept alcohol to a minimum, and, more important, my propensity to keep things in perspective minimized my stress. A good sense of humor also helped. My parents, most of all, taught me early that one could make a good meal from leftovers and beautifully decorate an old trailer with used paint. These are good rules to abide by as I look ahead to the next chapter of my life, when I hope to apply my accumulated knowledge to the advancement of whatever community I choose to be a member of. A good pitcher, after all, can be just as effective as a great pitcher. Or as Satchel Paige once said, "Ain't no man can avoid being born average, but ain't no man got to be common." It's just a matter of perspective.

8 Dance until the Music Stops

TANSIN BENN

Much literature equates sportspeople with dancers in terms of not only the social, psychological, and physiological requirements but also the way in which the body is perceived.[1] So being included in this book on the ageing athlete is a welcome space to write about the place of dance in my life. I have participated in many forms of dance, including ballet, modern, creative, ballroom, Latin, and dance as exercise for the health and well-being of older people. I built up qualifications and taught and developed dance in junior high and high schools, the community, and higher education. But I have never been a professional dancer in the high-performance career artist sense, although I learned much about that role along the way. My career took the route of education, teacher training, higher education, and researcher, with dance as a key focus but not the only focus, and perhaps having different key interests is important in adjustments to the shifts in identity that accompany life's path. Understanding the meaning dance has had in my life for the sixty-nine years to date requires knowledge of how dance has been entwined through my childhood and career stages that led to the retirement I currently enjoy, so each stage has a section in this chapter. The contextualising of "Ageing in the UK" underpins the "Retirement" section, and it is the context in which I have lived my life. The reflections that conclude the chapter are drawn from the process of writing it, and I have been grateful for the opportunity.

Childhood and Early Learning

I was born on Friday the fourteenth of March in 1952 to Mavis and Donald Shallish (born 1925 and 1921, respectively); a sister, Linda, was aged 2 at that time. We grew up in a monocultural white, relatively working-class seaside town in southwest England. Mum and dad had met at the start of World War II and sustained a courtship by letter writing in the years dad was away with the army. They married in 1947 when rationing and economic struggles were common features of everyday life. Mum and dad were both part of big families, with eight children in each, so we grew up in a large extended family, and holidays were spent with aunties, uncles, and cousins distributed, conveniently, in lovely places! By the time my sister and I came along in the early 1950s, dad was a builder. In 2009, at the age of 88 years, he died of cancer at home, but we can still enjoy seeing his "legacies" around my town and region. These range from older peoples' blocks of flats, to housing estates, shopping centres, and schools. Mum stayed at home when we were young to look after us, but as soon as we were both at school, she took jobs that could fit around the school day, such as hotel work and social care.

At the age of 5 I was encouraged to join my sister in a local dance school that taught us ballet, tap, and other forms, no doubt triggered by Mum's enjoyment of acrobatics and dancing in her youth. In 1939, at the age of 14 years, she had been part of a duo, with her best friend, that joined a variety show to entertain the troops, as acrobatic and tap dancers in their home county of Cornwall. Later she moved to London and, with her friends, enjoyed the famous dance halls there and the joie de vivre that strangely coexisted with the bombs and destruction of war. Mum remembers the war years as some of the happiest of her life. By the 1950s our family had a rented two-bedroom council home, with a big garden, on a new post-war estate. Mum taught me to tap dance with her on a small tap board in the kitchen. I knew that the ongoing dancing lesson bills contributed to my parents' financial struggles, but for as long as we wanted to learn, the lessons continued. My sister "retired" at 12 years of age, but I continued until leaving home for college to train to teach physical education, which included dance; at 18 years I already had a qualification to teach ballet. As will be seen, these preparations in dance were just the start of a myriad of ways in which dance has permeated my life, and at 69 years of age I am still dancing . . . and will continue to "dance until the music stops."

Besides dance, I enjoyed other movement experiences as a youngster; Mum and Dad made sure my sister and I learned to swim and playing outdoors with friends was normal. Being adventurous in school and on park playgrounds, I relished the opportunities for swinging, climbing, and freedom of movement. Physical education experiences at school were positive. My sister excelled at athletics, and I found that I could succeed in different sports, for example, making the netball team and coordinating the step patterning for hurdles with no problem. Joining a school gymnastics club at 11 brought the right level of challenge and success where, as in dance, practising skills, repetition, and mastery were required to get that special joy of moving with ease, fluency, and control that was its own reward.

Dance, in all its diversity, has been a sustaining thread throughout my life. It gave me most of the confidence and skills I used in all other sports and physical activities and in life generally. Those dance lessons taught me movement mastery, discipline and creativity, perseverance, the ability to cope through failure and success, and the ability to perform. I learned that practise paid off, and I grew up with like-minded friends who shared those times of struggle and success in working for festivals, competitions, and shows. Perhaps key to my lifelong engagement was developing an intrinsic value and respect for physicality, especially in aesthetic sports where the form of the movement, the how, is essential to skill mastery.[2] I also learned, by experience, that visualisation was an easy way to practice movement patterns as I sat on a bus, walked to school, or lay in bed before dropping off to sleep. I gained a keen kinaesthetic sense, deep movement empathy for the appreciation of skill as a spectator, and above all, a joy in the pleasure of getting lost in the dance that continues today.

The Years In-between—the Career

I enjoyed a thirty-eight-year career in lecturing, research, teaching physical education, and collaborating with my peers through the International

Association of Physical Education and Sport for Girls and Women (IAPESGW).[3] All of these roles have been fulfilling. I had wanted to be a teacher of physical education to maintain and develop my love for dance and gymnastics. I never aspired to a career in higher education nor to the opportunities and rewards that such a career offered. Serendipity, hard work, perseverance, and the drive for success took me down that path.

My early teaching career enabled me to make positive contributions to the lives of many people in the city of Birmingham, United Kingdom, where I spent most of my career. I enjoyed not only the creativity of the dance-in-education model, derived from the work of Rudolf Laban, but also seeing the impact it had on children in schools and later my students in teacher training. They became more skillful, creative, and confident through making and performing dances and developing skills of appreciation. The Birmingham Youth Dance Company, which I started as a performance outlet for children from my own school, won a place at the first National Youth Dance Festival in the 1980s. The group continues today, and the movement for youth arts groups has grown strong in dance and music. With a successful career in schools, I was encouraged to apply for a post in teacher training at the local college, the Anstey College of Physical Education, Birmingham. The brief time spent there, before it was amalgamated with a larger institution as part of government closures of all UK women's teacher training colleges, was a valuable steppingstone. I moved on to more teacher training at Westhill College and eventually to a long career in the University of Birmingham's School of Education. During this time, I contributed to archiving memorabilia from Anstey College, and that process led me to a greater appreciation of the role of these women's colleges in the preceding one hundred years. In 2018 I published a paper on some of my research from the archive as a tribute to the pioneers who had paved the way for so many women to follow and many more children to benefit.[4] These were the women who challenged gender hegemony, Victorian ideas of womanhood, and traditional male-dominated sports, thus opening visions of possibilities for women to participate in physical activities of their choosing. Slow and incremental though these changes were, they contributed to a higher level of accepting women's physicality here in the UK.

One of the most prestigious programmes I designed, and which I led at the University of Birmingham for fourteen years, from 1997 to 2012, was a customised, part-time master's programme in applied dance studies for professional dancers of Birmingham Royal Ballet Company. It was a world-first partnership that required vision, commitment, creativity, and perseverance and turned out to be one of the most interesting delights and challenges of my career. The international makeup of the four cohorts that participated in the programme demonstrated a work ethic and hunger for education that surpassed anything encountered with other students. They recognised this special opportunity because most had not followed traditional paths into secondary schooling but had been in specialist ballet boarding school environments from the age of 11 years. Perhaps because I had experiential knowledge of ballet training and therefore appreciation of how demanding the lives of the dancers had been in reaching the company, there was a personal determination to make this work. I knew about the challenges of skill learning, the risk of each new performance, the uncertainty of every tomorrow, and the rewards when everything comes together. I respected their enthusiasm to embrace higher education amongst their dressing rooms, touring lodgings, wings of theatres, and every other space they found to complete their degrees. Some dancers required additional help with language (most had learned English as a second language), study skills, and time management in extraordinary lives. Their ability to embrace all the requirements at astounding speed led to outstanding work, as noted in 2001 by Christopher Bannerman, the first external examiner of the course: "I know of no other analysis of dance practice which is equal of breadth and depth, either nationally or internationally. This has been made possible by the involvement of practitioners, who have been empowered by higher education, and who have now provided scholars with an unparalleled insight into the world of dance."[5]

I enjoyed learning with the students as they researched facets of their lives that had interested them for years; for example, issues of career transitions and personal identity. One principal dancer had retired, completed his training as a pilot, but always felt like a "dancer in uniform." He returned to the company, took the degree opportunity, and has since developed a second career as artistic director of a prestigious ballet school. Another dancer explored her lifelong struggle with maintaining a slender body and undertook research into eating disorders amongst dancers, from which a paper was published.[6] In addition to working with Birmingham Royal Ballet, I was a director on the boards of an Indian dance company and an African dance company in the city. All of these experiences illustrate how I was extending my understanding and appreciation of the nuances of dance, music, culture, identity, and the preservation of heritage through dance.

Appreciating my own freedom to choose my life's path and to participate in any physical activities was something I took for granted. One day, in the multicultural city of Birmingham, my work brought me face to face with the lives of Muslim women and their views on the body, gender, and physicality. This encounter would shape my research career over the middle course of my life. In the 1990s I was head of physical education teacher training for the primary sector, where teachers are generalists teaching all subjects including physical education. I was approached by a group of Muslim women who wanted to discuss the short training programme they were about to undertake. They could not participate in mixed-sex practical sessions, wanted to wear different kit (clothing), could not swim where we had male lifeguards or large windows, and would not attend sessions on Friday afternoons, which is a religious day for them. With the best of intentions, the college had embarked on a project to increase the number of ethnic minority trainees coming into teaching, and an unforeseen consequence was the tension that arose as we worked to understand the cultural needs and requirements of some Black and ethnic minority students to participate and complete their training; the Muslim women were one such group. With the help of the Islamic studies department staff, I started a small-scale master's research project that continued into my PhD and subsequent sixteen-year-long research career with the focus on better understanding the lives and experiences of Muslim women in physical education and sport.[7]

The research journey, first in the UK, then internationally, over the following years was mind-opening as I came to understand more about women who chose a religious, faith-based commitment by which to live their lives.

Islamic practices affected deeply how they viewed their bodies and the body's physicality, for example, as a private, not public, entity, therefore requiring modesty of dress codes. Perhaps the closest concept I developed in searching for understanding came much later, after a myriad of events in Oman, Syria, Libya, and Egypt, and with colleagues interested in the same issue around the world: that of "embodied faith."[8] I still believe this concept is worth developing and applying to the embodiment of culture, which embraces us all. There is a need for increased knowledge and understanding of people's choices of difference, of identity, for example, in dress codes and behavior that become embodied, that is, learned through socialization and what Bourdieu called the development of habitus and cultural capital.[9]

Dance forms are often used to express embodiment of religion or culture; for example, I worked closely with the South Asian–Chitraleka Dance Company, in Birmingham. They promote classical Bharatanatyam Indian dance and have an academy of 250 children learning the style and cultural context of the art form in the UK city. As an expression of the Hindu origins from which it grew, the movement patterns often use the postures on the ancient Hindu temples of South India and a complex language of gesture and facial expressions through which many Hindu legends are recounted. Performances embody, through makeup, costumes, and movements, the perpetuation of their religious and cultural identity. The more that is understood about the language of their intricate hand gestures, the more enjoyment a spectator can gain from the storytelling and expressive side of the art form. Through dance in education, young people can gain some exposure to such riches and opportunities to engage with the complexities that result from migration patterns, globalization, and diverse cultures in multicultural city lives.

Through such opportunities and others gained in travelling, I have learned of significant differences in how physicality, and thus movement forms, are shaped and valued, especially amongst indigenous and diaspora communities. Distinct sport and dance forms spring from diverse ways of valuing movement and use of the body that contrast with dominant sport and dance forms in western societies. In dance most of these have religious or spiritual connections.[10]

Such encounters have led to reflection, for example, on the place of faith in my life. I was raised as a Christian, and my shifting understandings have been influenced by developing awareness as a social scientist living in multicultural Birmingham and having close friends from different faiths. My education and life experience have contributed to my increasing interest in and knowledge of people, their lives, and the role of religion and spirituality. While I do not have a strong faith, I would defend the right of others to have a faith and to be allowed to follow that faith. Inevitably that statement raises debates about cultural sanctioning of harmful deeds in the name of religion that I would never condone. For the majority of people, faith helps them to lead lives with similar codes of behaviour towards themselves and others, with the goals of peace, humanity, and a spiritual search for meaning. In many ways I admire those with faith strong enough to carry them through the most difficult journey, dealing with the death of loved ones. Life experience and ageing have helped me to cope with the pain of these moments and simultaneously have acted as stark reminders that life is short and should be experienced fully each day because the only certainty is that our time on earth is finite.

Choosing a path when meeting a crossroads, for example, in making a career choice, was not always easy but has led to productive, fulfilling years. If I had pursued dance performance when I had the choice at 18, I would always have struggled with maintaining a dancer's preferred body shape, but that anticipated difficulty was not the reason I entered teaching. My parents wanted me to take advantage of the chance to go to college to train for a career, and I had enjoyed physical education throughout school. There are no regrets about entering teaching because there has been so much pleasure and diversity in the life I have lived. I now benefit from the security in retirement of being able to do what I choose to do (a certainty that professional dancers do not have in their lives).

Similarly, my husband had the chance to make a professional gymnastic career when he was invited to join a world-famous professional acrobatics company at the end of his schooling. Like me he was persuaded to take up his place at college, and thereafter his life took a different but interesting, diverse, and fulfilling path. We met through the sport of gymnastics when he needed more coaches and judges in the City of Birmingham Gymnastics Club and I arrived in the city for a teaching post with those skills to help. From the day Barry concluded his long career of seven-days-a-week commitment to training, coaching, and managing a spectrum of gymnasts from young recreational to high-performance men and women who were national and international competitors, he never looked back. The transition to retirement for both of us was unproblematic, perhaps because we were in control of when and how we finished those careers, had no identity dilemmas, and were ready for the next adventures.

The Third Age—Retirement

The UK Ageing Society Context

In the UK the visual and media representation of being an older person is often negative and derogatory: deteriorating health, an increasing drain on public services, and rising eligibility ages for state pensions to offset national economic issues. Certainly, awareness of loneliness and social isolation is real and growing, and "social prescribing" for places in gyms or in social activities is emerging as a better solution to the care of the elderly than medicalisation has been. That said, the acclaimed National Health Service is breaking, and "bed-blocking" by elderly patients is often blamed for its problems. There are some positives: for example, the concept of "active retirement villages" is growing, and laws have been introduced to remove discrimination in ageing, such as barring compulsory retirement from work at 65. The dominant view in the media is of ageing as a social problem, and as life progresses, the realities of ageing bodies and minds are faced by all of us fortunate enough to grow old. The facts of prevalent age-related health conditions such as joint and bone ageing and mental health mean that active ageing has to be managed against these realities. Being able to accept such inevitabilities, to understand that life presents different opportunities at different stages, and to stay optimistic about what one can do, rather than what one has lost or cannot do, can contribute to lives well lived. We in the UK are fortunate to live where a range of clubs and activities are available for those who choose, and can afford, to participate. Understandably such optimism fades among those faced with constant pain, life-limiting conditions, or the stark realities of nearing the end of life and needing care.

International research and travel have given me insights into social issues of difference, including poverty, poor nutrition and housing, and lack of education. Such deprivations remain sharp in my mind from visits to, for example, parts of India, China, and South Africa. These memories serve to increase appreciation of the life I have and the realisation that the happiness and contentment I often saw on the faces of children and adults living in those contexts was not necessarily dependent on the factors we might claim essential in the UK.

The Centre for Ageing Better recently released the UK report *The State of Ageing in 2019: Adding Life to Our Years*, which states that twentieth-century advances in public health, nutrition, and medical science have brought the gift of longevity, but it is enjoyed differently according to health, wealth, ethnicity, and geographic location.[11] Demographically, the 65-plus age range is the fastest growing age group, projected to increase by 40 percent in the next twenty years. By 2036 one in four of the population will be over 65. Factors that enable quality of life include the ability to work in flexible and empathetic contexts, to live in appropriate homes, and to manage health issues related to smoking, alcohol, obesity, and lack of physical activity, most of which are evident amongst the poorest sectors. Appropriate homes, good health, the option for work, and connected communities rank highly in maintaining quality of life. Unsurprisingly, social status made a difference, with the most positive outlooks on ageing being amongst those who had been in professional occupations. "Health is more than just the absence of disease. It is the capacity to do the things we want to do."[12] People from the Black and other ethnic-minority communities had the greatest risks of poverty, poor health, and shorter lives. The report called for greater government intervention for change to improve quality of life for older people: "Ageing is inevitable, but how we age is not. Our current rates of chronic illness, mental health conditions, disability, and frailty could be greatly reduced if we tackled the structural, economic, and social drivers of poor health earlier."[13]

The Unexpected Gift of Caring

My husband and I moved back to my seaside hometown on retirement eight years ago, leaving a long career in education at the University of Birmingham. As with most towns near the sea, there are a plethora of care homes; residential, nursing, and dementia homes; care agencies; stay-at-home and live-in support possibilities for older people; and other options, all at extortionate prices. These are self-funded by anyone who has life savings over £23,000, and that figure currently includes all the capital in one's home. After this source is depleted, care is state-funded. Currently there is a shortage of care workers to staff the wide range of support services, and those who do contribute to this essential profession are poorly paid, making retention problematic. Finally, a national hospice movement is mostly funded by charitable giving. Consequently, fundraising is the constant economic basis of support for people to die with dignity, either in hospice or at home with the support of hospice professionals such as palliative care consultants, nurses, and community practitioners employed by the charity.

Perhaps the fact that my husband and I have become carers is part of our shared destiny. My mother, through ageing, lost her once highly capable physicality, is now unable to walk, and has declining mental health. The timing of the family crisis when my mother could no longer live independently coincided with our retirement back to my hometown to be nearer to our extended family. We moved into our bungalow by the sea and fortunately discovered it to be ideal for wheelchair living. In 2014 we decided that Mum, our only surviving parent, would end her days living with us. In that year she had fractured her left femur, then her right one, in successive falls, leaving her unable to walk again, and she already had a diagnosis of Alzheimer's disease. Taking her home from the hospital with us was the right decision for everyone. At the time she was given three months to live by her consultants, and almost seven years later she remains with us. Her kidney and heart conditions gradually improved, and, once stabilised, she has continued to lead a healthier, happy, contented life. A contributor to her stabilisation has been nutrition. She enjoys the balanced, healthy diet that has been a normal part of our household, with freshly cooked food and plenty of vegetables daily. Socially, Mum is surrounded by an extended five-generation family who live within eight miles and visit regularly to support us all. We will soon celebrate her 97th birthday with the family, including her three great-great-grandchildren, who currently live in Mum's house, where my sister and I grew up.

Although living with Mum has been an unplanned and unexpected chapter in our lives, it has taught us many things. We enjoy sharing this precious time and valuing the moment in which Mum lives each day. We continue to learn new skills in caring, often requiring physical and mental effort. We admire the way Mum manages her own challenges of not being able to move without assistance, to do the smallest thing, or join in conversations. She has found acceptance, peace, and contentment through immense perseverance, and spends most of her time smiling as she enjoys watching the buzz of life around her and the activities we share. We watch the cruelties of Alzheimer's disease stripping her of yesterdays. We listen to her rare but real dark moments of lucidity, when she can say how helpless she feels, how much she appreciates what we do for her, but how much of a burden she must be. Sometimes she wishes she were dead, but these episodes are rare and most of the time she is happy and contented. A wheelchair-adapted car enables us, or her granddaughters who are a much-valued part of our care team, to take her on trips, for rides in the country, or to coffee shops, town, music concerts, my exercise classes for a local charity, or the many social tea dances that Barry and I attend. We see her nodding her head to the music and enjoying the couples twirling around the floor with a pleasure and empathy clearly derived from her own dancing days long ago.[14] With the family, we work to keep Mum connected to us all and the world around through a range of strategies, often using photographs of family, siblings, people, and places that have been important in her life.[15] Through such reminiscence activities she still knows us, a little of the life that has brought her to this point, and, we are certain, the love we all have for her.

Barry and I utilise our disciplined skills of care organisation to weave our lives together and make time and space for each other, Mum, and ourselves. Barry enjoys bowling, playing in a brass band, and dancing, and he contributes to the running of the clubs offering these activities. I volunteer as a teacher of seated and standing music-and-movement classes for older people through a local charity, Age UK Somerset. That activity has required more training courses, and now I contribute to the training of other volunteers. In my classes we "dance," whether we are sitting or standing, solo, in pairs or a large circle. We experience the joy of dancing as we move to the rhythms of the music, build movement patterns together, and systematically move all the muscles and joints old age allows.

On reflection, the unexpected chapter of early retirement whilst caring for Mum, with all its challenges, has been a gift. It certainly changed our retirement plans, but we have woven ourselves into the life that unfolded. To share this with Barry has brought a close relationship ever closer. I have always known that my husband is a special person, but it takes an extra step to follow this road with my mother. When we met through gymnastics over forty years ago, we found many similarities, such as our social backgrounds growing up, teacher training and physical education teaching experiences, and Barry's history in artistic gymnastics paralleling mine in dance, except that he reached greater heights to which I could never have aspired. He represented Great Britain in six-piece competitions, won the bronze medal at a world tumbling championship in the 1960s, became an honorary UK national coach in 1975, and travelled the world as an international judge and coach. I had taken a humble pathway into gymnastics, but my dance background enabled me to make a major contribution towards the achievements of the gymnasts in the club where I joined Barry as a volunteer coach, choreographer, and international judge for over twenty years of our relationship. I was also developing my career in higher education, designing programmes, lecturing, researching, publishing, attending conferences, entering senior management, and gaining international awards in recognition of my work. I also took on the presidency of IAPESGW from 2009 to 2013 as part of my contribution to the executive board from 2005 to 2017, finishing with an honorary life membership. Such additions to the day job had the wholehearted backing of Barry and brought strong friendships across the world, potential for collaborations across organisations, and solidarity of efforts to improve the situation in physical education, sport, and dance internationally.

Barry and I have supported each other in everything life has presented to us since we met, from the difficult rehabilitations after his spinal and toe joint fusion operations (yes, gymnastics was responsible for that) to overcoming the pain following the loss of loved ones, and to the joys of new arrivals in our extended family. My sister has now been married fifty years and had two daughters who had six children, and now the next generation is coming along. We remain a close, supportive family. The presence of Mum and an open front door ensures that our house serves as a permanent meeting hub for the family. Barry and I are taking this path with Mum together, knowing each day is precious, and that these memories will form part of our next chapter in life, wherever that may lead. A positive attitude to ageing and life's unexpected twists and turns have brought us new experiences, skills, and appreciation of life and strong connections with those who make our life more meaningful.

Ongoing Productivity—a Retirement Project

On our retirement, I persuaded Barry to take up ballroom and Latin American dancing as a hobby. Nine years later we are still enjoying a lesson a week, often attending afternoon or evening social dances locally. We have made many friends in the social context of dancing, most of whom are older than us and an inspiration as they keep dancing regardless of the realities of ageing and inevitably failing bodies. We take occasional short dance holidays with good friends. It is important that we hire the local community hall weekly so we can practise the many movement pattern combinations across the ten dances that constitute ballroom and Latin, sticking to our promise to keep this activity a hobby, avoiding the competition scene and medal chasing. Nevertheless, we strive to dance well rather than just be content to move around the floor; there's a touch of the perfectionist in both of us there.

Research has shown that social dancing is an excellent activity for older people.[16] The challenges presented are physical and mental, notably in the constant need to have and extend a movement memory, the focus required when dancing to be able to manage space, other dancers, music, and many movement patterns. The hobby has provided a new dimension to our partnership. Ballroom dancing challenged us differently because we had to work as one, to be dependent on each other for remembering the steps, keeping the timing and style of each dance, embodying the musicality, and working in synchronisation. For two people who had enjoyed mostly individual activities before this, other forms of dance for me and elite-level gymnastics for Barry, it proved challenging, but we are still enjoying learning and improving. When we are practising or out together social dancing, we are completely in the moment.[17]

Janet Carlson in 2008 used her reflections on ballroom dancing as a metaphor for life. An Amazon book review highlights that, for her, dance contains

the secrets to life and love: the give-and-take of dance, two bodies in rhythm and harmony, . . . the reciprocity of human relationships. Total trust between partners is as vital on the dance floor as it is within a marriage. And yet, both partners—in dance and in life—must stand on their own two feet. The unadulterated joy Janet feels as she intuitively moves to the music speaks to the kind of absolute, whole-body happiness we were born to have. On the dance floor, she finds resolve in the waltz, self-confidence in the tango, and passion in nearly everything.[18]

Carlson had once been a competitive ballroom dancer before a long break to raise her family and therefore had the capacity to reconnect at an advanced stage on her return to the activity. In our experience, such reciprocity and reflection can only be found once there is a level of mutual skill acquisition gained through repetition, practice, and movement mastery. Only then is there the freedom to enjoy such moments. No doubt our previous development of a "bodily-kinesthetic intelligence" has helped us to accelerate our skill learning, but we had so much more to learn to be able to enjoy ballroom and Latin dancing together that it continues to be well worth the effort.[19]

Another new project and challenge was teaching myself the basics of keyboard playing in my late fifties, inspired by my mum and husband, who could both play music. After many weeks of frustration with so many notes and uncooperative fingers, and trying to read music with eyes that found the dots rather tricky, I managed to play a recognisable tune. I found that first moment of producing recognisable music as incredible as performing our first waltz with good technique and skill efficiency so that it looked as fluent as it felt. Both moments were about journeys of perseverance, commitment, and application to the activity.

A famous saying by the American pioneer contemporary dancer Martha Graham suggests that "it takes ten years to make a dancer." Although we do not have time to master all things in life, it is good to know that it does not take ten years to learn enough to understand why someone might wish to devote themselves to such a pursuit. Learning by doing, or the gaining of experiential knowledge, has increased awareness of the skills of others, appreciation of different movement forms, and a richer life. The ability to respond to life's challenges has enabled us to enjoy a retirement that did not go to plan but opened new avenues of sharing a fulfilling life.

Concluding Reflections

The pleasure of writing this chapter, if perhaps indulgent, was in the opportunity to reflect on my life, how it has been shaped and reshaped by life's unique encounters. Currently volunteering for the Ageing Well department of Age UK Somerset Charity and caring for my mother has given me insights into the future that give me no fear. Ageing continues to be a positive experience, and for me it has been about

1. being immersed in an activity for its intrinsic value;
2. being content, knowing that there will always be those better and worse off than yourself;
3. giving to others, for example, through caring, volunteering, and joining community groups;
4. sharing life with loved ones, friends, and family and finding time to stay connected;
5. accepting life's inevitabilities and the unexpected;
6. appreciating each day and the freedom to choose how to spend it;
7. taking risks and embracing challenges because they bring new experiences;

8. reminiscing, remembering the life I have lived and the significant people and places that have made me who I am; and
9. dancing until the music stops.

Finally, how do I address the editor's question about legacy? For me, what matters is how I live my life, not what I leave behind, but I hope to be remembered by those who have known me for as long as memories last. I hope to have made a positive difference in the lives of some other people through the things I have done in teaching, research, volunteering, and sharing my life with special people. For some of my valued colleagues and friends around the world, for example, those in or from Australia, Austria, Bahrain, Bosnia and Herzegovina, Brazil, Canada, Costa Rica, China, Dubai, Egypt, India, Iran, Iraq, Japan, Germany, Greece, Morocco, Norway, Oman, South Africa, Syria, Turkey, the UK, the United States, and Venezuela, they will remember productive and memorable times together and the tangible outcomes. Together we contributed to activities, publications, and declarations that will live longer than us and will make a contribution to the understanding and aspirations of others. We hope that others may learn from our journeys or use them as springboards for their own. For my loved ones, they will remember another me. Most understand little of my career that happened in a city one hundred miles from our seaside hometown, or my activities in other countries that they will never visit; even elements of this chapter may come as a surprise. But they continue to be the people in the centre of my world. I would like them to remember the happy times we created together over the years and to know that I am grateful to have shared my life with them. Remember me as Friday's child—loving and giving.[20]

NOTES
1. Yiannis Koutedakis and Athanasios Jamurtas, "The Dancer as a Performing Athlete," *Sports Med* 34 (2004), 651, https://doi.org/10.2165/00007256-200434100 -00003; reprinted in C. G. Shell, ed., *The Dancer as Athlete: The 1984 Olympic Scientific Congress Proceedings*, vol. 8 (Champaign IL: Human Kinetics, 1986).
2. David Best, *Feeling and Reason in the Arts* (London: George Allen and Unwin, 1985), 157.

3. International Association for Physical Education and Sport for Girls and Women (IAPESGW) is a research and advocacy network to improve opportunities for girls and women in physical education, sport, and dance. The events of its quadrennial congress have formed an important part of building international networks for me, from my first attendance as a demonstrator for the UK in displays of dance and gymnastics whilst a student at college in 1973 in Tehran, Iran, to being president and an executive board member. The IAPESGW (www.iapesgw.org) started in 1949 and celebrated its seventieth anniversary in 2019 in Madrid.

4. Tansin Benn, "A Collective Biography: Women Pioneers of Physical Education at Anstey Physical Training College, United Kingdom," *International Journal of the History of Sport* 34, no. 16 (Europe regional issue, 2017), 1739–59, https://doi .org/10.1080/09523367.2018.1492555.

5. Bannerman quoted in Tansin Benn, "Reflections on a Degree Initiative: The UK's Birmingham Royal Ballet Dancers Enter the University of Birmingham," *Research in Dance Education* 4, no. 1 (2003), 5–16.

6. Tansin Benn and Dorcas Walters, "Between Scylla and Charybdis: Nutritional Education versus Body Culture and the Ballet Aesthetic; The Effects on the Lives of Female Dancers," *Research in Dance Education* 2, no. 2 (2001), 139–54.

7. Tansin Benn, "Muslim Women and Physical Education in Initial Teacher Training," *Sport, Education and Society* 1, no. 1 (1996), 5–21.

8. Tansin Benn, Symeon Dagkas, and Haifaa Jawad, "Embodied Faith: Islam, Religious Freedom and Educational Practices in Physical Education," *Sport, Education and Society* 16, no. 1 (2011), 17–34.

9. Pierre Bourdieu, *Distinction: A Social Critique of the Judgement of Taste* (London: Routledge, 1984); and Pierre Bourdieu, "The Forms of Capital," in *Handbook of Theory and Research for the Sociology of Education*, ed. John Richardson (New York: Greenwood Press, 1986).

10. Chris Shilling, *Changing Bodies: Habits, Crisis and Creativity* (London: Sage, 2008).

11. Centre for Ageing Better, *The State of Ageing in 2019: Adding Life to Our Years*, accessed September 27, 2021, https://www.ageing-better.org.uk/sites/default /files/2019-04/The-State-of-Ageing-in-2019.pdf.

12. Centre for Ageing Better, *State of Ageing in 2019*, 25.

13. Centre for Ageing Better, *State of Ageing in 2019*, 5.

14. Music is important for many people with dementia, and the centre of the brain that processes music stays intact longer than other parts. See, for example, National Health Service, *The Dementia Guide: Living Well after Your Diagnosis*, accessed August 26, 2021, https://www.alzheimers.org.uk/sites/default/files /2020-03/the_dementia_guide_872.pdf.

15. Reminiscing is a vital strategy to support people living with dementia in all its forms. See, for example, M. Downs and B. Bowers, eds., *Excellence in Dementia Care: Research into Practice* (Maidenhead, UK: Open University Press, 2008).

16. M. Connolly and E. Redding, *Dancing towards Well-Being in the Third Age* (London: Trinity Laban Conservatoires of Music and Dance, 2010); T. Vella-Burrows, A. Pickard, L. Wilson, S. Clift, and Sidney De Haan Research Centre for Arts and Health, *Dance to Health* (Folkstone, UK: Canterbury Christ Church University, 2017).

17. The experience of being totally absorbed or immersed in an activity can happen with anything, for example, running, writing, and playing music. Such experience can be theorised by the concept of "flow" and the autotelic personality type. But the appeal of this chapter has been in reflecting rather than theorising.

18. Abstract from Amazon.com review of Janet Carlson, *Quick, before the Music Stops: How Ballroom Dancing Saved My Life* (Crown, 2008).

19. Howard Gardner, *Frames of Mind* (London: Fontana Press, 1993), 206–37.

20. Wikipedia, s.v. "Monday's Child," last modified July 14, 2021, 16:16, https://en .wikipedia.org/wiki/Monday%27s_Child. The nursery rhyme, handed down through generations and first recorded in 1838, predicted babies' personalities according to day of birth.

9 Carpe Diem

LUCIANE LAUFFER

I was born on August 23, 1969, a cold Saturday night in Porto Alegre, the capital city of the southernmost Brazilian state, Rio Grande do Sul. The end of August is usually the coldest period in the Brazilian winter, and I have always felt the cold intensely. I don't have much to say about my biological background except from what my DNA results show. I was given for adoption at birth, and soon after, I was adopted by a family that wanted to look after a baby girl.

I grew up in a family of German descent. Curiously, my dad's German ancestor who immigrated to Brazil came from the same region in Europe that appears on the results of my DNA test, a triangle encompassing parts of Germany, France, and Switzerland. My adoptive family raised me in the Lutheran faith, and I still adhere to it. I was able to attend private schools, usually run by Catholic nuns, as there were no Lutheran schools close to our home.

The house I grew up in had been built next to my father's tile factory on a large plot of land with plenty of fruit trees, a lake, and animals. Some other houses were built for our factory workers. The house closest to ours had been built for my paternal grandmother. We lived there until I was about 19 years old. I was able not only to pick fresh fruit from—and climb and, of course, fall from—the trees but also to mingle with birds and sometimes cows and horses. Because of our geographic isolation, I mostly played with boys, sons of some of the factory workers, something that changed only slightly once I started attending primary school at the age of 5.

In school, I was introduced to only a few sports, such as running, gymnastics, volleyball, and Newcomb ball—a variation of volleyball. I also joined ballet in school, but that didn't last long due to cost. Later, during my teenage years, I started taking jazz dance lessons, but again the cost, as well as the travel involved, stopped my dreams of becoming a professional dancer.

Being adopted by a family that had fair skin and blue eyes, while I have olive skin and green eyes, meant that I would always feel different. When I was growing up, I remember some of my mother's friends referring to me as *filha de criação*, an expression in Portuguese that translates literally into "the daughter that you raised." I only started making sense of that phrase when, at the age of 7, I was told by my mother that I had been adopted at birth. Only a few years later I tried to find out more about my story, but mum just told me that my biological mother had died four days after my birth. Since then, I have not discussed the issue with her.

But that doesn't mean I stopped trying to find out about my roots. Sometimes, after becoming a mother, a woman's feelings change, and perhaps for me, my sense of identity needed to be rescued, so in the past few years I have become more active in trying to find more about where I came from. My search has been quiet and assisted by not only people who share the same problem but also those with access to the more advanced technologies such as DNA matching tests. Only time will tell if they will actually help. So far, I have been able to find distant cousins, some of whom have also been adopted at birth. Adoption seems to run in the family.

Once I was told about my origins to some extent, I started feeling that I didn't belong either in the house or to the people that I had always known. I didn't belong physically to that family and didn't fit into what they expected from me. Perhaps part of the problem was what my mum wanted for me: to learn to cook, to sew, and to look beautiful for a future husband. My dad seemed to give me more freedom, just wanting me to study and succeed in whatever I chose to do.

Despite my mum's and society's expectation, I didn't want to conform to the gender norms—especially those in Brazil—and struggled during my teenage years. I avoided groups of female friends who were mostly concerned with improving their cooking and sewing skills or just wanted to chat about recipes and the next crochet course in our church. That could have been the reason why I chose to attend a school in Porto Alegre, where I could pursue more than just a high school qualification as a primary school teacher. That move expanded my horizons, and even if I had felt a sense of displacement, I was creating my own space and starting my own path. Curiosity and a sense of adventure have always attracted me to other countries. Australia was one of them. Fascinated by Sydney, I first visited there in 1996. I fell in love almost at once and promised myself I would come back to stay. By 2001 I had managed to save enough money, alongside my partner at that time, to undertake a master's degree program in Australia for two years. The relationship didn't last long, but my stay did.

Despite having left Brazil, I still love to dance, just as most Latin Americans do, but there are few venues where someone close to my age can feel welcome without being confined to ballroom dancing or sixties music. Whenever I catch up with some of my girlfriends, we go out and dance

I love reading nonfiction, going to the movies, and traveling, which is perhaps my top interest. But in terms of physical activity, my passion is football (or soccer), another Brazilian element, along with dance, that is engraved on me. As a woman raised in Brazil, I was confined in a way to being only a supporter of football, but once in Australia and looking for a physical activity after pregnancy, I joined a community football referees' association and become one of them. I am now among one of the group's most active women—though there are still very few of us—as I am also a member of the executive committee, their only female instructor, and one of the few referee assessors, or evaluators. I have also joined a local team and play five-a-side football over the summer with other mums. I guess we give the term "soccer mum" a proper and active definition.

The perception of ageing depends on gender and geographic location. In Brazil, a woman is considered old at around 35–40, about the age when her reproductive system begins to slow down. I may never forget meeting a Brazilian man in Fiji while holidaying with my family. He told me he had recently divorced at age 40 and was happy to announce he was going back to Brazil to party, now that he was "free" again, and would go out with as many women as he could. But he specifically said, with a grin on his face, that he was referring to women under the age of 35, because "women over 35 are dead." Those words seem to sum up the way men see women not just in Brazil but in most Latin cultures, where male values are dominant.

In Australia, things can be quite different, to some extent. Older women are visible and celebrated on TV as reporters and presenters. They are and can also be CEOs, managers, prime ministers, and state governors—but when it comes to positions of power, women are more challenged than men are. A recent documentary about the first female prime minister, Julia Gillard, exposes this reality and the contradictions in which access and opportunity do not mean inclusion and acceptance.

In terms of ageing, there are big differences between countries: while in Brazil the elderly are still maintained as part of the family and looked after at home or in their own space, in Australia most elderly people are sent to aged care facilities, which have been multiplying, seemingly by the hour, around the country. I believe a difference in the sense of community sets the countries apart. With the ageing population growing in most countries, I believe it is imperative to keep the elderly in society rather than set them apart from it.

The process of ageing has definitely accelerated since my pregnancy, which happened at the age of 38. The brutal transformation of my body was not foretold in ads or magazines when I was planning to have a baby. During pregnancy, I developed preeclampsia, which is high blood pressure that classifies pregnancy as a high-risk condition. Because medication wasn't keeping my blood pressure at normal levels after the eighth month, I had to give birth through induction a week earlier than planned.

About six months after my daughter's birth, my blood pressure went back to normal levels, but two or three years later, the problem reappeared. The changes in my body have become permanent. Losing weight was very difficult, and the stress of raising a baby without close family support accelerated the greying of my hair.

Being able to take part in sport has been a big life change and a huge benefit to my health and general well-being. I had struggled to shed some extra kilos from my late pregnancy through mainstream physical activity and other measures. Wanting a high-intensity activity, I decided to go more radical and become a football referee.

Suddenly, I had access to special training and more help with keeping fit, and I enjoyed the fast-paced and challenging environment of men's and women's football. Since beginning to referee, I have been exposed to a new network of people. On many occasions, I was asked to join women's teams, but at first that activity would have interfered with my refereeing schedule, so for months I said no.

But when I came to see playing football as a new challenge, I accepted an invite and joined a team of ladies over 35. Most of them were also mums trying to get back in shape after having children. This activity revealed a world I had never known before, and physical activity brought me joy I didn't think was possible at a later stage in life.

I definitely feel a sense of accomplishment—but I am not done yet. Unlike my parents, who barely finished primary school, I was able to attend university and am now undertaking a PhD candidature, which few people among my extended family and friends network have ever done. And I am completing it in a second language and at a later age than most.

I guess my ambition and determination may be credited for my success, but also defying those who said I couldn't do it makes it even more worthwhile. I am determined, and even stubborn at times, and I follow my dreams. No one should ever stop dreaming.

Ageing brings greater wisdom. Only time gives you experience and the opportunity to learn from it. I have lived many joyful moments so far and expect to have many more of them—so I hope to put together a book about my story someday.

In regard to fears, I wonder how my body will cope with ageing—being less agile and more fragile—as I start slowing down. Ageing is socially magnified for women: a woman with grey hair is old, while a grey-haired man is charming; for women, the ageing process is said to begin when they can no longer be child bearers, while for men, it starts much later. With the growth of the ageing population, I hope that wisdom and experience will start to count. There seems to be an overemphasis on youth these days.

Of course, no one lives a perfect life. I have had occasional setbacks that may have happened because I don't like to wait for things to happen to me but rather chase the new. In 2007 my then fiancé and I moved to Canada to start a life together, but for over a year we were unable to find stable professional jobs in our fields. We may never completely recover from that year of emotional and financial losses. Many other migrants to that part of the world have gone through similar experiences, but I wonder how many of them would readily acknowledge their failure.

Soon after our return to Australia, I fell pregnant. It was a joy to have my little girl in my arms, but raising a child was difficult while my husband worked full-time and I struggled to establish a career in a new city. We had chosen to move to New South Wales, instead of returning to Western Australia.

My life has been a course of many ups and downs, but I look forward with hope. To find positives among the difficulties, one must take on the obstacles. Luckily, I have never had major health problems, which I link to a positive outlook.

I am an optimist. And I am resilient and determined; though sometimes stubborn, I will always engage in activities that challenge me.

I rarely engage in nostalgia. The past belongs where it is, but lessons from it help me function today—and that's why my experiences are so valuable.

Key friendships have been important throughout my life. Though having grown up in one country and then moved to another later in life made keeping friendships a bit challenging, I have many friends in my native country and maintain those relationships with the help of digital technology. In Australia, close friendships have taken longer to develop due to cultural differences throughout the years and considering my many moves. Some of these people seem to have much more in common to share now, after all my different experiences, while others seem to be stuck in the past and less relevant to the person that I have become.

The fact that family is so very important to me is probably a South American characteristic, and I contact my parents and relatives often. I have also travelled extensively and lived in two other countries, so I have friends spread around the world—from Thailand to Germany to Mauritius to Canada. I tend to travel to wherever I can visit or meet some of those people.

I have few regrets, but among them is having said no to opportunities just because of fear of failure or disappointment. I tend to live every moment well and think through my decisions, but I cannot always get it right. I cannot change my past, so I try to learn from it. Having achieved most of what I wanted in life, I can say that I have more of a sense of fulfillment at this stage. And I am waiting for more!

I hope my main legacy will be the example that I set for my daughter and perhaps other girls and women who know me. I hope they are inspired to pursue their dreams. Female friends in Brazil have expressed admiration for my courage in moving to another country and starting a new life from scratch.

As I restart my career after moving to other countries and becoming a mother, I have much to look forward to. I'm not close to the end, nor am I waiting for life to happen. I expect another fifty years of living life to the fullest, ignoring the social norms surrounding age so that I can do what I want. "Carpe diem" is my motto, and I make the most of each day. That's how Brazilians perceive life: enjoy the present, as no one knows about tomorrow.

10 Aging as an Adventure

M. ANN HALL

How long we live and how well we age are, in my opinion, a crapshoot. In other words, they're risky and associated with unpredictable outcomes. Sure, we have some control over the process, but however you think about it, there is still much left to chance. Presumably I have some good genes, at least on my mother's side, because she died naturally just a few months short of her one hundredth birthday. My father, on the other hand, died at 72, a mere two years after being diagnosed with ALS, better known as Lou Gehrig's disease. I hope I've dodged that bullet. I have a younger sister, but all other immediate biological family members passed away some time ago. Neither my sister nor I has any children, so our branch of the family comes to an end with us. As I write this, I have just celebrated my seventy-ninth birthday.

I am being a bit facetious when I call aging a crapshoot because I have spent a lifetime believing that sport and physical activity might help me age better and stay alive longer. They have certainly provided me with a life full of physicality, adventure, camaraderie, and just plain fun. In many ways sport and physical activity, through both first-hand experience and writing about them, have been my life and still are. What follows is an account of this life.

I was born in Toronto, Canada, in 1942, but after a few years I moved with my family to Ottawa, where I went to school. Both my parents were medical professionals—my father a radiographer and my mother a nurse—which meant that my sister and I grew up in a comfortable middle-class family. For most of my childhood, our house was at the bottom of a spacious, dead-end street with several empty lots that provided an enormous playground—at least it seemed so at the time—for us to roam, climb trees, create forts, and use the street for ball hockey in winter and pickup baseball in summer. When not in school, I was outside playing with the neighborhood boys and, rarely, girls, whom I often considered too prissy and fragile for my liking. I was, in other words, a classic tomboy and proud of it. My parents indulged my never-ending pleas for a new hockey stick or baseball glove, and when I was a bit older, they relented on the subject of a bicycle. I was so proud of that first bike—a secondhand, postwar CCM (Canada Cycle and Motor)—which my father fixed up and painted, complete with a racing stripe down the back fender. It was truly my "freedom machine" as I explored the larger neighborhood, rode to and from school, and visited my friends.

Summer vacations were usually spent with our mother at a Girl Guide camp, where she was often in charge. My favorite was Camp Woolsey, just outside Ottawa, where my days were spent on or near the water. It was there I learned to swim, row and canoe, and be safe and comfortable on the water. As soon as I was old enough, I became a Brownie, then a Guide, and finally a Sea Ranger. I learned camp craft skills, went on canoe trips, and could take care of myself and others in the wilderness. When I was 16, I acquired my own canoe, a sleek Peterborough cedar strip, with money earned from babysitting and working as a lifeguard during the summers at Brighton Beach on the Rideau River in Ottawa. I became a camp counsellor, then waterfront director, and later a trainer of camp leaders. In fact, from the time I was 5 until I was 25, I spent part of every summer at some camp or other.

Sportswise, I was a decent all-around athlete. In the late 1940s and the 1950s, at least where I lived, there were no organized sports programs for girls. I learned, from playing with boys on the street, how to throw a ball properly, how to shoot a puck, and how to run fast. I learned to skate on a nearby playground, flooded in winter, where a winter carnival often took place. In 1948 Ottawa-born Barbara Ann Scott won an Olympic gold medal and the world figure skating title. A tumultuous reception awaited her upon her return to Canada's capital. Children were let out of school to watch and wave as she toured the main streets in a car strewn with spring daffodils. I remember seeing her as she passed by but was too young to understand who she was or what she represented. I had, however, no desire to acquire a Barbara Ann Scott doll, complete with skates, fur-trimmed dress, and tiara, because to do so would seriously damage my tomboy image. Like millions of other young girls of my generation, I took up figure skating but secretly longed for black hockey skates, hoping one day to play with my real heroes, the stars of the Toronto Maple Leafs or the Montreal Canadiens, knowing full well that I could never be, indeed did not want to be, like Barbara Ann Scott.

There were no organized leagues for girls to play ice hockey or baseball, or any sport for that matter in those days. Opportunities to compete were limited, but that situation changed somewhat when I entered high school in the midfifties. Here, for the first time, I encountered properly trained physical education teachers, who organized intramural and extramural sport programs especially for girls. I was able to join a team and try out for the junior and, later, the senior school team in several sports—basketball, volleyball, and track and field. I loved it, basically becoming a gym rat, since we were encouraged to help run things through the Girls' Athletic Association. I had decided that I would become either a doctor or a scientist—probably influenced by my parents' professions—but as my high school years came to a close, I realized I could continue doing what I truly loved if I trained as a physical education teacher.

I went off to Queen's University in Kingston, Ontario, for a four-year program that would grant me both bachelor of arts and bachelor of physical education degrees. For three years, mornings were spent in academic courses and afternoons completing PE courses. The final year was devoted to finishing the more theory-oriented PE courses. I did well, graduating and winning the gold medal in 1964, which gave my father some consolation because he was concerned about how I would continue to teach PE when I got "old." At that time, no one fully understood where physical education was headed as an academic field. While at Queen's I played intercollegiate volleyball for a couple of years and basketball through all four years, although at that time in Canada there were no national championships for any women's intercollegiate sport. We were limited to competing against teams in several Ontario and Quebec universities. That limitation too would soon change. Nonetheless, it was exciting and fun to travel for away games, and to be coached and trained properly.

After another academic year in Toronto to acquire my teaching certificate at the Ontario College of Education, I was ready to begin my career as a high school physical education teacher. Jobs were plentiful in those days because new schools were opening to accommodate the postwar baby boomer generation. I chose to return to Ottawa where I expected to land a job in one of the new schools. Instead, I ended up in the third-oldest school in the city because the principal, who had been the vice principal of the high school I attended, requested me for his staff. I suppose I should have been flattered, but the job turned out to be a nightmare. I was shocked at the blatant discrimination and impossible conditions under which I was expected to teach and encourage young girls to acquire an interest in physical activity. As the only PE teacher at my school, I was working around the clock preparing lessons in three subject areas, administering an intramural program, coaching all the girls' teams, and teaching my lessons in a small, dingy gym while my three male counterparts, having taken the best facilities and equipment, lounged about just waiting for me to crack up. I found some solace by playing in a women's recreational basketball league.

My solution at the end of the school year was to leave and return to university. No one ever asked me why I was leaving the school, and those awful memories stuck with me for a long time, fueling much of what I did and thought from then on. I was accepted at several universities, and wishing to remain in Canada, I chose the University of Alberta, arriving there in the fall of 1966 to begin my master's program. I played for the Pandas, the women's U of A basketball team, for one year, all that was left of my eligibility, but I was not a success. In Ontario universities, we played the six-a-side, two-thirds court, and limited-dribble women's rules, whereas in the west, universities had long since switched to the five-a-side, full-court, unlimited-dribble men's rules. They are entirely different games, and I had difficulty making the adjustment. Nonetheless, it was good to compete and be part of a team again. Also, my downhill skiing ability improved significantly with access to the marvelous ski resorts in the Rocky Mountains. I earned money both during the academic year teaching skating to first-year students required to take a PE course, and in the summer teaching beginner tennis classes for the city's recreation program. Life was good.

I completed my master's degree in the requisite two years. At 26 years old, I was pondering what to do next when I was called into the dean's office and unexpectedly offered a job in the Faculty of Physical Education at the University of Alberta. Put simply, was I immediately available to take the place of a female faculty member who had unexpectedly become pregnant? Of course, I said yes, hoping that I was also qualified for the job. I taught a variety of courses those first years on staff—secondary school PE, history of sport and PE, comparative sport and PE, and the usual activity courses like aquatics and skating. In 1969 the Faculty acquired a brand-new PE building that had been added on to the old one. In addition to new offices and research labs, it also came with six squash and six racquetball-handball courts. In a place like Edmonton, which was freezing cold and covered in snow for six months of the year, having an indoor space for new sports was a huge plus. I took up both racquetball and squash, loving them both. In North America at that time, the standard squash game was hardball— played with a hard rubber ball that certainly hurt if you got hit with it. By the 1980s, however, we had switched to the international version of the game. Our courts had to be widened slightly, and we used the smaller, soft squash ball. It was certainly more fun, easier to teach, and safer. I competed recreationally in both squash and racquetball, and at one point won the Canadian women's novice racquetball championship. I was also jogging regularly to improve my stamina. I ran a few 5Ks for fun but never contemplated a marathon.

After three years of teaching in the Faculty of Physical Education, it was clear that the next step educationally was a doctorate. I had become friends with the British sport sociologist and educator Peter McIntosh (*Sport in Society*, 1963) when he visited the U of A to give special courses. We also met up on the squash court. Through him I investigated the possibility of going to a British university to continue my education, and I arrived at the University of Birmingham in the summer of 1971 to begin my doctoral studies. To my knowledge, I am the first Canadian, and probably the first North American, ever to complete a PhD in physical education in England. This made me an oddity because the area was not fully recognized in Britain as a legitimate university subject. My degree was earned entirely by research, and I had taken to England a straightforward question: Why do some women make physical activity an important part of their lives and others do not? Given the freedom to explore where I was heading intellectually was both exhilarating and frustrating at the same time, because although I had a wonderfully supportive supervisor, I was basically on my own for much of this time. I've written more expansively about this period in my formal education in *Feminism and Sporting Bodies: Essays on Theory and Practice* (Human Kinetics, 1996).

More important for this essay is that I took up squash far more seriously than ever before. I joined a private club in Birmingham and took lessons from Nasrullah Khan, a member of the famous Pakistani family that ruled the squash world for fifty years. I played at the club and for the University of Birmingham, although the team was not very successful. Nonetheless, it was fun, and I improved sufficiently so that I taught squash courses when I returned to the U of A, and indeed for the next twenty years. My most serious athletic injuries also came from playing squash: a complete rupture of my left Achilles, which was repaired and has not since been a problem, and rotator-cuff tendinitis in my racquet arm, which still bothers me today.

I returned to teaching at the U of A in 1974 with my newly earned doctorate. Researchwise, I knew that "women in sport" was the general focus but was undecided as to which disciplinary perspective to take. The social sciences and humanities interested me the most, but would it be history, sociology, psychology, or social psychology? I had little formal training in any of these areas. This dilemma also corresponded with what was happening in physical education as it seriously began to transform itself from a profession into an academic discipline or, perhaps more accurately, a series of subdisciplines now readily identified as the history of sport, sociology of sport, psychology of sport, and so forth. Coupled with the growing rise of the feminist movement and academic feminism, it became clear that I could help shape the sociological study of women and sport. To gain a better understanding of my intellectual life at this time, one can read *Feminism and Sporting Bodies*.

From the mid-1970s to the early 1980s, I was extremely busy through teaching several courses, doing administrative work in the Faculty, publishing my research, attending and speaking at conferences, and volunteering for work related to feminism, such as establishing a national organization devoted to feminist research or a women's studies program at the U of A. I did, however, try to keep reasonably fit through regular squash and jogging, and the occasional downhill skiing trip to the mountains.

In 1983–84, I was granted a one-year sabbatical from my university, and I decided to spend the first few months at my alma mater, Queen's University in Kingston, Ontario, where I had graduated almost twenty years earlier. I drove across the country, stopping off in Minnesota to join a canoe trip organized by a group called Woodswomen, one of the first adventure travel companies serving women exclusively. Advertising a "trip for women who have done wilderness canoeing and want to develop more skills in making [their] own route decisions, map-reading, and navigation," the company also pointed out in its brochure that the expedition would be strenuous, with rain, hard portages, clear lakes, some rapids, and beautiful scenery. I had not been canoe tripping for a while, and this jaunt was a wonderful opportunity and privilege. Over two weeks, eight women canoed along the Boundary Waters of Minnesota and then into Quetico Provincial Park, a large wilderness area in northwestern Ontario. A highlight was discovering the ancient pictographs, or rock drawings, on the side of a cliff in Darky Lake, deep in the Quetico wilderness. We bonded as a group, and I promised myself more wilderness canoe trips, something not easy to accomplish in landlocked Alberta.

At Queen's University, I had been appointed a Queen's Quest Visiting Scholar in Physical Education and a scholar-in-residence through the dean of women. I taught a couple of courses and lived in one of the student residences with four hundred undergrads, who were free to consult me if they wished, although not many did. Kingston, Ontario, was then, and still is, primarily a university city, but both the university and town had grown enormously since my student days. A strong Canadian women's movement was also emerging, and Kingston was no exception in developing a vibrant and supportive women's community. It was through this network that I met the woman who has been my partner for the past thirty-eight years. We had little in common through life experiences because she had previously been married and had four children. At the time, Jane's youngest was still in high school but the others were well on their way to establishing their own lives. She had earned her teaching degree and was working as a special education teacher. We shared two interests primarily—a love of books and reading as well as a love of physical activity and being outdoors, preferably canoeing on a lake in summer or skiing in the mountains in winter. We spent many a happy time exploring Frontenac Provincial Park just north of Kingston.

After another four months in Toronto studying at the Ontario Institute for Studies in Education, I returned to Alberta. Before the term began in September, Jane and I decided to join a monthlong canoe trip down the Noatak River in Alaska, again organized by Woodswomen. Above the Arctic Circle, the Noatak National Preserve protects the largest untouched river basin in the United States. We flew to Fairbanks, where we met the six other women on the trip including our trip leader, and from there went on to Bettles, in the Gates of the Arctic National Park. After a day or so of waiting, a float plane took us and our gear to Pingo Lake in the Brooks mountain range and very near the headwaters of the Noatak. It was stunningly beautiful.

We soon learned that canoeing on a river is not at all like canoeing on a lake. The Noatak is slow-moving and gentle for most of its 425-mile course, carving out a striking, scenic canyon that serves as a migration route for plants and animals between subarctic and arctic environments. It is also fed by a relatively large watershed, which means that rare but severe rain events can result in temporary rapid inundation of normally dry river bars often to a depth of several feet. If you were camping on one of these gravel bars, you could easily be swept away and drowned. This meant that every night, after we had chosen our camping spot on the tundra, we had to haul our various watercraft—two canoes, a folding Klepper kayak, and a rubber dinghy—a good fifty feet up the banks of the river. As the trip went on and we used up some of our supplies, the boats became lighter or perhaps we simply got stronger. Navigating the occasional rapids was something we got better at as we progressed through the route, but it was always a thrill.

Our small group functioned in true feminist fashion. There were no rules (except for boat hauling), and through consensus we let our bodies, weather, and the river decide when and how long we should be on the water each day. Some days we rested and explored the tundra or climbed up a shale mountain, hoping to catch sight of a caribou herd or an elusive grizzly. We were being unobtrusively watched by the locals and our progress on the river followed, something we learned when we reached the tiny village of Noatak at the end of our journey. For Jane and me, the trip cemented our resolve to live together, which would not be easy given that our abodes were over two thousand miles apart, and Jane still had family and teaching responsibilities. It took us two years to figure it out, and in the summer of 1986, we moved Jane, along with her canoe and horse, Bucky, to Edmonton. We settled into a lovely, refurbished old house in the Mill Creek area, where we still live, with access to miles of trails for biking and walking.

True to his name, Bucky was a handsome buckskin. Jane had acquired him several years before because she wanted to ride regularly and to teach her children proper equitation. For this activity, he was the perfect horse—gentle, kind, athletic, and forever patient. When I visited Jane in Kingston, I rode Bucky on several occasions even though I knew absolutely nothing about riding nor had any experience with horses. When Jane and Bucky arrived in Edmonton to begin a new phase in our lives, I was 44 years old and Jane had just turned 50. It had not occurred to me to start a whole new athletic career, but that is exactly what happened.

Around Edmonton are a number of private riding stables where for a monthly fee you can board your horse. The stable help is responsible for feeding the horses, cleaning their stalls, and putting them out in paddocks, whereas grooming, riding, and maintaining the horses in top condition are up to the owners. We found an appropriate stable for Bucky, who at this point was getting on in years. Jane soon acquired another horse, which meant I could ride dear Bucky, but it became clear that if I was going to take up riding seriously, I needed a horse of my own. At the stable was a young, chestnut "grade" (heritage unknown) named Aries, which the owner had found in northern Alberta. He was being used to teach children vaulting or gymnastics on horseback. Obviously patient and kind, Aries was suggested as the horse for me, which became a reality in the summer of 1988. I also acquired my first riding coach, Otto, a precise German with years of experience, who no doubt wondered if I would ever learn to ride properly. In those days it was possible to roam around the countryside unimpeded by fences, which meant we took the horses on long trail rides through the bush. Jane also helped to train Aries by riding him in the indoor arena and teaching him basic dressage movements. She also competed with him in local horse shows, where they did well. I was slowly gaining more confidence, but admittedly riding was the most difficult sport, indeed the most technical, I had ever tried. Riding also gave me an enormous sense of empowerment, perhaps more so than any other sport. It was thrilling to learn how to control something infinitely stronger than me, but it was pointless to try and physically overpower this animal because I was never going to win. Riding is all about subtleness and timing.

I was granted another sabbatical leave in 1990–91, and we decided to spend the first four months in Germany, where we had friends in Münster, one of whom was a professor at Westfälische Wilhelms-Universität. Jane and I pursued our riding interests, although without a car we were forced to travel to a stable and back by bicycle. Jane was looking for a new horse, which she found in Feudale, a beautiful Westphalian mare bred specifically for dressage. Her newly acquired horse stayed in Germany for the next six months while we went off to Perth, Australia, where I taught at the University of Western Australia.

Back in Edmonton, our horses—Aries and Feudale—were now at a small, private stable called Beckwith, along with a dozen or so other horses, all with women owners who rode daily. We decided it would be challenging and fun to work up a "quadrille," which involves any number of horses (in our case, eight) who perform a series of dressage movements in a pattern to music. We worked diligently all fall and winter creating the routine and practicing every Saturday. In the process, we got to know each other, and we certainly became familiar with the foibles and quirks of each other's horses. We called ourselves the Beckwith Belles, which we considered hilarious because most of us were well past middle age and anything but "belles." We had originally wanted to include everyone who rode at the stable, but several dropped out for a variety of reasons—their horse went lame, they did not have time, or they simply found it too difficult. Most, however, were involved in some way, such as transporting horses, helping find the right music, and lending moral support.

By spring, we decided that we were ready to show off our efforts. Getting ready for a quadrille performance takes a great deal of time and effort. Boots and tack must be polished, horses bathed, and their manes braided. Then the horses are loaded onto trailers and transported to the performance site, usually another stable in the area. We performed our quadrille mostly in indoor arenas and usually as an exhibition event at a regular dressage show. It consisted of fairly simple dressage movements such as turns and circles, shoulder-in, haunches-in (travers), half-pass, and extended trot. But the most difficult parts were keeping the horses in sync and persevering when one or more decided to act up. One of our most exciting performances was outside at a well-attended jumping show featuring international jumpers, and we were elated at how well it all went. The Beckwith Belles have long since disbanded, but some twenty-five years later, several members are still riding and we get together occasionally as a social group.

In the summer of 1993, Jane and I decided that we wished to purchase a summer cottage in Ontario. Although it seemed crazy given that we lived in Edmonton, Jane's immediate family, most of whom lived in Toronto, was increasing as her children married, and there was now one grandchild. Also, my sister still lived in Ottawa. Rather than disrupting their lives by staying with them while visiting, we wanted a place where the ever-increasing family could visit us. We laid out some criteria—the main one being location on a lake in the Canadian Shield, with its iconic rocks and pines, and relatively close to Toronto and Ottawa—and contacted a real estate agent. We found what we were looking for on a small lake about an hour north of Kingston, an hour and a half west of Ottawa, and three hours east of Toronto. White Lake is environmentally protected because it is home to an important fish culture station on the highway side. No craft are allowed on the lake except canoes, kayaks, sailboats, and electric-powered boats. There is absolutely no fishing. Since 1994 we have spent every summer at this cottage, which has welcomed our extended family, now including ten grandchildren, and many friends. We sold it a few years ago to one of Jane's sons, but we retain a long-term lease and plan to enjoy it for several more years.

In 1997 I decided to take early retirement from the University of Alberta. Although only 55, I had been there for thirty years, and probably more important, we were offered a handsome financial package. The province of Alberta is financially dependent on its nonrenewable resources, primarily oil and gas, and it regularly goes through periods of boom and bust. We were experiencing an economic downturn in the late 1990s, and universities were looking for ways to buy out their most expensive staff. It had not occurred to me to retire at that stage, but I realized that I could continue to do what I loved most about being at a university—research, write, and publish—without the distractions of teaching, graduate students, committee work, and so on. As long as I had my library privileges, I would be fine. To this day, however, I still give a few guest lectures to various classes. I have also published seven books and numerous papers since retiring.

Of course, retiring from the university also gave me more time, although not necessarily more money, to pursue my riding career. Aries was still going strong, and both of us learned to be better at dressage. But by 2002 he was almost 20, and we decided it was time to retire him. He had been such a faithful horse, and I did not want to lose him entirely. Very close to our cottage in Ontario was an experienced horsewoman, who specialized in competitive trail riding, but she also had a large property with a sand ring where she gave lessons primarily to children. We told her about Aries, and she agreed to take him. She used him occasionally for lessons, and several of Jane's grandchildren rode him when they visited the cottage. Eventually he was put out to pasture with other horses, and when I visited and he heard me call, he would come thundering out of the bush to retrieve his carrot treats. He had a good retirement and lived until he was 26.

My second horse, Winston, was a sturdy grey purchased from a breeder in Carp, Ontario. Although we got along fine, dressage was not something he really enjoyed. We eventually tested him at jumping and he seemed a natural, but I was not interested in taking up that aspect of riding. After four years, I sold him and bought Alaska, a beautiful, pure white American Hanoverian, who ironically was bred to jump but hated it, and was being retrained as a dressage horse. Alaska was certainly more horsepower than I had ever ridden before, and it was magic when he went well. I even entered a local horse show with him, but without much experience, we both found it stressful. We continued to work away together, but despite excellent veterinary care, he was showing signs of not wishing to perform any longer. By 2013, I was over 70 and had ridden consistently for some twenty-five years. I gave Alaska away to a good home where he could be a schoolmaster to someone with less riding experience. I put all my riding gear in storage and decided to think about it for a year.

Jane's riding career had its ups and downs. After she retired Feudale, she had several horses which for one reason or another did not work out. In 2002 we went on a horse-buying trip to Germany where she bought Elli, a lively warmblood mare. Jane was in a riding clinic in Edmonton with Elli in the fall when she was thrown and seriously hurt—broken femur and shattered ankle. Elli was shipped immediately back to Germany and never seen again. By spring of the following year, Jane was ready to look for another horse. She found one in Kenzo, another German warmblood but trained to the highest level of dressage. At the time, Kenzo was in Ontario at Franklands Farm in Brockville. Since we were coming to our cottage for the summer, I shipped my horse Winston to Franklands, and Jane and I both took lessons from Gina Smith, a former Canadian Olympian. Both horses were shipped to Edmonton at the end of the summer.

Kenzo was a wonderful horse for Jane, and she competed in quite a few shows with him. Unfortunately, he had to have emergency colic surgery, which he survived, but it was difficult to bring him back to his former self. Jane retired him and he lived until he was almost 30 just being a horse. She bought a couple of other horses, trained them, and then gave them away. (Jane turned 85 this summer, and is still very much involved in the local horse world.) I never did return to the sport but am surrounded by wonderful memories from my time as a rider. Not surprisingly, I have more time and certainly more money.

Pilates is a physical fitness system named after Joseph Pilates, who developed a series of mat and equipment exercises designed to develop stability and mobility throughout the body. He came to the U.S. after World War I, opened a studio in New York City, and began teaching classes, often to dancers. I had some experience with yoga but found it boring, especially the meditation, and it did not seem to do much for my body. Even when I stopped riding, I wasn't experiencing any bodily issues, but I knew that I needed to so something to keep agile and fit. Jane had been going to our local Pilates studio for some time, and I decided to give it a try. That was eight years ago, and I'm still taking classes several times a week. Due to COVID-19, and the restrictions of in-person classes, our studio switched to an online version that has worked extremely well.

Pilates uses precise movement sequences to develop stability and mobility throughout the body. The first thing I noticed was how uneven my body was, right side versus the left. When I lay flat on a mat with my legs outstretched, I could feel that my left side was jacked up higher than my right side. I am right-handed and play racquet sports with my right hand and arm; thus, over the years, it has become my dominant side. One of the things about riding is that you cannot have a dominant side in that you need to be able to move your hip forward evenly on both sides; in other words, you need to be symmetrical to signal exactly what you want the horse beneath you to do. I had trouble with riding because I was not nearly as strong and effective on my left side. Several years of Pilates exercises have changed this inequity, but my body is still a work in progress.

I have never been particularly flexible, especially through my hip flexors and hamstring muscles. I don't feel that I have become more flexible through Pilates, but the problem certainly has not become worse. The supposed benefits of Pilates are to add strength without compromising joint function, to lengthen muscles to improve range of motion, to correct structural imbalances, to reduce joint compression, and to improve balance, control, and coordination. I can say without doubt that I have benefited and seen improvement in all these areas, but progress has come slowly, almost without me noticing. In large measure this success has been due not just to my perseverance but mainly to the excellent instruction we receive at our studio. Our classes are small; the instructors intimately know our individual bodies and capabilities; and they are continually learning and experimenting in their own Pilates practices. I see no reason why I can't continue practicing Pilates well into old age. (The Canadian government typically classifies people aged 65 and over as "elderly," at which point they are eligible for federal benefits such as the Canada Pension Plan and Old Age Security payments. Also, older members of Indigenous communities, who are respected for the wisdom they have gained during their long lives, are often called "elders.")

Although Pilates exercises provide for overall physical fitness, and proper breathing is an important aspect, they do little to improve cardiovascular fitness. I needed to play a sport that required running around and use of my racquet skills and court sense. Pickleball was the perfect choice. It combines many of the elements of tennis, badminton, and table tennis. Like miniature tennis on a badminton-sized court, it uses a plastic ball the size of a tennis ball, a paddle twice the size of a ping pong bat, and a badminton-like scoring system (you can score only when you are serving). It can be played indoors or outdoors. Since it has become so popular, and courts are at a premium, most people play the doubles game. I took a series of beginner lessons to learn the fundamentals and have been playing ever since, mostly indoors in the winter at one of Edmonton's large recreation centres. I team up with women and men of different ages, although most are retired, and it's soon evident who is playing "smart" because they simply can't run around as much anymore. I'm slowly learning how to play smart too. Unfortunately, COVID-19 temporarily put an end to my pickleball activity, but it was replaced by luxurious hikes throughout the trails in Edmonton's river valley.

I began this essay with the notion that aging is a risky and unpredictable experience, over which we have little control. Some of us have lucky genes, and some of us do not. In fact, if you read books like Barbara Ehrenreich's recent *Natural Causes: An Epidemic of Wellness, the Certainty of Dying, and Killing Ourselves to Live Longer*, you learn that our body is subject to randomness and even outright conflict at the cellular level. Our body can attack itself, and rather than protecting us, our immune system can nourish cancer cells. There is little one can do about it. At 76, Ehrenreich considered herself old enough to die and refused annual physicals, Pap smears, mammograms, cancer screenings, and the like. "Not only do I reject the torment of a medicalized death," she states, "but I refuse to accept a medicalized life." She does, however, keep up her weekly gym workouts because they make her feel better and less grumpy.

To a certain extent I agree with Ehrenreich. I see my physician only when I have a problem and not to undergo a series of pointless tests. Nor do I read self-help books about "active aging" or "successful aging," or even worse, about "antiageing" or "reverse-aging." My diet has changed little over the years, and since I do most of the day-to-day cooking in our household, I choose our menus carefully and prepare almost everything from scratch. We eat well with no dietary restrictions.

Writing this essay has forced me to think about aging, which I realize I rarely do. Of course, I know that my body is aging because I can see it in the sagging skin and muscle loss. No amount of physical activity is going to change those aspects of aging, but it does make me feel good in the trying. I don't pine for my younger self because that is pointless and wishful thinking. I do not engage in nostalgia. Compared with most women my age, I don't think that I look younger, but people are sometimes surprised to discover how old I am. I find it amusing when people ask if I am still working, which given my research and literary output over the past twenty years, I suppose that I still am.

I don't see much changing as I continue to age, providing of course that I keep my good health. It should be clear by now that I don't believe I have much control over that aspect and all I can do is to keep doing what I am already doing. The adventure continues!

11 An Antiaging Sporting Life in an Aging Society

KOHEI KAWASHIMA

The Past

I am a Japanese man who was born in Tokyo on August 29, 1961, the same day in August that Michael Jackson, a hero of my young days, had been born three years earlier. My father, Isamu, was born in 1928 in Kasukabe, Saitama Prefecture, just north of Tokyo. He was the first son of an employee of a small hat manufacturing company, which was one of the major industries in the area. While the lineage of Isamu's father can be traced to a local wealthy farmer, that of his mother can be traced to a low-ranking samurai in Iwatsuki, a city near Kasukabe. My mother, Kayoko, was born in 1934 in Shinagawa, Tokyo, to a father who was a timber trader and a mother who was a purveyor of tofu to the nearby Sensoji-Temple—a position my mother often proudly recalls as "goyo-dofu," meaning a respectable merchant. The lineage of Kayoko's father can be traced to a farmer in Kanagawa Prefecture, just south of Tokyo. Kayoko's grandfather left for Tokyo in search of fortune during the Meiji era (1868–1912) and established a successful lumber business.

Therefore, my ancestors include a samurai, a wealthy farmer, a respectable tofu merchant, and a resourceful lumber businessman, each of whom must have reached middle- or upper-middle-class status during the Meiji and Taisho (1912–1926) eras. Their descendants, however, lost that status through the depression and wartime years of the early Showa (1926–45) era. My maternal grandfather's lumber business went bankrupt in the early 1930s. He sought a new fortune in Seoul, Korea, which was then a colony of Imperial Japan, but lost everything when the nation was defeated in the Pacific War. Nearly penniless, he returned to Japan with his wife and five children, sought refuge in his close friend's hometown, Matsuyama, Ehime Prefecture, and began a new life. Ehime Prefecture is on Shikoku Island, which is the smallest of the four major islands.

My paternal grandfather's fortune also declined during the Showa depression. His employer, a hat manufacturer, paid a family wage that could barely cover the costs of daily necessities. Thus, my father did not receive enough support to pursue an education, despite the advantage of being the first son, and was forced to enter a national aircraft crew training school. Following Japan's defeat, he struggled to support his family and found an opportunity through a job offered by a Tokyo printing company.

Protestantism served as an important tie between my parents. When the wave of evangelism originating in Yokohama reached Kasukabe, my father's grandmother converted to Christianity and discarded her family's Buddhist altar in the river behind her house, thus beginning a multigenerational family of Christians that includes my elder brother. My mother converted to Christianity at a church in Matsuyama in her adolescence when her family suffered in the postwar poverty-stricken economy. The two young Christians met at a church in Ueno, Tokyo, and married later. Unfortunately, their faith was not transmitted to all their children, and I remain a black sheep although I am approaching *musoji* (sixty years old). Fortunately, however, I seem to have inherited the Protestant work ethic, which significantly influenced my education. After finishing elementary and intermediate education at local public schools, I was able to enter the nation's top-ranking high school and undergraduate and graduate programs at the University of Tsukuba. It was my diligence and industriousness cultivated in the Protestant ethic, I believe, that allowed me to pursue such an educational path; I studied for one year at Georgia State University and five years at Brown University during graduate school. One factor that led to pursuing education in the United States was my vague yet broad interest in American culture that was induced by my parents' Christian faith.

My father, Isamu, is a product of the physical education program instituted by Imperial Japan. Prior to World War II, the national policy was oriented toward cultivating a stronger nation; the assiduous training of his mind and body from early childhood to become a strong soldier also yielded the practical advantage of scoring high on the training school entrance exam. He ran along the Ura-Tone River in Kasukabe and strengthened his body with push-ups and pull-ups. His brawny upper arms and sculpted abdominal muscles seem to have been a source of pride for him for a long time since, and when I took a public bath with him, I too felt proud of the dynamic movement of his body. His position as a salaried worker at a hat manufacturing company, however, did not allow him to take advantage of what I would later understand as the first golden decade of modern sports in Japan—the 1930s. At the time, American sports such as baseball, basketball, and American football had steadily influenced the leisure activities of Japan's elite population, but my father was unable to play most ball sports. As a member of the postwar mass society, he enjoyed watching professional wrestling, boxing, sumo, and baseball.

I seem to have inherited my father's sporting habits. I am not certain of his awareness of his class position, but as a son in a working-class family, I was taught the importance of being healthy and having a strong mind and body. Because my legs were weaker than those of my friends as a child, my father took me mountain climbing and hiking. I was also encouraged to practice karate as a younger teen and join the high school volleyball club as an older teen. Before entering university, I was able to develop a healthy five-foot, ten-inch, 180-pound body. But from college to my forties, I was involved in sports only as a spectator. It was only when I faced the crisis of my fifties that I relearned the importance of playing sports.

As a man born and raised in Japan, I belong to the ethnic majority and the traditionally privileged gender. From the perspective of an American social history researcher, my position could be viewed as one that is mainstream. Looking back on the lives of my parents and my own life through the lens of the discriminator-discriminated dichotomy, I see that some degree of discrimination still exists.

First, my family was subjected to socioeconomic discrimination. My working-class paternal grandfather, by marrying the eldest daughter of a higher-class local industrialist from the Kawashima clan, established what is called a branch family. As a branch family child, my father could not expect great financial assistance for his own higher education, while his cousins in the main family could. He had to abandon his hope to attend the Kasukabe Technological High School. My mother's family lost nearly all their property aside from a backpack with personal possessions for each member during their evacuation from Korea, while my mother's aunt (her mother's elder sister), who was married to a wealthy jeweler, returned to Japan in a chartered ship with almost all their property. My mother's family had to wait until the late fall of 1945 to return to Japan, while her aunt's family was able to return in late August, immediately after Japan's surrender, due to their abundant financial resources. Moreover, growing up as a son of a printing company employee who eventually became the owner of a small printing office, I found myself on a lower rung of the socioeconomic ladder, even when the famed Izanagi economic growth of the 1960s and 1970s led to greater class mobility for many people. During this time, my elder brother often went to elementary school without wearing socks. His concerned homeroom teacher called my mother to school to give her a warning. My friend from a rich neighboring family was able to drive on the Tomei Expressway, completed in 1968, which was a luxury that my family, without the second set of "three sacred treasures"—a car, a color television, and an air conditioner—could never hope for. Listening to my friend joyfully recounting his experience—"We drove on the To-mei!"—I misunderstood "To-Mei" (Tokyo to Nagoya) as *to-mei* (meaning "transparent") and believed that the car would become transparent when speeding up.

Second, the neighborhood in which I grew up was "Kita-ku," or the North Ward. Metropolitan Tokyo, like many other Japanese cities, developed region by region—first the south, then the west, and finally the north—and Kita-ku was in the district that developed last and most slowly. The difference in living conditions among these districts was well known by Tokyo residents. Although I may not have noticed this difference during childhood, a time of immersion in local life, I came to recognize the north's substandard status when I was in high school and interacted with students from all areas of Tokyo.

Third, as a second son, I suffered from the legacy of the prewar primogeniture system in which the eldest was granted respect and privilege. My maternal grandfather, living under this legacy, always called my brother by his first name while he called me "young brother," a practice that could hurt a small boy deeply. Of course, compared with racial discrimination in contemporary American society, my suffering was trivial. Furthermore, in an increasingly democratic and meritocratic postwar Japan, I expected to attain upward social mobility through hard work and academic accomplishments. I could, in college, continue to make up for the handicaps of my family's socioeconomic conditions with the help of an economic equalization agent, such as the Rotary Foundation and the Fulbright Foundation, which funded international exchange programs for young men and women in undergraduate and graduate programs.

As the second son of the craftsman class in Tokyo's north district, I was subject to restrictions by class and locality, but it was not like the estrangement and extreme poverty due to deep-rooted discrimination against the Buraku people, at the bottom of the old feudal caste system, particularly in western Japan. It seems that I uncritically shared the postwar pro-American liberal ideology of my parents, who were satisfied with the increasingly improved material conditions brought by economic growth. I inherited the values of discipline and diligence from my father and the virtues of intellectual curiosity and positive thinking from my mother. While extreme leftists horrified the nation with violence at the University of Tokyo and the Asama Lodge, I lived a relatively secure apolitical life, maintaining faith in the equality of opportunity in which individual effort always mattered, and I always sought the best educational environment I could attain.

The path to elite athleticism was closed to me, a slow runner. I was keenly aware that my choice of sports was limited. I liked both playing and watching sports but intentionally avoided playing major sports, such as baseball and soccer, that relied on athletes' running speed. I preferred to play games that required dexterity and physical strength, such as table tennis, volleyball, and basketball. I even gained popularity among classmates by showcasing my skill in these games. My favorite game was volleyball. Because the Japanese men's and women's national teams won medals consecutively from the Tokyo Olympiad of 1964 through the Montreal games of 1976, I was encouraged to participate in clubs in junior and senior high school, where I served as the attacker and captain during my senior year.

I loved to watch baseball and sumo. These sports accrued many Japanese followers during my childhood, as reflected in the popular saying about the nation's three favorites: "the Yomiuri Giants, Taiho, and *tamagoyaki*," which refers to the greatest professional baseball club; the strongest *yokozuna*, or highest-ranked sumo wrestler; and the favorite egg dish of the time. The Giants won nine consecutive Japan Series titles (1965–73) with team manager Tetsuharu Kawakami, while Taiho recorded forty-five consecutive wins, then the second-longest winning streak in sumo history. I was also a fan of Ikki Kajiwara, who wrote the comic titled *The Star of the Giants*, which described the glory of the Giants with a small but hard-working and relatable fictional pitcher, Hyuma Hoshi, as its protagonist. I also enjoyed the comic titled *The Fanatic Life of One Karate Man*, which was the life story of Masutatsu Oyama, a real, legendary karate master who developed the globally known karate dojo (practice school) Kyokushin-kai. Mostly due to Oyama's influence, I joined Kyokushin-kai and practiced karate for one year (1972–73), striving for a black belt although I obtained only a yellow one. I quit Kyokushin-kai and began playing volleyball in a school club. My dream for the black belt was abandoned early in my karate training, but my experience became the foundation of my long-lived interest in martial arts, which has persisted to the present day.

My school-age sports experience comprised only a marginal proportion of my leisure time, so it was impossible for me to predict my future as a researcher in American sport history.

A collecting mania consumed most of my leisure time. For example, collecting coins was central to my elementary school hobbies. Nonetheless, my collection was just a small-scale one, with inexpensive, old, and valueless national and foreign coins that could be purchased with a boy's small savings from regular allowances, New Year's stipends (*otoshi-dama*), and birthday gifts. It was not intended to satisfy the interest of my aunt, who was my father's younger sister and the most materialistic of my all relatives, always asking, "Does it make money?"

I was deeply interested in collecting Kamen Rider cards. Kamen Rider, meaning "Masked Motorcycle Rider," was the superhero of my childhood who beat monsters dispatched by the evil corps Shocker. A Kamen Rider card came with the purchase of each Kamen Rider snack, produced by the Calbee Company and priced at twenty yen, or about five cents, per package. I made a huge investment in gathering the entirety of the first series, numbers 1–105, while scattering around the neighborhood unopened packages that contained cards already in my possession. In one of the most memorable, soul-trembling moments of my childhood, I finally came across the card that completed the series.

I also began a collection of tickets, pamphlets, and other memorabilia that I received at sea and mountain resorts during school tours and excursions, and family trips and vacations. I preserved them in a neatly arranged order in albums. I also kept a diary every day from third grade to the end of high school. In retrospect, my hobbies were fundamentally those that required the least money but the most patience and commitment, which was a product of my social class handicap in comparison with my wealthier and more hedonistic friends, who enjoyed a life of yachting and boating at resorts such as Enoshima and Shonan. Concurrently, however, the hobbies of my younger years may have prepared me for my future athletic participation in long-distance swimming, marathons, and bicycling, all of which demand steady and consistent effort. Still, in those days, I could not even imagine that my hobbies would influence my future endeavors in sports.

The Present

Though potentially a common phenomenon in industrialized countries, it is particularly common in Japan—a rapidly aging nation—that the word and concept of "aged persons" are considered somewhat obsolete. In my perspective, the body ages and declines but the mind remains the same once one reaches adulthood. There is an old saying that "the mind is young for life"; this is true for many of us. Still, if the definition of "aged persons" stands, one can determine when that stage begins according to two criteria: one is the point at which one can no longer perform their regular job (due to the system of mandatory retirement in the case of Japan), and the other is the point at which health fails. The loss of a regular job leads to the loss of security in economic life, while health failure leads to the loss of physical and mental security. Japan maintains a mandatory retirement age, which was previously 55 years old but has been extended to 60, 65, and beyond. Japan's average healthy life expectancy is approximately ten years shorter than actual life span, thus being in the seventies depending on one's gender, region, and related demographic factors. We find, therefore, that the age at which one is considered an "aged person" is sometime in their seventies when they can no longer perform their regular job, begin to lose their health, and are deprived of functioning as an independent person.

In Japanese society, various services are provided to aged people. Pension systems provide some economic security. Depending on the type of employment, one can be covered by the national pension, corporate pensions, or mutual aid pensions throughout retirement. Unifying different pensions continues to undergo trial and error without any end to the controversy over who pays what amount and who receives aid due to the differences in systems, careers, and fund reserves. For people over 70, local municipalities offer free or low-cost public transportation. Depending on the degree of dementia and disability, the national and local governments also provide medical care, leisure, and amusement services. Moreover, one can participate in radio gymnastic exercises every morning in neighborhood playgrounds, which are organized by local communities and facilitate social and recreational interaction among residents. There are grounds and facilities for gate ball, a Japanese ball game that resembles croquet, which is very popular among aged people. I have personally investigated welfare systems and services in several municipalities such as Tokyo, Fukushima, and Shizuoka in search of the best choices for my parents and relatives. I have observed the level and content of their services, which convinced me that, despite these services' bad reputation as a cause of the nation's debt, tax money has not been wasted.

I first realized that aging had become a personal problem around my fiftieth birthday when, having experienced life as an opportunity for upward mobility, I suddenly recognized a downturn: menopause, or syndromes relating to it. Menopause and related syndromes in Japan are typically considered a women's health issue and thus irrelevant for most men. But menopause is increasingly seen as affecting men, and I was one of them. After entering my fifties, I began to feel as though I was losing concentration and reading comprehension. Writing and understanding foreign languages such as English became painfully fatiguing. I was beginning to be deeply worried about men's menopause and consulted several specialists in urology and psychosomatic medicine, but I could not find a solution. For a scholar, the inability to think and write presented a particularly formidable obstacle. I was then at the peak of my administrative responsibilities, and the stress from that position may have been a factor in my declining health. I sought refuge in drinking and overeating, which led to a weight gain of ten kilograms. In retrospect, I suffered from melancholy, symptoms of which, as I can recall today, included unstable sleep and depression in the early morning.

To address the crisis in my early fifties, I took several initiatives that can be divided into two groups. One is focused on my difficulties with reading and writing in English, and the other involves what I saw as a decline in my general ability and skills for academic activities such as reading, writing, and thinking. I applied different measures to each. For the first group, I found offense, not defense, more effective. Rather than struggling with English, a skill I developed considerably during the nearly half-century since my first year at junior high school, I opened the first pages of textbooks in two new foreign languages, German and French. I had been longing to master these languages, and I expected to find significant room for personal development. I would soon realize that it was an excellent decision. As an introduction,

I established a correspondence program for each language by the Kumon group, one of Japan's major educational corporations, which suited me very well. I won the first prize in the progress rate for both languages after six months of learning. For more than fifty years of my life, I had never won first-place honors; these certificates were a source of unexpected pride. They still occupy a corner of the display shelf at my university office. As acquired skills and knowledge in second languages are fated to wane without regular use, I have not been able to maintain them at a practical level. But these accomplishments in two European languages have become the foundation on which I set clear goals of further learning and traveling in my retirement life.

To address my more general intellectual slump, I found little room to further develop my mind, so I turned to my body, the energy and strength of which I had not cared much to employ since my college days. This change of direction led to my struggle with my weight and rediscovering sport and exercise.

Specifically, I attempted to pursue three courses of action: diet therapy, fun, and sport and exercise. Participating in a tie-up program by phone with a health care and diet expert sponsored by the Promotion and Mutual Aid Corporation for Private Schools of Japan, I was given four assignments, all of which were concerned with order and choice while eating. I was instructed to eat vegetables before any other foods. Second, I was to limit the amount of meat I ate to the size of my palm. Third, I was to eat no more than a small cup of rice. Fourth, I was told to refrain from drinking alcohol at least one day per week. As I learned from subsequent experience, these four assignments comprise basic knowledge in dietary and health care therapy, and they were very effective. By assiduously adhering to the rules of these assignments while simultaneously doing light exercises at the gym, which would later develop into full-scale sport participation, I lost ten kilograms in about two months, which was one-third of my original target of six months. My phone partner congratulated me on my success in a tone of marvel and awe.

My second course of action was what I termed "fun seeking," which functioned as a necessary intermediary between diet therapy and full-scale involvement in sport and exercise. Experience has taught me that human behavior may be roughly classified into two categories: actions resulting from desire and those resulting from principle. Having faced a crisis in my early fifties, I came to identify one of its causes in the way I had lived, which was a principle-based life. I had made many decisions and always acted from what I believed I should do: which university I should enter, which country I should study in, which graduate program I should choose, which job I should take, and so on during my twenties, thirties, and forties. Entering my fifties, I grew exhausted and disgusted with my principle-based life. It is likely that I was at a stage that any principle-based person would, perhaps inevitably, reach at one time or another. Having lost sight of direction in my life during this crisis, I sought a solution in making this new phase of my life not principle-based but desire-based.

How can we identify what we want? I first sought an answer to this question in the Japanese tradition of the "three pleasures of men": drinking, womanizing, and gambling. To what extent, however, was a married man ethically allowed to engage in these behaviors? To answer this question was far beyond the ability of a social historian, but I was able to take advantage of the intellectual training I underwent as a PhD student by engaging in meditative activities that situated myself hypothetically in the practice of the three pleasures. After spending several months in this practice, I reached a conclusion: drinking would destroy health, womanizing would destroy the family, and gambling would destroy the household. After all, I concluded, I should not simply do what I want but do what I should, thus understanding that a principle-based person could never become a desire-based person. A sense of resignation accompanied this conclusion, but it also gave me strength, which compelled me again to take an offensive, not defensive, position and opened my eyes to the importance of adhering to the principle-based life that I had been living nearly all my life.

Thus, I was convinced that I should engage in exercise and play sports. To counter my intellectual slump, I focused on training my body, which had significant need for development due to years of neglect. The question remained—which kind of exercise and which sport? The question was a matter not of what I wanted but of what I should do. Thus, I chose an exercise that even a couch potato could easily begin, which is walking. I contracted with a major entertainment conglomerate that operates a gym in my neighborhood, where I began walking on a treadmill. Soon, however, I was inspired to move a little faster, a little longer, and in a fresher space with cleaner air. My walking shifted from indoor to outdoor, from my neighborhood to beyond it, and from my municipality to outer municipalities. The desire for speed compelled me to shift from walking to fast walking, and then to jogging, which greatly increased the distance I traveled. To accelerate further, I sought machine intervention and invested in a rather expensive road racer, which led to my engagement with the world of cycling. My average speed increased from three to four miles per hour by walking, to six or seven miles per hour by jogging, to twenty to thirty miles per hour by bicycling. My aspiration for speed also made me dream something preposterous, a triathlon, in which I would strive for the joy of transforming myself into a nonhuman species—moving like a fish in water (swimming) and like a bird in the sky (bicycling)—and then returning to human form on land (jogging). My goal, however, would be scaled down from full triathlon to half triathlon, which became a dream itself for a reason I explain below.

Another factor that intensified my enthusiasm for exercise was the prospect of participating in official competitions, including marathon races in Chiba and Toyama, and hill climbs in the Noto Peninsula in Ishikawa, the Nasu Heights in Tochigi, and Tsumagoi Village in Gunma. My race times were less than mediocre, but the camaraderie with other runners and riders consistently facilitated my involvement in the sport craze throughout my early fifties. Yet, despite the great pleasure that these experiences brought me, I began to view my physical activity from a different perspective, which stemmed from a simple question that emerged while I was negotiating with my legs, searing with pain, during a Toyama marathon race: "Am I strengthening or damaging my legs?" When I was convinced that the answer was "damaging," I forced myself to cool down my sporting fever, scale down my dream of triathlon to half triathlon, and impose a limit on my aerobic exercise. Since then, the focus of my exercises has shifted to muscle training.

Around this time, I came to be infatuated with golf as well. It began with joining in a four-month beginner class at the gym to master the basics. This class climaxed with the horrible experience of my debut on the course, but I survived it, though miserably. I went to a driving range whenever I had the time, practicing with all available clubs. Again, though, my overwork backfired. The same question arose: "Are you strengthening or damaging your arms?" A specific cause for restraint, however, arose in this case: a dull pain in my right elbow, which is said to be the area that golf beginners typically injure. I went to an orthopedic surgeon and was eventually forced to cease practicing golf to this day. Thus, I have not achieved my goal of playing golf with my high school friends. Still, golf occupies a secure position as one of my lifelong sports. Along with mastering German and French, it has provided me with a challenge for my future life. Golf is suitable for both socializing and exercise, and there is no doubt that it is suitable for aging players. In that sense, my affair with golf has just begun.

People often ask if there are joys and fears that accompany aging. We generally assume that no joy accompanies aging, which is likely true for many people. On the other hand, aging incites a variety of fears in most people. The loss of health and economic security can be counted as among the worst of them. To improve the well-being of aged people, it is essential to eliminate any likelihood of experiencing these pitfalls. Exercise and moderation in eating are perhaps two of the most effective measures against the former, while saving money and spending thriftily protect against the latter. If we avoid these losses in our late lives, it may be the case that death is no longer something to fear but something to embrace as a liberation from life.

What role have friendship and love played and will continue to play in my life? In one stereotypical view of aging in Japan, a man becomes a wolf while women form flocks. It is likely that aged men often act by themselves, while aged women go out and get together. This contrast holds true not only in Japan but also in many other societies, as it reflects social and cultural gender differences that transcend national boundaries. I am aware that I am solitary more often recently, but I am also well acquainted with the value and role of friendship. I meet regularly to dine and drink with friends, colleagues, and alumni to maintain companionship. Eventually, golf competitions will be added to this list.

What about love? Ideally, it should be the bond that is shared by those in relationships and among family members. It is also desirable that loving relationships exist between generations. But it cannot be denied that love is sometimes abandoned for the sake of happiness. Furthermore, the form of love may differ as one ages. There are testimonies that after one's fifties, the meaning and form of love are transformed in one's sixties and seventies in a way that was not foreseen. I hope that this experience of change based on continuity is common throughout human society.

In Japan, there is a saying that wisdom grows with age. Whether this is true depends on how wisdom is defined. In one way, wisdom does not grow with age, because memory generally declines while knowledge increasingly becomes uncertain and blurry. Assuming that wisdom is based on memory and knowledge, it is in no way strengthened or increased with age. Experience, however, increases with age. As our experiences widen and vary, we acquire the ability to view things from different perspectives, take other persons' points of view, and anticipate and prepare for reactions to an action. It is possible to make a decision that one would otherwise be unable to make with less experience. Therefore, depending on the definition, it can be said that wisdom increases or does not increase with age.

Now that I am approaching an age from which I can look back on my fifties, I can say that I was able to respond relatively well to the late-middle-age crisis. Resorting to dieting, pleasure seeking, exercising, and playing sports, I thought and meditated, reflected and acted, consulted experts, deepened my understanding, and made informed choices and decisions. Physical aging has steadily come upon me, but I have learned to deal with it sufficiently and appropriately. Of all the experiences I have had, rediscovering the value and effectiveness of exercise and sports is the most rewarding. Having been long forgotten from my twenties to forties—when I was at the peak of health and physical strength—exercise and sports now comprise my primary interest and activities. As I realize that there are many people in my generation who have not acknowledged this truth, I feel obliged to share the story of my active life with my contemporaries.

The Future

What will my legacy be? I want to be remembered as a researcher who made an unlikely transition from history—a discipline considered the most bookish in Japan and in which I completed a doctorate program at a U.S. institution—to sport studies, a likely antithesis to history. History is an academic subject that is hard, memory-based, and requiring learning at one's desk, while sport studies is a practical one with soft, action-based, experience-oriented content. Throughout my transition, I reconfirmed the significance of learning the arts of both the pen and the sword, and the positive role and effect of sport on the lives of aged people. In a modest way, I was able to put into practice what I had learned. In doing so, I began to pay attention to the practical utility of sports while maintaining distance from the faster, higher, stronger ideology of modern sports that is generally propagated by the media. I will continue to run, ride my bicycle through the hills, train my muscles, play golf, and encourage my family, friends, community members, and our overall society to exercise and play sports through lectures and seminars, publications, and the media.

I have several concrete goals in the areas of work, health, and leisure. In work, I aim to write a survey book of American sport history, which has not been written in Japanese for several decades, and to teach others about the relativity of modern sport ideology. In health, I plan to continue training my muscles to develop a sculpted abdomen, eating with my own teeth, and walking on my own legs for as long as possible. Finally, in leisure, I hope to visit Germany and France with a fluent working knowledge of their mother tongues. All these count among the top priorities. I hope that after completing all of them, I will be liberated.

12 Going Strong

GARY OSMOND

The category of old hardly does justice to the many ways that the meanings
of the later years resonate with experiences earlier in life.
—Jaber F. Gubrium and James A. Holstein, "Beyond Stereotypes," in *Ways of Aging*

Jaber F. Gubrium and James A. Holstein, introducing their anthology on
aging, argued that the later years of an individual's life "can only be understood in relation to times of life that came before."[1] In this equation, key
contextual factors for interpreting meanings of aging are "historical circumstances, cultural backgrounds, and biographical experiences."[2] My
view on my own aging process can be pictured as a fishing cast net frozen
in midair as it leaves an angler's hands and hovers above the sea, visually
defined by parabolic billows and troughs. High domes dominate the shape,
representing my positive attitude to my aging self. The small, wavy dips
punctuating the contour define those sagging moments that to deny would
be self-deceptive. The source of this outlook is multifaceted and mutable,
a complex combination of cultural and historical background, personal
experience, and personality as predicted by Gubrium and Holstein. As I
think about this combination of factors—itself a net or a network—several
feel salient. I am, among other things, an Australian Canadian, a migrant,
an academic sport historian, a gay man, a midlife convert to exercise, a
social being and friend, and, without doubt, an aging human being. I will
reflect on these various aspects of my identity in this chapter.

I Am an Australian Canadian

I am an Australian Canadian, more accurately an Australian Canadian Newfoundlander. Newfoundland, where I was born in 1962, joined the Canadian confederation in 1949. As a result, I grew up a bona fide Canadian, but I was marked culturally by the fact of my province's history. That background had several manifestations, including dialect, accent, customs, and diet, for example, but it also affected my views on living and aging. Even today Newfoundlanders see themselves as a distinct brand of Canadian, but in the 1960s and 1970s when I was growing up, being Canadian was a secondary identity to my primary national affiliation as a Newfoundlander.

Three of my grandparents, coincidentally all born in 1901, left their small, remote fishing villages and headed to the eastern seaboard of the U.S.A.— the "Boston States"—in the 1920s. Settling in the New York City borough of Brooklyn, they were part of a Newfoundland diaspora in that region: a 1946 clipping from a Brooklyn newspaper makes reference to an estimated seventy-five thousand first- and second-generation Newfoundlanders in the Brooklyn area.[3] Each of my grandparents had returned to their island home by 1930 to establish families, to reconnect with home, and to escape the urban blight of the Great Depression in economically weakened New York City. None were formally educated beyond grade school level, but by dint of hard work, determination, and intelligence established solid, respectable lives, and all encouraged their grandchildren to become educated in ways unavailable to them as young people. One grandmother also encouraged us to "see the world," to experience life to the fullest before "settling down." This advice was anathema to my parents, sensible people who grew up in the postwar industrialized 1950s for whom life's formula was more cookie-cutter routine than was their parents'. I listened to my grandparents and combined study with as much international travel and work as I could.

As I was growing up, my aging grandparents thus had a profound effect on my outlook, and I never saw them as old-fashioned or as old people whose ideas were out of step with modern life. Their experiences at the start of the twentieth century directly influenced and reinforced my life decisions toward the century's end. They also directly influenced my view on aging itself. All were proud, self-sustaining older people who remained living in their own homes until the last possible minute. And those homes, breezy and comfortable in summer on lakes and ocean frontage, were exposed and underheated in winter. I, and my generation, would struggle to live there under those conditions today, but my grandparents were acclimatized. They were physically active, which may have helped. My grandfather Ambrose skated across frozen lakes for exercise, hunting, and fishing, but mostly the elders' exercise was what we would call incidental activity—achieved in the routine duties of growing vegetables, cutting grass with scythes and manually powered mowers, tramping through woods and bogs to pick berries by the gallon load, hunting and fishing, and shoveling snow. As a child I wasn't always attuned to these various activities and their associations with healthy aging—they were just a way of life—but as an adult I have often reflected on this realization and taken great delight in some of the recollections.

One memory stands out. My 93-year-old, independent-living grandmother Gladys insisted on shoveling the snow from the walkway to her front door. The distance wasn't huge—probably eight meters, but the volume of snow that regularly fell made this task a daunting one. For my father, who lived nearby, his mother's snow clearing seemed perilous. His was a practical concern—he was less worried about her exercising per se (he knew her strength and determination—she was "still going strong," as the expression put it) than he was anxious about her slipping on the ice and breaking a hip. Fair enough, but this concern didn't stop Nan. One day, her shovel disappeared from its handy parking spot outside her front door. This problem was bad timing for Nan, as a blizzard was bearing down. She rang my father, explained the situation, and asked him to drive her to Canadian Tire, the big hardware store, so she could buy a replacement. Dad, who probably wished he'd thought of stealing the shovel himself (and possibly did), refused: "You're too old to be shoveling snow. It's high time you stopped. I'll come clear your path." Determined, and knowing her son well enough, she announced that if he wouldn't drive her, she'd walk there herself. "Off you go, then!" said Dad, and triumphantly hung up the phone.

His victory was short-lived. As he sat back down in his chair, he glanced out the window at the swirling snow and blowing trees, and realized that she was likely to be as good as her word. Cursing under his breath, as was his wont, dad drove off to her apartment, which was empty. Rerouting towards Canadian Tire, his car the only one on the blizzard-blurred street, he saw a tiny figure in the distance trudging along the snowed-in sidewalk. Cursing louder now, as he recognized the walker, he pulled up. Nan got her shovel that day and continued to clear her walk for several more years.

I tell this story because it makes me smile at my Nan's resilience and character, and because it's typical of many tales about her that I treasure now that she's gone. But I also relate it because of what it says about her own view on aging and how it influenced my own perspective as I creep up there in age myself. There were many older people in my life growing up who saw aging not as something defeatist, or something to be defeated, but as one more thing to take in stride as they carried on with living. There's nothing unique about Newfoundlanders, of course. Age is valued and respected in many societies worldwide, and in Newfoundland the attitudes of aging people themselves, and to processes of aging, were as much practically based as they were philosophical. And not everybody I knew or know there matched Nan's gumption and robust health. Nonetheless, there is something special in my memories about my exposure to unconventional aging that I can attribute to my Newfoundland childhood.

I Am a Migrant

I introduced myself as an Australian Canadian Newfoundlander because my national identity is plural. I am also a migrant. At 24 years of age I moved to Australia, where I have remained for over thirty years. I had lived in Canada proper—what we Newfoundlanders call "the mainland"—for only seven years. I was a student during that time, and not particularly attuned to aging except as it applied to my own development from teenager to adult, so being Canadian (as opposed to the specific identity of being a Newfoundlander) didn't have any discernible influence on my sense of age and aging. Becoming an Australian has had greater bearing.

I came to Australia on what was called a working-holiday visa, a short-term migration category to facilitate holiday visits of up to one year that permitted young visa holders to work. I arrived knowing very little about Australia or its history and culture. In my decades of living here, I have grown and learned as well as simply aged. I began my full-time working life in Australia, did doctoral study, changed careers, built new relationships and friendships, and consolidated my identities. As an immigrant, I have also been able to draw comparisons between my adopted country, my country of birth, and other countries and pass judgment on Australia as a place in which to age.

My judgment is kind. Australians in the main, or at least in my experience, embrace age and do not let advancing years pin them down. The climate, while mostly hot, can be oppressive, but locals have adapted to it. The standard of living is high, food is plentiful and affordable, and health care is largely free. In Australia, the average life expectancy has grown dramatically since the Australian colonies federated as a country in 1901: a girl born in 2014–16 can expect to live to the age of 84.6 years, and a boy would be expected to live to 80.4 years, compared with 50.8 and 47.2 years, respectively, in 1881–90. Comparatively, this places Australia fifth, behind Iceland, Japan, Switzerland, and Norway, in life expectancy among member countries of the Organisation for Economic Co-operation and Development.[4]

I do not want to paint too rosy a picture. While Australia can be a place for the healthy aged and aging to thrive, the same is not always true for those who are ailing or incapacitated in their old age. As I write this in 2019, a national Royal Commission into Aged Care Quality and Safety is about to commence.[5] This enquiry, initiated by Federal Parliament, was prompted by reports of widespread abuse and neglect in nursing homes and aged-care homes.

I acknowledge that my perspective on healthy aging and how Australians age healthily is influenced by my own personal experience. For one, I work in a university department of human movement studies, perhaps better known internationally as kinesiology or human kinetics. My colleagues aim to keep fit. I see vibrant older clients milling about the hallways as they come and go from experimental exercise classes. Many of these are aimed at cancer survivors, often older people with an uncanny and likely atypical zest for life. I realize that this environment colors my view. So too does my own pattern of physical activity. I swim regularly in an outdoor pool that is open year-round, starting early to beat the damaging sun. Both the fifty- and twenty-five-meter pools are full at 6 a.m., many lanes with leather-skinned men and women in their seventies and older. This is typical of Australian pools, especially at an hour when teenagers are still typically abed. At my gym, I am the second-youngest by far in my twice-weekly training group. Any preconceptions that I might have had about the stamina, strength, and endurance of aging people went out the window long ago.

What I witness in the pool and in the gym is not typical, I know. Largely, Australians are not sufficiently physically active. Between 60 and 70 percent of the Australian population was sedentary, or had low levels of physical activity, in 2011.[6] While my perspective may be biased, however, it serves me because the older people whom I observe living active, healthy lives act as inspirations to me. There is a direct link between them and my own physical fitness levels, and my motivation to continue exercising.

Australian government policies heavily influence national attitudes towards aging and life choices for the aging. One area that interests me in particular because of my age and career stage is retirement. It is rare for people here to work beyond 65, and many people retire in their fifties. In many areas, retirement is compulsory at particular ages. Judges, for example, must retire at 70: the specter of the elderly justices such as those on the Supreme Court of the United States is unknown here. For decades, Australia has had a national system of retirement funding, what we call superannuation. Employers must contribute a percentage of an employee's annual salary or wages, and employees must make mandatory contributions themselves. This system is imperfect—generous superannuation schemes of the past have tightened. Men were privileged over women. In the growing gig economy where people work casually and often irregularly, retirement savings often fail to stack up sufficiently. But this system does allow working people to end their careers at an earlier age than in some other countries.

One impact of this system is that many people can retire relatively young, or at least can afford to do so from a financial perspective. Most leap at this opportunity, but not everybody does. I know several people who, having retired either because it made no sense financially to continue working or because the thought appealed to them, later struggled to adapt to postwork life. This might be considered a first-world problem, but it has caused genuine anguish for some of my friends and colleagues. The lesson offered is universal—have a retirement plan up your sleeve—but the uniqueness of Australia in terms of trends to early retirement make this an aspect of aging that cannot be overlooked.

The optimistic scenarios of aging that I may have conjured do not apply to everybody. One of the biggest gaps in terms of aging exist between white and Black—between non-Indigenous Australians and Aboriginal and Torres Strait Islander people. This historic and cultural problem is linked directly to government policies and has drastic real-life consequences, to which I will return below.

I Am a Sport Historian

My own sense of aging is partly informed by these racial realities because I am a sport historian whose current research focus is Indigenous Australian sport histories. For several years, my research colleague, Murray Phillips, and I have had the privilege of working with the Aboriginal community of Cherbourg in our home state of Queensland, funded initially by the Australian Institute of Aboriginal and Torres Strait Islander Studies and propelled since by tremendous enthusiasm within that community for exploring and documenting their own sport history. This collaboration has led to several research outputs, strong bonds, and deeper insight on my part into Aboriginal communities. Currently, I am in the fortunate position of holding a four-year Future Fellowship research grant (2017–21) from the Australian Research Council to co-narrate community sport histories with four other Aboriginal and Torres Strait Islander communities in Queensland. This ongoing project is deepening my knowledge and insight. Since starting it, I have also become a member of a second research team that is working with Aboriginal communities in other states of Australia to document, analyze, and digitize their sport histories.

These research opportunities have granted me unique insight into the past—close-up exposure through intimate contact with community members and special access to archival records normally under public embargo. The past, or at least the colonial past, has been a grim experience for many Indigenous Australians, whose traditional cultures were destroyed, populations decimated, languages lost, and lives controlled. Most Australian states legislated so-called protection acts in the late nineteenth and early twentieth centuries following crimes, massacres, economic and sexual exploitation, and other depredations committed against Indigenous people by settler-colonial populations. Queensland, the focus of most of my research to date, had the worst of these acts, which were far more restrictive than legislation in other states. The Indigenous population of this state was subject to draconian legislation, first enacted in 1897 and continuing in various names and acts until the 1980s, that controlled most aspects of people's lives. A large proportion—over 40 percent—of Aboriginal people were forcibly removed from traditional lands, communities, and often families into government-run settlements and religious-administered missions; the remainder of the population, even if legally exempt from the legislative frameworks of control, were subject to removal to these reserves at any time.

The "inmates" of settlements and missions, as they were called in official parlance, had little control of any aspect of their lives. Permission, which was required to travel off the reserves temporarily or to receive visitors, was frequently denied at the whim of superintendents. Food was rationed. Punishments were meted out for any transgression, real or perceived. Families were separated, both between the reserves and within them, where many children were taken from their parents and sequestered in dormitories. Inmates were not free to marry without permission. Traditional languages and many other such practices were forbidden.

Western sport was permitted, and often encouraged, within the reserves, and was Janus-faced. While sport was sometimes wielded as a tool of oppression, with opportunities for advancement curtailed, for example, it also offered Indigenous people rare opportunities for limited autonomy and freedom, for identity building at individual and community levels and occasionally for resistance. Indigenous Australia, including the Queensland

Aboriginal settlements and reserves, produced a significant number of notable athletes across many sports, and sport is a treasured legacy of the past in these communities today.

In discussing this legacy, I have gained new insight into aging among this often overlooked Australian demographic group. The traditional authority of elders was usurped by the state, yet within Aboriginal culture, elders remain greatly respected, as are their achievements. I have frequently been surprised at the depth of knowledge and respect for elders in conversing with members of Queensland Indigenous communities. Sporting memories run deep. When I visit the former reserves, I expect recollections of well-known athletes from the past—and there were many—but I am regularly amazed at reminiscences of sportswomen and -men whose names rarely or never made it into the newspapers but whose memories as elders are cherished within the communities today. These include supporters like chaperones and women who sewed and laundered uniforms, people whose roles in broader sport history are rarely celebrated. Recently in Woorabinda, a former Aboriginal reserve in the central highlands of the state, I was regaled with stories about Auntie Alice Barnes, an elder in the community parlance and "an old stager" in officialese, who won a draft horse derby at a rodeo held on New Year's Day in 1951. I was able to confirm this story, which had otherwise not been reported widely, and was able to share specific details with the community in a gesture of reciprocity that underlines the intentions of my research project.

Today's elders are also greatly respected within the community, and a gesture of respect that is mandated within and expected from outside these communities is to call an older man or woman "Uncle" or "Auntie," respectively. For outsiders, like me, these terms are difficult to grasp fully and even to use. They have a folksy quality, these monikers, but they are less terms of endearment than they are titles of authority and respect. When I began visiting these communities, I felt awkward using them, maybe because in white cultures they are familial terms. I wasn't always sure when to use them—many people whom I met appeared to be my age or not much older—and I feared insulting them by using the titles inappropriately. Nobody challenged me when I used the honorific titles, and if anyone thought the less of me or doubted my sincerity, they did not openly reveal it. Over time, I learned to appreciate these titles, and now use them as a rule rather than as an exception. This valorization of age has eased my entry into communities and helped reinforce my slowly building relationships and bonds as a white outsider.

These research opportunities have also granted me insight into present realities. The oppressive state apparatus has, over several generations, damaged self-esteem for many Indigenous people and their communities, enhancing the significance of respect bestowed on age and elders. Health and life expectancy have also suffered: the life expectancy for Aboriginal and Torres Strait Islander people is roughly ten years lower than the national average.[7] The irony of this inequity is that in many such communities, I would be an elder. I am the same age as many of the people that I interview. In this context, then, I am not a person who is aging but a person who has aged. This is perhaps less ironic than tragic, but it does focus my mind on aging as a relative process. While I do meet septuagenarians and octogenarians, their ranks are few and certainly smaller than in the general population. Many people my age suffer prematurely from significant health problems. Just as arresting, our lives have paralleled chronologically but not in experience; as late as the early 1980s, when I was studying at a Canadian university and traveling the world unfettered as a young white man, my Queensland Aboriginal contemporaries on the settlements were still subject to legislative limits on their ability to roam and to thrive.

These specific experiences as a sport historian clearly have shaped my perspective on aging, but there are others not related to reflecting on my Indigenous fellow Australians. I was a latecomer to academia, having worked as a schoolteacher and then as a university administrator before returning to doctoral study in my forties. I was 44 when I completed my PhD in sport history and commenced my university career as a full-time lecturer and researcher. The pathway to that degree was challenging in terms of my age, not because I struggled with stamina or in any direct way as an older student but because I was the eldest by far of my school's doctoral cohort. I am not sure precisely why this was challenging, but it reminded me of my age and of the risk I was taking in forgoing paid employment to study with no clear career pathway in sight.

At the same time, those challenges were liberating. I had taken an opportunity to do something new, a kick in the face to naysayers, an affirmation of my belief in the power of lifelong learning and a chance for career rebirth. It was enjoyable, but it was also a reminder of the kernel of truth in the chestnut that age is a state of mind and not a limitation. Throughout my early years as a doctoral student and newly employed lecturer, I was buoyed by the regular presence in the school of a nonagenarian colleague, a man who joined the faculty after his retirement as a scientist to advise graduate students on computer programing. Dr. Alf Howard, born in 1906, was a figure from the fabled Age of Discovery.[8] As a young graduate student in chemistry in the late 1920s, he had joined the joint British Australian and New Zealand Antarctic Research Expedition in 1929–31, organized and led by Sir Douglas Mawson, as a water scientist. In his late nineties, he remained intellectually, physically, socially, and culturally engaged, and was an inspiration to many graduate students. Alf (as he liked to be called, without formal titles) was an inspiration to me as a "mature-age student," as we like to say in Australia, undertaking doctoral studies. I was conscious of being older by two decades than most of my fellow students, and Alf reminded me that age really can be a state of mind.

I Am a Gay Man

The Irish novelist, essayist, and academic Colm Tóibín, writing in his forties of his own homosexuality, reflected that a part of him "remained uneasy, timid, and melancholy" as a result.[9] I relate to this—skeins of unease, timidity, and melancholy accompanied me for several decades like invisible companions. Although I came out to my family, friends, and colleagues in my early twenties, and moved to Melbourne at 24 to be with my Australian partner, the constant and wearying process of coming out in each new social encounter was destabilizing. This is an experience that is shared by many LGBT people, and it constituted a dis-ease for me. Sometimes I chose not to out myself, or at least not immediately, which reinforced my natural timidity. I was never miserable, and certainly not depressed by this situation, but Tóibín's mention of melancholy has made me realize that for many years I have been wistful about the decade of adolescence and young adulthood during which I was closeted and about how that experience shaped my life.

As I age, however, this regretful mist has lifted and my unease and diffidence are sloughing off (I am writing this, for example). Some people speak of a freedom that comes with aging, but I think they often mean the attainment of a stronger sense of not caring or of not worrying what others think and the concomitant liberty to be themselves. There may be a healthy spoonful of defiance in that attitude. My experience is different in the sense that I do not feel particularly defiant, and do still care what people think, but aging is giving me a greater self-awareness and, more important, a self-acceptance that previously felt stifled or capped.

This self-acceptance may be a common experience of aging, but in my case it is linked directly to my sexuality. One great gift—and there were many negatives—of being a young, out gay person in the 1980s was that it freed me from the often restricting confines of social expectation. There were no role models, and no set way to be. I was able to pursue a life that wasn't altogether conventional, and it gave me the confidence to continue to choose paths less traveled as I aged.

Sport was one of those pathways. As a school pupil, acutely aware that I did not fit into standard or valorized masculine roles, I was shy of competitive sport. Team sports were the only options in my school and town—ice hockey, basketball, baseball—and I didn't play any of them. I did enjoy running events at the annual school sports days, I loved cross-country skiing, swimming, skating, cycling, and being physically active in general, but these came with no social capital and counted for little communally. Nobody told me the physical, emotional, or psychological value of these activities, but I knew instinctively and experientially that I enjoyed them. Had anybody told the 17-year-old me that the 57-year-old-me (itself an unimaginable idea to my teenage self) that I would be physically active as I aged, I would simply have shrugged. No surprise there. But if that clairvoyant adviser had told me that I would be an academic sport historian, I would have dismissed them as a crank. For the emerging unsporty gay me, such a career would have been inconceivable—homosexuality and sport were, in my mind as in the minds of some people still, mutually exclusive.

My decision to pursue a doctorate in sport history, and my subsequent academic career, were possible only because being gay had liberated me from that blinkered mindset. There was, for me, a pleasing irony to that study and work choice; for others, such as my nongay colleagues, it seemed less incongruous, which has shown me that my thinking remained a little rigid. As I age and move towards eventual retirement, my career and sexual identity coalesce nicely in my academic setting of sport history research and teaching. In particular, I find sport history an ideal setting in which to reflect on and critique hypermasculinity, homophobia, and gender stereotyping—some of the very factors that prevented me from being able to appreciate competitive sport as a physical activity when I was young.

Age and experience have also given me an appreciation of the cultural and political times and settings in which I have lived as a gay man. I have been a beneficiary of liberal social attitudes and progressive government policies, bolstered by stable economies, that have helped me live a fulfilling life and to be able to live openly as gay. This was not the case in either Canada or Australia when I was a child or teenager, nor was it the case in much of the world, and it remains a fact that in most other countries, my temporal twin would not have the options that I have had. Homosexuality was illegal in seventy-two countries and punishable by death in eight in 2017, and civil rights do not extend to the range of spheres that they do where I live.[10] In 1987 I was able to migrate to Australia owing to my same-sex relationship with an Australian citizen: this right was not one that Canada afforded at the time and I think very few countries then recognized same-sex couples in migration matters. While Australia did not allow formal same-sex marriage until 2018, this step was largely symbolic, as the country had long before legally recognized same-sex relationships in most other spheres, including inheritance, property, and taxation, along with immigration. I have watched these changes unfold, have played a small activist role where I felt I could, and recognize that my choices in life have been eased by these larger contextual factors.

Changing times and cultures have helped me as a gay man in one other fundamental way. I have become a biological father, a donor dad, to two children, with whom I have a strong, loving relationship. They live elsewhere in Australia, and while I see them regularly, I have no parental role in raising them beyond simply "being there" and providing loving support. Fatherhood via sperm donation is not an uncommon experience for gay men in many western countries but it was very rare when I was younger. I think I knew of one lesbian couple in the early 1980s who had a child, but I do not know if that child had any knowledge of, or relationship with, a father or donor. As a result, contributing to the making of a rainbow family was not in my imagination as a younger person. The likely absence of fatherhood was not a negative influence on me, but the opportunity to become a donor dad, once it arose, was a profoundly positive gift. Coming as it did since my midforties undoubtedly helped me maintain a more youthful identity, rather than an aging one, although the lived experience of *romping around* with children temporarily does remind me that I am aging. It links to my identity as an aging man in other ways too—as a reminder that having no set pathway as a teenager starting out in life was ultimately a great advantage, and as a prompt to reflect on the social, cultural, and legal changes from which I have benefited.

I Am a Midlife Convert to Regular Exercise

Working in a school of human movement studies and with sport and exercise as a common, daily professional backdrop, I have moved beyond simply appreciating physical activity to understanding its benefits at both population and individual levels. As I entered my workplace this morning, I noticed a poster aiming to recruit participants aged 50–65 for a study on exercise and cognitive ability, just one of many studies on physical activity and its benefits undertaken in this and similar research institutions. I need little convincing of this co-relationship, based on my observations of colleagues and on my own participation in sustained, regular exercise over the last decade or so.

In a school that is focused on physical activity, sport, and health, it is not surprising that most people are active. Several of my colleagues and students have been or are athletes at elite, international, or national levels, and many more participate in sport or regular physical activity at community and club levels. There is a passion for sport, and a critical approach to its interplay with culture and society. There is an even greater respect and appreciation for physical activity and its benefits, and an active engagement in improving knowledge of the dynamics and limits of exercise. For an exercise neophyte like me, this is an ideal environment because it not only encourages physical activity but also fosters understanding.

That understanding also extends to nutrition, which along with exercise and health is part of my school's area of responsibility. I mentioned diet above as a cultural byproduct of being a Newfoundlander. While the diet of my childhood encouraged plenty of fresh berries and fish, it also pushed sugar. Newfoundland was not unique in its sugar consumption, but in a sweet Olympics I have no doubt that it would have punched well outside its weight. I reduced my sugar consumption long ago but remain vigilant not only because of its long-term associated risks but also because I can feel that it does me almost immediate harm after the initial buzz of pleasure. Alcohol is similar. I didn't discover it until I was virtually middle-aged, and love a drink now, but I am a careful drinker. As with exercise, I sense instinctually and feel corporeally the benefits of a healthy, balanced diet and suffer the negatives of excessive sugar and alcohol; working in my school reinforces my own lived dietary experience.

I came to this school nearly two decades ago as a graduate student who felt like a rank outsider in terms of my participation and knowledge of sport. I was not physically inactive by any stretch—as I noted above, I cycled, swam, skied, and walked recreationally from an early age and had developed an intuitive appreciation of the benefits of such activities. But as I also noted, these nonsporting pursuits had little social capital, and I entered my graduate program in sport history acutely aware that in social terms, at least, sport appeared to trump exercise. I no longer hold that view, in part because of my immersion in a school that values all physical activity but also because aging has given me a new perspective. This perspective is informed by my observations of the damage that sport has wrought to the physical bodies of many athletes, is shaped by my developing knowledge of the benefits of sustained regular exercise of all sorts, and is confirmed by my own experiences with physical activity in a noncompetitive context, in particular swimming and gyms.

As a child in chilly Newfoundland summers, I took swimming classes offered by the Red Cross at our town's outdoor pool. Swimming was serious business. Many elderly Newfoundlanders feared the water, which had claimed the lives of thousands of fishermen, skaters, boaters, and bathers over the centuries. My father grew up right on the lakeshore, and my mother a stone's throw from the sea; neither swam. My grandfather Ambrose had watched his own father drown when he fell through thin ice just before the First World War, and my mother's cousin had drowned one sunny summer's day while playing with friends in shallow water. Cold waters deterred others. Modernity came to my town in the form of a swimming pool when I was a child, and my father resolved to take swimming lessons not only to conquer his own aquatic ineptitude and anxieties but also to serve as an example for his children. We duly took lessons, and I learned to swim. This gift, along with a bicycle when I turned five and my precious toboggan, were among the most important things given to me by my parents because they instilled in me a love of exercise.

In Australia I discovered a whole new swimming culture, and taking the lead from my work colleagues at the time, I taught myself to swim laps, building up endurance and learning breathing and stroke technique. Later, I was in a relationship with a former elite swimmer, who encouraged me to swim. This engagement with exercise and love of water, introduced when I was young and fostered for nearly thirty years in Australia, has been life changing in a literal sense. First, my love of swimming led me directly to my PhD studies and a dissertation on the contributions of Pacific island swimmers to Australian aquatic sporting cultures. Second, my experiences as a casual lap swimmer at my local pool have changed as I have aged. When I was younger, swimming was about cooling down, having fun, and burning off excess energy. As I have aged, these benefits continue, but I now appreciate how swimming up and down lanes also stretches out my tired limbs, calms my overcrowded mind, and gives me energy and strength. This has led me to better appreciate exercise and encourages me to try other activities.

As a sport historian I know that gym cultures are as old as the hills. Eric Chaline's 2015 book *The Temple of Perfection: A History of the Gym* (London: Reaktion Books, 2015) offers a global overview of the institution and its associated cultures. I am also aware of the loose transformative phases in western culture over time, from the masculinist bodybuilding cultures associated with individuals like Eugene Sandow and Charles Atlas to the Weider empire that began in the middle of the twentieth century. A more recent phase is the "globalisation of gym culture," which is distinguished by the "development of more diverse training techniques, multidimensional fitness gyms, less gendered and more individualized spaces, and the increasing appearance of fitness professionals, such as licensed and fully-trained personal trainers and group fitness instructors."[11] I have vague memories of the mid-twentieth-century Weider-era cultures, which were peripheral to my direct experience but of which I caught occasional glimpses. For a young gay man who was secure in his essential masculinity, those spaces of grunt, sweat, and testosterone held little attraction.

My aging has corresponded with the globalization of gym culture, which I first watched with mild distaste and then increasing academic and, later, personal interest. Gay culture was an early convert, and I observed the growing and now virtually mandatory obsession in my community. For several years I admired how gay men in the Marais district of Paris held out, maintaining a lean and unmuscular look while the rest of the western world seemed preoccupied with getting ripped. That resistance has now changed. I see several of my younger male colleagues and students obsess with gym workouts and am aware of the growth in male body dysphoria. This was a culture that worried me. I did experiment with gyms, but my early forays were not adequately supervised and led quickly to injuries.

Aging has changed that. Swimming had exposed for me the benefits of regular exercise, but my joints were stiffening and I was aware of my growing physical inflexibility. The direct catalyst was a stretch class offered by a small, local gym studio, and the quick remedy offered by simple exercises. My partner was a regular gym goer, and I decided to give it another shot. Eight years later, I too am a regular, rising at 4:30 a.m. two days a week to work out with three others under the supervision of our vigilant and supportive trainer. The benefits have been enormous—in terms of fitness, flexibility, and strength, of course, but also in terms of overall energy, health, and mental resilience. What I had not considered beforehand was the social benefit. Skipping a session for no valid reason is a no go, largely because I know that three other people will be waiting in a dark parking lot counting on the full-group esprit de corps to sustain them like it boosts me. The experience has also influenced my attitudes to aging and activity: one of my gym buddies is in his midseventies and, largely as a result of his fitness accumulated over decades, recently astonished his medical team by the speed of his recovery from major surgery. Another is similarly much fitter and healthier than most women her age. I am not naïve about this—another older but fit member of our gym is suffering from advanced cancer that no amount of exercise would have prevented—but I am encouraged by these friends as physically active role models. I have also been influenced by them as friends and see the social spin-offs as vitally important in my life.

I Am a Social Being

Working in a school of human movement studies has reminded me of, and educated me in, the importance of exercise, physical activity, and diet to health and well-being. What is not stressed is the role of social connection in healthy aging, which appears to be a factor in the global phenomenon of "blue zones," geographic concentrations of people who lead healthier and longer lives than average and boast higher concentrations of centenarians than elsewhere. Recently I have noticed a number of media stories on the links between social engagement and healthy aging, and cite Julianne Holt-Lunstad, a professor of psychology and neuroscience at Brigham Young University: "We now have substantial evidence that social connection has a protective effect on health and longevity and, conversely, that lacking connection is linked to risk."[12]

I am convinced of this value at a population level, and on reflection on my family know how social activity aided some relatives. My irrepressible grandmother (she of the snow shovel incident above) was, I'm certain, my healthiest and happiest relative, and lived well until her hundredth year. She cultivated a broad social circle. When she was widowed, she moved from her village into my larger hometown. My father, her son, installed her in her new apartment and worried about her all that first night. Early the next morning he went to check on her, but she didn't answer the door or phone. She wasn't there—she was next door, where she'd gone the evening before to introduce herself to the young neighbors and spent the entire night playing cards with them. I realize now that many of my favorite family stories revolve around aging and what to me, growing up, seemed like amazing feats for older people. As I age, I see these stories less as astounding exceptions and more as examples of personal agency, a determination to live life as full as possible and not to be limited by external notions of what older people should or should not be doing. These people inspire me nonetheless.

I am aware of the limits to the wonders of social connectedness at an individual level. My own father, like his mother, thrived on social contact and was a much-loved neighbor, friend, and work colleague to hundreds of people. He was also physically active and healthy all his life, but he died young nonetheless after a short and shocking battle with cancer. Social connectedness, I am reminded, is only one of several factors contributing to health and longevity.

I am a social person too, but also love isolation and quiet. On the Myers-Briggs personality indicator scale, once in vogue in workplaces, I repeatedly fence-sat between extroversion and introversion. I believe in balance, and know how and when social contact helps me. As I age, I seek out social contact, not cynically as an insurance policy for good health but because it's a good thing for me—and only at times when and if it's a good thing.

As a migrant, I have lost touch with many old friends from Canada, and I have moved several times within Australia over three decades and left friends behind each time. Social media, cheap travel, and improved communication help at one level, but they are no substitute for regular face-to-face connections. As a migrant, then, I am especially aware of the importance of cultivating friendships and not taking them for granted, but this goal isn't always an easy thing. Even at home, professional demands and personal commitments (like early-morning gym sessions) limit my spare time available for social gatherings and connecting with friends. Of course, my workplace is a social environment, and it is one of the things that I value about work. My pleasure in the gym, too, as I have described above, is anchored as much in the friendships it has cultivated as in the physical activity and challenge.

I Am Aging

As we know, the body is "central to aging experiences" and in most cases, an individual's fifties is "a decade of aging reminders."[13] As Anne E. Barrett and Clayton Gumber have shown through their research, older identities are partially predicated on the experience of regular physical problems or the required consumption of reparative or preventive medicines.[14] Borrowing from S. R. Sherman's notion of the "retrospective self," they posit that "frequent aging body experiences may generate older identities through their provision of frequent comparisons with the 'retrospective body.'"[15]

I am certainly aware that I am aging, but I am unsure how much that is connected to bodily reminders. There are physical signs of aging that would be futile to ignore completely, but so far at least these have been minor. Yes, my "retrospective body," the younger me, was more supple, less creased and, well, *younger*, but in many ways I am more bodily grounded and in better shape now through my participation in physical activity and greater attention to my physical well-being generally than when I was younger. Physical change can happen in two ways: suddenly, through accident, trauma, or disease, or incrementally. I have been fortunate to have had experienced only incremental change, which like the metaphorical frog being slowly boiled, I hardly notice.

The reminders of aging for me come from elsewhere. My partner has retired, several of my close friends have done the same, and I have started to imagine, if not actively plan, my own retirement from work. Working with young students shreds most of my illusions of lingering youth. Iconic sporting events or figures of what seem to me recent vintage are outside their realm of experience. The Sydney Olympic Games in 2000, for example, and Australian runner Cathy Freeman are historic signposts rather than personal memories. Teaching these students, however, doesn't make me feel old, as such, but keeps me young by requiring that I remain vigilant to events, people, and topics that are on their radar rather than just in my own memory banks. For me, as an historian teaching students who wish to better understand the past, this dynamic is a healthy one; for a person who is aging, interacting with young people provides a connection with current events that I might otherwise struggle to maintain.

I recently read an interview with an author who described his age as being "between 55 and death." The remark made me laugh with its in-your-face attitude and confrontation of reality. Of course, everybody who is alive is literally somewhere between their age and death, but when the comment comes from somebody in their sixth decade or beyond, it is more than a statement of fact. I assume the speaker wasn't depressed by his own observation, as some people might be. For me, the quote sizzled with vibrancy. It provided a reminder to reflect on my own six decades of lived experience rather than dwell on what might lie ahead. The process of reflection on the historical, cultural, and biographical circumstances of my life to date, as sketched out here in this essay, has offered me a key to better understand my own aging process, experiences, and attitudes.

NOTES

1. Jaber F. Gubrium and James A. Holstein, "Beyond Stereotypes," in *Ways of Aging*, ed. Jaber F. Gubrium and James A. Holstein (Oxford: Blackwell, 2003), 8.
2. Gubrium and Holstein, "Beyond Stereotypes," 7.
3. For an excellent fictional account of this history, see Trudy J. Morgan-Cole, *By the Rivers of Brooklyn* (St. John's NL: Breakwater Books, 2009). For a broader scholarly study of this diaspora, see Jennifer Bowering Delisle, *The Newfoundland Diaspora: Mapping the Literature of Out-Migration* (Waterloo ON: Wilfrid Laurier University Press, 2013).
4. Government of Australia, Australian Institute of Health and Welfare, "Deaths in Australia," July 18, 2018, https://www.aihw.gov.au/reports/life-expectancy -death/deaths-in-australia/contents/life-expectancy.
5. Government of Australia, Royal Commission into Aged Care Quality and Safety, *Final Report: Care, Dignity, and Respect*, accessed January 19, 2019, https:// agedcare.royalcommission.gov.au/Pages/default.aspx.
6. Australian Medical Association, "Physical Activity—2014," June 18, 2014, https:// www.ama.com.au/position-statement/physical-activity-2014#Anchor%2010.

7. Government of Australia, Australian Institute of Health and Welfare, "Deaths in Australia," July 18, 2018, https://www.aihw.gov.au/reports/life-expectancy -death/deaths-in-australia/contents/life-expectancy.

8. Helen Wolff, "Alfred (Alf) Howard [1906–2010]," CSIROpedia, February 12, 2020, https://csiropedia.csiro.au/alfred-howard/.

9. Colm Tóibín, *Love in a Dark Time: Gay Lives from Wilde to Almodóvar* (2001; rpt., London: Picador, 2010), 2.

10. Pamela Duncan, "Gay Relationships Are Still Criminalised in 72 Countries, Report Finds," *Guardian*, July 27, 2017, https://www.theguardian.com/world /2017/jul/27/gay-relationships-still-criminalised-countries-report.

11. Jesper Andreasson and Thomas Johansson, "Globalised Fitness: The Franchising of a Physical Movement, Fitness Professionalism, and Gender," *Leisure/Loisir* 42, no. 3 (2018), 303.

12. Julianne Holt-Lunstad, "Why Social Relationships Are Important for Physical Health: A Systems Approach to Understanding and Modifying Risk and Protection," *Annual Review of Psychology* 69, no. 1 (2018), 452, https://www.annualreviews .org/doi/full/10.1146/annurev-psych-122216-011902.

13. Anne E. Barrett and Clayton Gumber, "Feeling Old, Body and Soul: The Effect of Aging Body Reminders on Age Identity," *Journals of Gerontology: Social Sciences* 20, no. 20 (2018), 1.

14. Barrett and Gumber, "Feeling Old, Body and Soul," 1.

15. Barrett and Gumber, "Feeling Old, Body and Soul," 4.

13 On a Meaningful Life with Sport as a Permanent Companion

ELSE TRANGBÆK

"The desire to give, the ability to do!"

Those were the words on a large stone standing outside my gymnastics clubhouse that I saw as a child on my way to training. They are words that have had much meaning for me over many years.

Danish author and philosopher Morten Albæk says that to feel the sense is "the sum of the life you have lived, the life you are in right now, and the life you are looking towards, in accordance with what is right for you."[1] For me, the various phases of my life challenged and added meaning in different ways, and when I think back, I've often thought of the words on the stone in front of my clubhouse.

But let me tell you a little about my home country. Denmark is a kingdom with a population of about 5.8 million. The signing of the Danish Constitution in 1849 initiated a more representative governance, in which parts of the population had the right to vote. In 1901 a parliamentary system was established, and in 1915 women's right to vote was recognized. In 1973 Denmark became a member of the European Community. In 2013 and 2016 Denmark was recognized as "the world's happiest country," but in 2018 it was only the third-happiest, after Finland and Norway. Every year, the United Nations delivers a report, called "World Happiness," which ranks 156 countries on, among other things, life expectancy, prosperity, the degree of corruption, and general confidence in government agencies and institutions. Denmark, like other Scandinavian countries, has a welfare model, which ensures universal care for citizens and is predominantly financed by the tax system. Thus, for example, education, medical care, and hospital visits are free for everyone. In addition, Denmark has a labor market, or flexicurity, model that combines flexibility for employers with several types of security rights for employees. Overall, it is a society characterized by great security, with limited inequality between rich and poor but a relatively high tax burden.

I was born on February 7, 1946, and that year not only had the largest birth cohort in Denmark but also was the first to follow the five-year-long occupation by German troops during World War II. A youth commission established at that time presented the obstacles that would be encountered by children born in the aftermath of the war. "There are probably no conditions of life or social area where the baby boomers will not meet any particular difficulties. They are too many, and the possibilities [are too] few. They have to live in congestion and increased competition."[2] The commission's fear was that the entry of a multitude of baby boomers into the job market would greatly increase the unemployment rate. Special subsidy schemes were created, and a set of initiatives employed, to counter the dire predictions.

During the first years after the war, Danish society transitioned from an agricultural country to an industrial society, which meant considerable social and economic changes, especially for women. While the economic crisis of the 1930s prevented many women from working outside the home, postwar economic growth and a resulting demand for labor made the employment of women necessary. Many women engaged in part-time work, and the Danish newspaper *Social-Democrat* wrote in January 1955, "Part-time work would give a man a happier wife." The statement must be seen in light of a report on part-time work, adopted by the Danish Parliament, which called for a labor reserve that could "be drawn on in the labor-poor periods." Entry of women into the labor market could be achieved only by transferring many of the skills used at home to new jobs in the social and health care sector. While the employment rate among women over 15 years of age in 1900 was 37 percent, it increased significantly throughout the twentieth century, reaching 75.7 percent of all women aged 16 to 66 years by 2017.

In the 1960s and 1970s there was more upheaval in relation to gender roles. As stated, women's participation in business increased significantly, which led to calls for equal pay, better maternity leave, and a fairer distribution of housework by the newly established and fast-growing women's movement and the Woman Workers' Union. The period was also characterized by conversation about sex and the body. The contraceptive pill came on the market in the 1960s, Denmark introduced it in 1973, and the country became the first in Europe to provide access to free abortions. These changes helped give Danish women greater self-determination over their own bodies and sexuality, and led to considerable interest in knowledge about one's body.

Housing standards rose, many families moved into detached homes and bought televisions, and the number of bicycles decreased as more men began driving cars. Most women, however, still rode bikes to work, thus maintaining a high level of fitness. Today the bike still plays a central role in everyday life in Denmark as a means of transport and leisure activity. Copenhagen has been acknowledged as the world's biggest biking city.

As a supplement to school gyms in Copenhagen, many new sports facilities were suitable for multiple activities, but especially team handball, a popular sport in Denmark. It was crucial for the development of sport that activities could move indoors. The new sports facilities proved to be important gathering places for young people. During the 1970s there was a boom in interest in sport, especially among women.

Economic growth went hand in hand with youth rebellion in the late 1960s and lasted well into the 1970s. Young people and women in many ways rebelled against parental and societal traditions, but positive change occurred only slowly within the established sports movement.

My Childhood

My mother told me that when Germany surrendered on May 4, 1945, thus ending that country's occupation of Denmark, I was conceived in a rush of happiness that night. I might not have been born otherwise, because my parents already had two children: my sister, who is nine years older than I am, and my brother, who is five and a half years older. I feel privileged because I grew up in a time when, despite a lot of shortages in the years after the war, many things were possible, perhaps especially for women.

About the Home

I grew up in a loving family and a home characterized by political engagement and dialogue based on political convictions. My father was a skilled workman and after many years had his own business. In the crisis of the 1930s, before I was born, he was often unemployed, became involved with trade unions, and for a time was a member of the Communist Party. In 1956 he withdrew from the party after Hungarians revolted against Soviet occupation of their country. When the rebellion was met with violence by Soviet troops, between twenty-five thousand and fifty thousand Hungarians and approximately seven thousand Soviet soldiers were killed. Many more thousands were wounded, and almost a quarter of a million people fled the country, including about one thousand who migrated to Denmark. In spite of my father's withdrawal from the Communist Party, I often later heard him say, "You must perform according to ability and enjoy leisure time as needed." It was his social mantra. My father died far too early at the age of 65.

My mother was born in 1915, the same year Danish women won the vote, in the Danish countryside to a family with nine children. Once married, she worked as a housewife, though she would have liked to have studied and worked outside the home in a challenging career. What kept her from that goal was her having only seven years of schooling, but she was a gifted, clever woman, a fantastic mother, and the nerve center of our home. When I came home from school, she often was there with hot chocolate and buns and had time to talk about what interested me. Later she helped my father for many years with financial statements for his company and similar work. In her later years, she lived in her own home until about a year before she died at the age of 91.

On Primary and Lower Secondary School

My years at the local primary and lower secondary school began in the 1950s and ended ten years later with an exam. When I think back to that time, one teacher, Mrs. Meta Ditzel, stands out. She was a fantastic woman and teacher who wanted students to make something of their lives. Later, as a member of the Danish parliament, she took on major problems such as world peace and the role of the United Nations. Under her and other teachers, my fellow students and I learned the universal language Esperanto, discussed gender issues, reflected on the political parties' programs, and held our own elections. Today when people talk about the refugee crisis, I think back to the 1956 arrival of Hungarian refugees in my hometown, Viborg. For the first time, I was confronted with the fact that my safe framework was a huge privilege, and learning about peace in school gave me a new perspective.

About the Association

I learned a lot in school and at home, but the gymnastics club, where I spent much of my free time, played a special role. I trained four or five times a week in the school's gym during the winter and at an outdoor gymnastics area at Viborg Lake in the summer. The club's dynamic chairman, who also was my coach, expected much from his gymnasts. When the summer season began, all members had to help with maintenance of the clubhouse. Each member was assigned duties, and I was only 15 when I became a member of the board of directors. The tasks I was given were relevant to my experience and abilities, however, and during daily training I was allowed to exploit my talent. I've had a full and active life in sport, which also sharpened my political and social commitment and strengthened my identity. Throughout my lifetime I have been engaged in sport as an active athlete, coach, and manager.

Home, school, and the Viborg Gymnastics Club together formed the framework of my childhood. Everywhere I met adults who engaged in conversation with me and helped me learn. Everywhere I felt involved and had duties and responsibilities to help manage things. By asking questions and taking an analytical approach to the challenges I met, I learned it was possible to have an influence on both a small scale and a large one. My active and engaged childhood taught me the essential meaning of life and gave me faith in its possibilities.

Youth–Olympic Games–Education

I left primary and lower secondary school after graduation in 1962, and at that time I had no desire for a high school education. So, I got a banking qualification that suited my active life in the gymnastics club. Through the club I had met the man in my life, Kurt, but he moved in 1963 to Copenhagen to study. I followed him in 1966. Both of us were on the national team in artistic gymnastics and met mostly in the gym and with common gymnastics friends. Most days of the week, I left home early in the morning, worked in the bank, and then went directly to training. Some days I trained children before my own training started. In 1968 I was selected for the Olympic Games in Mexico, where I was to participate in the artistic gymnastics combined events. But before the Olympics and at just under 22 years of age, I married Kurt. We'd been offered an apartment, but a requirement was that we be married. Since then, the property has changed several times, but the man in my life has remained the same. In 2018 we celebrated our golden wedding anniversary. But at the time of our marriage, we were part of a group of newcomers to Copenhagen who gathered in a gymnastics club in Rødovre. We trained there many hours a week, and I trained at other clubs in nearby communities in my spare time.

The 1970s were not only a period of youth rebellion, the women's movement, and the peace movement but also a time for asking questions about the democratic structure of sports organizations and the increased commercialization of sport. My husband participated in an activist group within the Danish Sports Association who fought for athletes' involvement in the decision-making bodies. I supported the initiatives during this period but was busy with my own education at the time. Approximately ten years later I joined the battle for greater influence by women in sports bodies. But first, my active sports career was a big part of my identity.

The Olympics as the Creator of Identity and Political Awareness

On October 12, 1968, I walked with other Danish athletes into Olympic Stadium in Mexico City for the opening of the Olympic Games. I was only a Danish female sports gymnast, not a star but one among the many other gymnasts who formed the "court" surrounding the real stars and helped set off their performance in appropriate relief. No Danish athletes would be sent off like that today. For me, sport participation sharpened my political and historical awareness of both sports and gender. Why should I as a female gymnast be subjected to a gender test? And why could I not accept an offer to train with the East German gymnasts? Why should we live in a "women's house" that allowed no male visitors? These were only a few of the things that gave me a stronger identity and strengthened my political awareness.

Gender Awareness and Doubts about Gender

I learned that it was many years before women even had access to the Olympic Games. The first Olympic village, where athletes could live together during the games, was established in 1924. The rights of women, however, were not taken into account. They could either be accommodated outside the Olympic village or be assigned to a special women's house where men were denied access. Neither could the women athletes visit the men's houses. Only since 1992 have women and men lived side by side in the Olympic village. The fact that gender standards have changed is evident from the 450,000 condoms, or forty-two per athlete, dispensed at the 2016 Olympic Games in Rio de Janeiro. The Olympic Games have undergone significant change, just as sexuality has defeated puritanism.

At the Olympic Games in 1952, the eastern European countries allied with the Soviet Union appeared, and the competition got more contentious. The Olympic arenas now had women who in several ways fit past prejudices about sportswomen, because some of them, especially the track and field athletes, looked masculine. The discussion revolved around whether they were biologic women or whether they were hermaphrodites or men in women's clothes. The sporting ideal of equality at the starting point and the suggestion of cheating meant that all female Olympic athletes from 1968 until 1996 had to verify their sex through a test. Therefore in 1968 I was subjected to a test consisting of scraping the oral cavity to collect cells that laboratory technicians and geneticists could quickly analyze. For my part, the test showed no abnormality. My test was administered in the women's house of the Olympic village, but the doctor of the Danish delegation followed me and the other three Danish female athletes to ensure that it would be proper. A Danish swimmer had already given birth to a daughter, but nevertheless she was subjected to the test.

Political Awareness

One of the sports mantras is that sports and politics should not be mixed. The Danish Olympic gymnasts numbered three, two men and me, and there was a coach only for the men, which was a huge problem for me. We arrived well before the competition began, to become acclimated to the thinner air in the high elevation of Mexico City. It's difficult to train without a coach, and I was happy when the East German team, one of the world's best, offered to let me train with them. That offer, however, was refused by the leaders of the Danish Olympic delegation, but, happily, I ended up training with the Swedish gymnasts. The reason for the refusal was because of a political situation. In the spring of 1968, the Czechoslovak president, Alexander Dubček, started a democratization process, which was supported by the young, the old, workers, and intellectuals. In August 1968, however, the Soviet Union and other Warsaw Pact countries invaded Czechoslovakia and destroyed what had come to be called the "Prague Spring." Thus, I had no basis for cooperation with the East Germans. I had personally found that politics was part of sport. It was not entirely about what you had to "play" with. I didn't protest, but it was not so quiet elsewhere, as two Black American runners, Tommie Smith and John Carlos, who won the gold medal and bronze medal, respectively, in the two-hundred-meter race, demonstrated the power of sport as a political statement. During their victory ceremony, they raised their fists into the air to show sympathy with the Black Power movement for equal rights. Without the media coverage, it would never have been global news and a historic event. The 1968 Olympic Games in Mexico were unique. Gender testing and racial rights were broadcast from the Olympics to the whole world, and the games became an arena from which a political agenda could be raised.

The New Study Program

After my husband had finished his studies, I also studied part-time for a short period, but in 1971 I gave birth to our first child, Mette. I participated in gymnastics in 1972, still on the national team, and had successfully performed the qualification requirements for the Olympic Games in 1972 but decided to stop. Supported by my husband, I enrolled in a course in 1972 to start a new study program. Later it resulted in a master's degree in history and physical education from the University of Copenhagen. After graduation, I gave birth in 1979 to another daughter, Lotte. My adolescence had been decisive for my adult life. I had been diligent, hard-working, and dedicated to gymnastics as well as my studies. But without strong support from my family and a certain amount of luck, my fortunes may have been much different.

Adult Life—Work, Family, and Leisure Activities

Working Life

Once I had completed my master's degree, I was employed at DHL (Danish Institute of Physical Education), which represented the practical part of sports education, while the University of Copenhagen provided the human physiological part of my work. My role consisted of teaching gymnastics and developing the humanities and social science research areas in connection with sport. It was interesting pioneer work. I was lucky enough to be granted time in my job to write a dissertation in history at the University of Copenhagen. I wanted to write on women and sports, but my supervisor didn't think there were sufficient sources on the subject. Therefore, the theme became gymnastics in the nineteenth century. Through my work on the dissertation, I became aware of many women and female pioneers in sport, which meant that in the future I got to work on not only school history, the history of organizations, and social welfare and sport, but also the history of women in sport.

As stated, I was asked, among other things, to develop the discipline of sports history. So, inspired by Professor Jan Lindroth of Sweden, I helped establish, in 1984, the Danish Sports History Society, which I chaired for the following twelve years. The society managed to create a Danish forum for dialogue on the development of the field, and every year it produced a yearbook, with articles addressing sport in a social context and promoting and supporting the dawning research. I became head of a research department at DHL, which initiated an upgrading of the workforce via PhD studies. The University of Copenhagen established a Center for Sports Research, where from 1992 to 1997, I was the daily manager. It was a center without walls to ensure cooperation between various research areas, including human physiology research. The many research-related initiatives were a contributing factor to the Department of Sport, which the University of Copenhagen created as a merger of DHL, the Center for Sports Research, and the Human Physiology Department. It has been interesting to have been part of this journey, the acquisition of various skills, and the development of professional and managerial qualifications. For many years I was a member of the Dansk Research Council of Sports, and from 1996 to 2000 I was the chairperson. At the same time, I was head of sports education in Copenhagen, and in 2007 I became head of the department until I chose to retire in 2012 and move to professor emerita status. In my many years of involvement with sport science research at the university, I was associated with many networks as well as Nordic and international colleagues. One of the networks that became important for me was the group of Danish women historians. As a historian focusing on sport, I have not always been considered a real historian, even though I had a PhD from the history department. Many scholars did not find the field of sport history fully acceptable, but female researchers I met supported me, as have my Nordic and international sports professional colleagues through the international associations HISPA/ISHPES (International Society for the History of Physical Education and Sport) and CESH (European Committee for Sport History).

The Choice of Research Topics and the Myths

My research commitment and curiosity are a result of my dedication to gymnastics and the sports world, where democratic, gender, and cultural discourses have been absolutely central. Thus, my master's thesis was on the German *turnen* gymnastics, and my PhD dissertation was on gymnastics in Denmark. But women's history has been my special focus and has resulted in many articles, books, and other works. Here are just a few examples.

The Myth of the Invisible Women

The many female pioneers who became visible to me through my dissertation studies provided the starting point for further work on women's history. Over the years, my research has resulted in many articles about pioneers, cultural builders, and cultural carriers in Danish women's sport. Many of these works were collected in the book *Women's Sport: From the Roots to the Top*, published in 2005.

The Myth about Sport Belonging to Men

One of the many themes I worked with before publishing *Women's Sport* was the importance of elite sports for women. When modern sport had its breakthrough in the late 1800s, it was seen as a transitional ritual for young men. By participating, men developed determination, self-control, courage, and willpower that were crucial to their ability to move into the public space. But what skills did sport give the women who ventured into sporting challenges? What could they use the skills for? In the 1990s I conducted a research project involving Danish women who had participated in the Olympic Games between 1924 and 1948. In many ways this research became a life history project, as the women were asked to assess the importance of sport during their adolescence. I compared them with women who cultivated sports and gymnastics on another level. The Olympic women were chosen because they represented not only the very best in their sport but also a well-defined group of female top athletes. The women completed a questionnaire, and many of them I interviewed subsequently. Common among them was that they had achieved strong personal competencies and had become good citizens, but not in the same way as men. The essential factor was that they had *the generational time* in common. So, the conclusion can be that it was not and is not the sport itself that provided opportunities during that era. When I retired, I decided to follow up with women in elite sports today. I used the same questionnaire and interviewed forty women who had participated in the Olympic Games since the 1960s and as late as 2018. The result was a new book: *Olympic Women: About Elite Sports and Women's Lives through 100 Years*. The women reported challenges, greater emancipation, and experiences that I gathered for a diverse and collective narrative about women in elite sports. In relation to the previous female Olympians *the times* are different, which gives both new opportunities and new challenges. But common to the early and the more recent Olympic women is that the Olympic Games are all about anything but their sport. One of the athletes said the special thing about the Olympics is that "when so many athletes throng together, it is quite natural to talk to any 'foreigner' who you meet. . . . It was a great experience of a multiethnic society where everyone respected each other as people of equal worth."[3]

Leisure Time and Visibility

I recently heard a lecture by a journalist who had written about the first group of strong female government ministers in Denmark. They were all born in the 1940s and became ministers in the 1970s. One of the speaker's points was that if a woman was "approved" at one place, she could largely be useful and influential in areas where women lacked visibility and influence. The promotion of some women may, in principle, block other women in the same field from rising up. As a top athlete, you are visible and thus approved in the world of sports, and if you then display a certain amount of curiosity and a critical approach to the absence of women in managerial positions, you are almost obliged to get involved. So I did.

As a 15-year-old, I was on the gymnastics club's board, where I learned about the importance of volunteer efforts in administering and organizing the sport. The club's chairman, who was also my coach, took me to the annual meeting of the Danish Gymnastics Federation so I could learn about the system to which I as a gymnast belonged. Since then, I have engaged myself in my clubs, the Gymnastic Federation, and the top management of the DIF. An important factor in my long involvement in sport was that in the early 1980s, a group of women and I pointed out the need for women in management at the DIF. At our request, the DIF set up a working group, and we hired a gender equality consultant and established courses to qualify women for election to managerial positions. Some women were elected, and in 1988 we managed to elect a woman as one of the two vice chairs. In 1994 she chose to withdraw because she did not think she was spending her energy and time productively. She asked whether she "can get to contribute something in a culture where it still seems . . . that too much energy is used to mark territory and less to act as jointly liable for the total organization."[4] In 2002 I joined the DIF's management board, which consisted of ten members. I remained there for seven years as the only woman until another was employed. Many times, we women had argued for a form of gender quotas, but the request was always rejected. We in Denmark, in contrast to our neighbors in Norway and Sweden, have found it difficult to discuss gender quotas in general. In many ways, progress toward gender equality in Denmark is lagging behind that of the other two countries.

Mainstreaming

While sports federations can operate without interference from the public, it is a little different with the elite organization known as Team Denmark, which was established in 1985 with the Elite Sport Act. The purpose was to develop Danish elite sport in a more social way. In 1995 the European Union adopted a new strategy for mainstreaming, which was to create equal opportunities for men and women. With reference to the Danish law on gender equality, the state required that both men and women be equally represented on public boards. Team Denmark is headed by a board appointed by the minister of culture, who is responsible for sport. The members of the board must represent different interests and areas of expertise, and live up to the state's objective on mainstreaming. Therefore, the board of Team Denmark consists today of an equal number of men and women. For eight years, from 2008 to 2016, I had the pleasure of sitting on that board. I was nominated by the DIF as a representative for research.

I have reflected on my experience of being a member of the boards of the DIF and Team Denmark. In the DIF I often felt that I expressed myself as a representative of my gender and not as the possessor of certain expertise and knowledge. In Team Denmark the equal gender representation (four males and four females) and the appointment on the basis of knowledge meant another meeting and management culture. It has been an important experience. My story about the rise of more female managers to the top sports hierarchy reveals a sluggish system, which is lagging behind greater gender equality in Danish society. There is still much to be done. Women are active on the sporting fields, but there are few female coaches and few women where the big decisions are made. Personally, it has meant a lot to me to be elected and appointed and to learn from working in different management operations. These opportunities have had an impact professionally as well as recreationally and have expanded many important social and professional networks connected to the knowledge of and interest in sport.

I stated the importance of visibility and approval. I feel I was "approved" and therefore could be and have been used in many places, but other women also could have filled the space. When I turned 60 years old, there was a small celebration for me, and one of the speakers pointed out that when I came to events or meetings, I often included a new woman. I was very pleased with her words, as many had helped me on the way, and there was a need for many more women to contribute to developing sport. In that way I introduced more women to the previously all-male sport hierarchy.

Family Life

In work and leisure, I have, of course, faced challenges, but the biggest challenge in my life was when one of my daughters was hit by serious illness, which weakened her body and required medical treatment for many years. This family crisis resulted in a period of challenges and reflections on my part about the importance of a strong family and a supportive employer. For more than ten years, my daughter depended on the hospital in different ways. The Danish welfare model, with paid hospital expenses, put no economic limits on the right treatment. Therefore, I never questioned the high Danish tax burden. We get value for our money, as exemplified by this health issue.

Many resources sometimes are required to maintain life during crises, and in this case, an understanding employer was there as the family stood together and became more closely linked. My husband's and my knowledge of the physiological area of sport science was a great help as we could meet with doctors to ask relevant questions and ensure follow-up practices. Our insight into training helped show some of the therapists that if there was to be progress, our daughter had to challenge and press the body's boundaries. Luckily, she developed into a healthy girl and woman who has given birth to two wonderful children. Together with the family, she is physically active with challenging hiking in mountain areas and skiing in the Norwegian mountains.

A strong family has been key in my life, and our all our members are interested in sport. We travel together on holidays and for the past thirty-nine years have gone to Norway to celebrate Christmas with skiing; the group now includes children, sons-in-law, and grandchildren, a total of eleven people. In addition, we live relatively close to each other and help and support each other with everyday life. Common to all family members are the joy of and interest in physical activity and sports such as skiing, tennis, running, and swimming.

Later Life

At the age of 66 years, I retired and accepted an appointment to professor emerita, but I am still affiliated with the university department, which I consider a great privilege. As I felt my desire to continue writing, I decided to follow up on my project with the older Olympic women, and the result was the book *Olympic Women: About Elite Sports and Women's Lives through 100 Years*. I continue to work on large and small projects. One of my ambitions is to write the history of my gymnastic club and assess its importance to local welfare in the municipality. The club will celebrate its one-hundredth jubilee in 2024 and is the municipality's oldest club. In addition to my research and writing, I enjoy the new freedom to decide for myself about the use of my time. My husband and I attend cultural events and often go to the theater; it is easier now that we do not have to get up early the next morning. We have time to spend with our five grandchildren. Nurturing grandchildren has made me reflect on the responsibility we have toward the world we pass on to them. Senior life has meant that we travel a lot, either alone, with children and grandchildren, or with friends. Living a healthy life with physical training and exercise on a daily basis is fantastic. We train through fitness exercises, tennis, skiing, and a lot of walking.

When I think back, I feel very privileged. I was able to work in activities that I have enjoyed all my life and have had opportunities and challenges that I had never dreamed of when I left primary and lower secondary school in 1962. My working life, leisure life, and family life have been connected, and I will paraphrase Morten Albæk's words in the introduction: "The sum of the life I have lived, the life I am in right now, and the life I look forward to, in accordance with what is right for me."[5]

The aging process and the move from one stage of life to another for me has meant that new opportunities and challenges are presenting themselves. I've never felt a loss of identity. I have never had only one identity. I have been able to see a red thread through my leisure life as athlete, coach, and leader in the world of sports to my working life and family life. Sometimes one area was fuller than others, but none of the areas have ever been on its own. But regardless of age, sport has been a central companion and so far, along with a little luck, has kept me healthy.

When I dream about the future, I hope that my grandchildren and other children and young people are allowed to grow up in times that create peace of mind and confidence, and in environments that promote responsibility for the world around us. As postwar children, people my age were not given many opportunities, but many earned opportunities perhaps because they received an upbringing that reflected the words on the stone in front of the clubhouse I went to as a girl.

NOTES

1. Morten Albæk, *A Life. A Time. A Human* [in Danish] (Copenhagen: Gyldendal, 2018), 30.

2. Jytte Hilden and Inge Dalsgaard, *On Track for the Year 1946* [in Danish] (Copenhagen: Frydendal, 2016), 10.

3. Quote from Else Trangbæk, *Olympic Women: About Elite Sports and Women's Lives through 100 Years* [in Danish] (Odense, Denmark: Syddansk Universitetsforlag, 2018), 179.

4. Quoted from Else Trangbæk, *Women's Sport Science: From the Roots to the Top* [in Danish] (Copenhagen: Gyldendal, 2005), 252.

5. Albæk, *A Life. A Time. A Human*, 30.

14 Making a Difference

JANICE J. CROSSWHITE

I am Janice Jean Steel, born May 2, 1944, in Melbourne, Australia, a female, now 75 years old. My parents are Australian. My mother, Jean Donnison, was a housewife, and my father, Howard John Steel, was a fireman and played senior Australian rules football for the Melbourne Football Club. He retired as deputy chief officer of the Melbourne Fire Brigade. My brother, Keswick John, is 4 years older than I am.

I was raised as a Christian and was confirmed in the Church of England but have no religious affiliation now. I attended University High School, then moved on to the University of Melbourne for a diploma of physical education and to the Melbourne Secondary Teachers College for a trained secondary teachers certificate (1962–64) and, later, an approved fourth year of training. I furthered my education in 1976–77 by earning a bachelor of arts in education from the University of North Carolina, Chapel Hill.

I was married January 8, 1970, to Perry Rothrock "Rocky" Crosswhite, who was recruited by the Melbourne Tigers basketball club from Davidson College in the United States; he was the third U.S. import to Australian professional basketball. He went on to play for and to captain the Australian basketball team at three Olympic Games: 1972 in Munich, 1976 in Montreal, and 1980 in Moscow.

My sports participation has been ongoing. I represented my high school in swimming, track and field, softball, and hockey, and represented the state of Victoria in softball, basketball, and hockey. At Melbourne University I won a Half Blue and a Full Blue (annual awards to outstanding individuals in their sport) for softball and was the Australian university hurdles champion. I was a basketball pioneer, as the sport did not start in Australia until the late 1950s. I was 21 years old when I started playing and have continued ever since, except when pregnant with our four children. I have played in local basketball competitions, both daytime and evening, and in masters basketball tournaments.

When I was growing up in Australia in the 1950s and 1960s, there was a societal bias favoring males in a patriarchal society, and being exposed to fire stations where there were no female firefighters, I somewhat accepted the bias as the norm. I can remember my aunt and uncle going to watch my brother's football games, but no one watched my softball games. And I was the better athlete!

Other than the bias noted above, I have not directly experienced any personal prejudice but have witnessed and experienced discrimination and acted against it. For example, when I started my teaching career at Preston Technical College, the boys' school had the use of a full basketball court while the girls' school had a small volleyball court as its PE teaching area. I was able to get permission to take my classes into the boy's gym when it was free, something that had not been done before. Over the years, I have stood up to discrimination, called it out, and supported others to do likewise. Unconscious bias and prejudice do explain a lot of behavior, especially in sport.

When I married, I could not continue my personal superannuation pension fund; it had to be cashed in. This law was not changed until 1977, when both women and men had the same rights to superannuation retirement pensions. In 1972, when my husband and I wanted to purchase a hobby farm, we needed a deposit of $20,000. No bank would give us a mortgage, as my salary, which happened to be higher than my husband's at that time, was not considered eligible simply because I was a married woman.

Due to such experiences and my temperament, I have been a volunteer activist for gender equality. I have been a board member of Womensport Australia; the founding president of Womensport and Recreation New

South Wales, of which I am a lifetime member; the founding president of Australian Womensport and Recreation (also a lifetime member); a member of the executive board of the International Association for Physical Education and Sport for Girls and Women; and a president of Manly Warringah Basketball Association (another lifetime membership). I have a strong sense of self and consider myself fairly confident and self-assured. I call myself a feminist. Regardless of discrimination, I got on and did my own thing.

I have often initiated things. At Preston Technical College I started up a softball club and conducted the first girls cross-country events in Victorian schools. I was the first PE teacher in Victoria to teach basketball and coach school teams in new competitions run by Basketball Victoria. I gave school staff and their families use of the gym one night a week and changed senior school sport (years 9–11) so students could try ballroom dancing, squash, tenpin bowling, rowing, and the Duke of Edinburgh Awards Scheme (based on personal challenges that are noncompetitive, to develop individual skills and recognise these achievements with awards), as well as the traditional school sports, to reduce absenteeism and to offer a broader range of choices.

In 1979, the International Year of the Child, I initiated, secured a government grant for, and organised the Panton Hill Festival, which is still running every October. The festival is now a theme-based weekend event that encourages creativity in arts, crafts, cooking, and other activities by awarding prizes. Local clubs and the fire brigade roll out activities, with the dog jumping competition a crowd highlight.

As president of the Manly Warringah Basketball Association, I established a company limited by guarantee, which is a private limited company that has guarantors rather than shareholders, so it's suitable for voluntary organisations, to construct a four-court sports stadium. To achieve these things, I worked with like-minded women and men, cooperating on a shared vision and achieving a common goal. I have not been afraid to take a leadership role, start up new organisations, and challenge authorities or the status quo on outdated views and rules, standing up for what I consider to be fair, honest, and transparent treatment for all.

I think sport, particularly team sports, can give you confidence through being part of a group that helps you learn to get along and cooperate with others, follow directions, accept feedback, and learn leadership. This learning extends to other parts of your life and can be of particular significance in a work or business setting.

During my leisure time I enjoy various craft activities, gardening, reading, and bushwalking. Over the years I have done pottery, macramé, patchwork quilting, spinning, weaving, knitting, embroidery, and cross-stitch. Currently I am doing cross-stitch pieces for our older granddaughters—using six-inch hoops, I am highlighting feminist statements, such as "The Future Is Female," "Nevertheless She Persisted," "Make History," "You Can Do It," and "Boss Babe." I read a book or two a week, a mix of fiction and autobiographies. I follow politics and keep up to date with current affairs.

Living on a small fifteen-acre hobby farm, I breed Murray Grey cattle, keep chickens, breed Labrador retriever dogs, and have two cats. I take very good care of our animals and get very attached to the cows, dogs, and cats. They are all part of the Crosswhite extended family. In another life, I think I could have been a vet. The cows are fed hay in the morning and afternoon, and often we collect "cow food" from a local greengrocer and a bakery—our girls will eat just about anything. Their calves are sold at market during the spring in transactions I always find difficult as the animals really are pets, with names and identities. Stupenda is chief cow and a bossy boots. She is smart, can open gates with her nose, and will push me with her body if she wants to get closer to the hay or a treat. Hazel is a daughter of Stupenda, and we have kept two of Hazel's calves, Carrot Top, who is red, and Bundoora, who is black. We suffer cow abuse, as all of them will moo at us as soon as we are seen outside the house. With a drought here at present, a round of hay costs $200, and it only lasts about four weeks. So, my cows are really an expensive hobby!

The chickens, or chooks, as we call them, usually number about twenty, plus a rooster, and produce enough eggs for me to sell three or four dozen a week to my gym friends. House food scraps go to the chooks, and the cleaning out of the chook shed and their run produces great compost, all part of recycling. Indeed, I use a five-and-a-half-horsepower mulcher to chop up prunings, weeds, fallen branches, and the like to produce bins of compost that I mulch down for the garden.

Since buying the farm, Rocky and I have always lived with one or two Labrador retrievers. Our children have grown up with them and have had a dog most of their lives. I am a registered dog breeder and usually breed a litter (both black and yellow) every second year. Jess, a black Lab, is 12 years old; Daisy, her daughter, is a yellow 7-year-old; and Coco, daughter of Daisy, is a black 4-year-old. Daisy and Coco will run off at times, returning with a kangaroo leg or tail in their mouths. They will disappear under a fence, swim in a few local dams, and then return home. After dinner all dogs come into the lounge room to sleep on their sheepskins near the open fire.

Skittles is the housecat, a pretty, long-haired tortoiseshell that stays near the house, coming in at night. She has lost three lives: snakebite, a mysterious poisoning, and being locked in a bedroom cupboard for nearly a week when we went on holiday. Tabby Cat found us. She appeared under our house and then moved down the paddock to the hay shed, where she spends her days controlling rats and mice. She is a lovely friendly tabby, requiring her daily nurses and pats.

With over fifty olive trees on the property, I can produce olive oil, and the large orchard supplies fruit for eating fresh or making jams and preserves. A large vegetable garden provides some of our food.

For fitness, I attend various classes at a gym five or six times a week, and on Tuesday mornings I play tennis with a friendly local group of "seniors." We have a swimming pool next to the house, so over the warmer months I can swim, and in the late afternoon we walk two dogs through a bush reserve across the road from our property.

I have always volunteered in sport and in my community, particularly supporting public education. I have been president or secretary of my children's school councils over a period of twenty-five years and served on ministerial committees for public schooling in Canberra and for Women in Sport in Sydney. I have served on various local council committees, and I am a regular contributor to local government consultations and policy initiatives. I currently serve on the Panton Hill Bush Reserves advisory committee.

In Australia one is not considered elderly until she or he is 80 years of age or older. Life expectancy in Australia was 82.5 years in 2019, averaging

80.4 years for men and 84.6 years for women, figures higher than those in the United Kingdom and the United States. Australian men and women can qualify for the aged pension at 66 years of age if their income and assets are below a certain level. Benefits are considerable: rent assistance, reduced cost of car registration, and other financial support.

Australia has world-class public and private hospital care. The Australian government offers free medical care (called Medicare) through life. But private health insurance allows one to choose doctors and hospitals without being on a waiting list. For public patients, there is no cost for treatment in a public hospital. For so-called elective surgery, that is, anything that is not immediately life-threatening, such as cataract surgery or hip or knee replacement, the difference between public and private care is the waiting time, as the public system prioritizes urgent care over anything deemed elective.

At 60 years of age, all Australians qualify for a seniors card that offers cheaper public transport and discounts to movies, various shops and businesses, attractions, and other benefits. A Seniors Week is held each year, and there is a free national seniors organization and newspaper. Local councils also offer many services for pensioners and the aged: cleaning, local transport, subsidized housing, and social events.

Australia is currently rolling out a National Disability Insurance Scheme, which will provide funding for supports and services to about 460,000 Australians aged under 65 who have permanent and significant disability. For many people, it will be the first time they receive the disability support they need. There are around 4.3 million Australians who have a disability. Funding goes directly to the individual for the particular services they require; it is not a pension.

My own aging body is one that needs looking after. I want to stay active and strong and continue to do all the things I enjoy, like playing in my 70-plus basketball team, so I need to look after myself and take care of injuries. My philosophy is, "If you don't use it, you will lose it." I continue to stay active and sometimes do push too hard, injuring myself while gardening or doing farm work. I will work too long or do too much digging, for example, which stirs up an old back injury (broken at thoracic vertebra 10 in a horse-riding accident). Looking after yourself is about understanding your body and managing its weaker points. I have a physiotherapist and a sports physician, both of whom are very good, and lately I have had more regular therapeutic massage.

My heart rate was decreasing a few years ago. Reluctantly, I had a pace-maker put in, and since then I have added an after-lunch rest or nap to my routine. I now eat smaller meals, as I do not want to carry any extra weight, though I consume three good meals a day. I like to cook, and we eat healthy and good-quality food. I shop at the Queen Victoria Market, where I know many of the traders, so we buy fresh, good-quality meat, fish, cheese, fruit, and vegetables.

I still play masters basketball with the Aussie Butterflies Club. We participate in tournaments and always play in the biannual Australian Masters Games and the quadrennial World Masters Games. I did play in local basketball competitions until my late sixties but have found masters games more enjoyable as I am playing with women closer to my age and skill level.

The Aussie Butterflies have been highly successful, with my age team progressing through the 45-plus, 50-plus, 55-plus, 60-plus, 65-plus, and now 70-plus age groups and winning Australian Masters championships and World Masters Games gold medals in Portland, Brisbane, Melbourne, Edmonton, Sydney, Turin, and Auckland. Most of the women have represented Australia or their state and have continued to play basketball. Along the way we have lost three teammates to cancer and some to injury. A nice feature is that at one time we played against each other in different teams but now need the numbers and play together. The Tokyo World Masters Games beckons in 2021.

We are a unique and feisty bunch of women, keeping in touch and playing with both former teammates and new teammates as we age. The important thing is to enjoy the competition, the friendships old and new, and the fun. And there is something extra special when a group of women get together and enjoy being female, talk a lot, dance, go shopping together, eat and drink together, and enjoy a sport that they are passionate about.

Despite my athletic accomplishments, I consider my major success to be raising, with my husband, a family of four children: Cara Jane, born in

1974; Julia Janice, born in 1978; Anna Elizabeth, born in 1980; and Ian Clyde Steel, born in 1982, all of whom have been successful in their education, work, and sporting careers and are now married or partnered and raising children. My husband and I have thirteen grandchildren, aged 2 to 15 years.

I had a very good teaching career in physical education, having been rated outstanding for promotion to senior teacher, which led to physical education advisory work and teacher training experience. I introduced basketball to the University of Melbourne physical education diploma after writing to the head of the department about the need for it, once women's basketball became an Olympic sport in 1976.

I did not work for twelve years while raising a young family on the farm but then moved into part-time administration for the Australian Council of Physical Education and Recreation and the Australian Sports Commission in Canberra and, later, full-time work in the Australian Capital Territory Government as the junior sport coordinator. I also did consultancy work in human resources: one full-time contract was to staff the new Parliament House in Canberra, chairing interview panels for jobs from store staff to architects.

We moved to Sydney in 1991 when Rocky took up the executive directorship of the Australian Olympic Committee, which had decided to bid for the 2000 Olympic Games. It was too hard for me to work full-time in Sydney, with four children doing very well in their sporting careers and having to be driven to after-school training and weekend games. They all represented their school, club, state, and Australia in basketball; two had Australian Institute of Sport scholarships and three had basketball scholarships to U.S. universities (Davidson, Oregon, and Virginia). In Sydney I did sport consultancy part-time with Rocky when we established Crosswhite Consultancy Sport and Recreation, and later I worked successfully as a recreation planner and consultant in local government.

Crosswhite Consultancy worked with sports associations and sport sponsors to deliver on special programs, such as a Sports Vision program for emerging athletes with Bausch and Lomb, a Canadian eye care company. An enjoyable and challenging contract for me was with Basketball Australia in 1994 to deliver on the OZ94 World Basketball Championships for Women, conducted in three Australian locations with the finals in Sydney. I did the accreditation program, the publications (official program and guidelines for teams, officials, and referees), and ran the VIP program. I remember having to add alcohol, only one drink, along with the usual choices of juice, tea, and coffee, to the drink allowance after briefing the international referees, as many were used to having alcohol with their meals, and we had not planned for that. We could not afford to have the referees upset before a game was played!

In 2004 we moved back to Melbourne (Rocky was now the chief executive officer of the Australian Commonwealth Games Association) and returned to the farm I had rented out for the twenty-one years we lived in Canberra and Sydney. My job was to renovate the house, the pool, the weed-infested paddocks, fencing, and other things, so I retired from my professional career to become a farmer, property manager, and renovator. I have renovated one of our investment properties and continue to manage some of our properties: a Melbourne townhouse and an ice cream shop at Noosa Heads, Queensland.

This has all been very satisfying. I have a sense of pride in what I have achieved and that I have been a strong support to my husband in his career (we make a good team!); a resilient mother and supporter of my children in their education, sports, and careers; and a loving grandparent.

Through Rocky's sporting and administration career, it has been a privilege to have attended or been involved in many Olympic Games and Commonwealth Games from the 1970s to 2018. Rocky is a member of Basketball Australia's Hall of Fame and the Sport Australia Hall of Fame and currently serves on the latter's board.

A memory that stays with me is of the 1992 Barcelona Olympics when Rocky was team manager for Australia and thus was in the athletes' village nearly all the time. I somehow had the job of selling tickets for the Australian versus U.S. basketball game (the first U.S. Dream Team at the Olympics), as unsold tickets would cost our team. I hid tickets in my shoes and nervously stood outside the stadium, having little idea what to do. I was mobbed, sold the tickets in a flash, and couldn't get away quickly enough. But I did it for the team!

At the 1994 Lillehammer Winter Olympics, wearing the Australian uniform, I inadvertently got to ski on the official course, for a little while; I did a day of downhill and a day of cross-country, getting lost and stuck in a snowdrift, as I was by myself but having a fabulous experience. The 2000 Sydney Olympics were amazing, highly successful in all ways and thoroughly enjoyed by us as VIPs with car transport to attend any event, day or night.

My successful qualities are basic: an efficient administrator, a good contributor, an organizer who is used to planning ahead, and a persistent and reliable leader. I am on time with meetings and deadlines, and can be relied on to do what I say I will do. I don't have a temper or get upset too much—I just get on with it and get around or solve the problem—so I am task-oriented. I understand cultural and language difficulties and can be sympathetic to others' values and find common ground. I think I have high standards and maybe expect too much of others on some of my committees. Then again, I am told I am a good role model and mentor for women in sport.

I think I am a realist and would classify myself more as a critical thinker than as a complacent person. On committees I am the one who asks the most questions and am usually the most active committee member. If you are a member of a committee, you are there to do a job.

As I contemplate growing older, I am not sure there are many joys in aging. From now on we more or less follow the same patterns we have established in life. We can look forward to more time to travel, to visit family interstate and overseas, and to enjoy the changing lives of our children and grandchildren. At 75 years of age, I know that probably three-quarters of my lifespan has been spent.

I stay in contact with girlfriends from school and work and stay connected with neighbors and activities in our local rural community. We want to stay on our hobby farm, and we will hire local labour to make it work.

In 1991 my husband and I had to make funeral plans for ourselves when the Australian government requested that it be done before my husband left for the African continent to assist in seeking votes from members of the International Olympic Committee for the Sydney Olympics candidature. So, our gravesites have been purchased. We have made wills, of course, and kept these up to date, as over the years we have lent money to our children for them to buy their homes and a farm.

As one ages, wisdom does not necessarily accumulate. Moving through life and being successful is about making good decisions and exercising sound judgment as options and opportunities come your way, making the best decision at that time after having looked at all of the information. In today's more technical society, wisdom and knowledge from years ago and knowledge learned through life's experience sometimes can be irrelevant! But what does not change is sound moral behavior and integrity of purpose, and doing good for others, the wider community, and not just for oneself.

I can't say that I have had personal setbacks or ever suffered from depression. I do get unhappy and annoyed with myself when I reinjure my back. I tend to become quiet and start treating myself with stretches, pain killers, anti-inflammatories, heat packs, and bed rest.

I am concerned for my husband, who has an inherited blood disorder, Von Willebrand disease, which caused him a few problems in later life when he had an ankle fusion operation and a liver abscess. We need to be sympathetic to each other's health needs and look after each other.

As I age, I am quite nostalgic and sentimental, and value history. We can learn a lot from history and use that knowledge today. History was one of my teaching subjects. I am the collector for the Steel family history. In 2002 I travelled to Northern Ireland, Edinburgh, and in later years to Manchester and the Lake District around Keswick to catch up on family history but without much success.

In our Melbourne houses (Carlton and Panton Hill) I have antique Australian furniture, along with modern pieces, and many old pieces and collections of pottery, silver, and glassware. On the farm I have collected old wares and have them around the house paddock: insulators, farm implements, and installations made of rustic pieces. My children tell me that I have enough of these things. I am not sure why I value these "old things." I do enjoy shopping in "op shops," or Goodwill stores, as I find interesting and different things, help charities, and recycle goods.

I am not complacent. I do believe that "if good people do nothing at times, bad things can happen." We have a civil and moral responsibility to look after ourselves, our families, our friends, and our communities.

I have been fortunate to have been brought up by good parents. My mother never worked outside the home, so her presence gave stability and consistency to home life. We lived in fire stations in inner Melbourne, as was the tradition in those years, so my father was also on site. He was more loving than my mother and was the parent who occasionally watched me compete at school athletics.

My parents and Rocky's parents did not demonstrate or talk of love in an open way, and as parents we are similar. Our four children and their partners are more demonstrative in their relationships with their children. We knew we had loving and supportive parents behind us, and the same applies to our children.

Our marriage was quite a love story. I had tickets to an American play, so I went to Rocky's high school, where he was teaching history and asked him to come to the show with me. We had met once before. After six weeks we were engaged, and we were married in another three months! He was 22 and I was 25.

I reflect on changes in generations. I used public transport, that is, trams, or walked to school and sport and was never driven. My parents were never involved in any capacity. My mother did complain about my dirty washing, however, particularly dirty softball pants from sliding into bases. And she questioned why I wanted to play basketball, as she believed one sport was surely enough.

My parents saw me play only one basketball game, when my team, Melbourne Comets, played South Korea at the Albert Park Stadium. They did attend one of my softball games, when their annual holiday coincided with the Australian Championships in Adelaide. I represented Victoria in softball from 16 to 25 years of age and played against Japan in an international series.

I was motivated to "do my own thing," and parental involvement was not something I needed or missed. Indeed, I tell my children that it is a good idea not to be around their children's trainings and games all the time, as children need to play for themselves and for their own reasons, not because they want to please their parents.

I was successful as a student and in sport. In primary school I was a sixth-grade school captain and did the same during years 7 and 8 at Hawthorn West Central School. At University High School I was a house captain and prefect, and was captain of the softball team, gymnastics team, and athletics team. A few years ago, University High School celebrated one hundred years of sporting achievement, and I was one of ten women named with ninety men to mark the centennial.

I was an all-rounder of a student, having a go at whatever was in season with sport and the same in the classroom. I feel very grateful that I attended an excellent public senior high school with a strong principal and teaching staff who were leaders in their field. For example, in year 11, I studied American history—the first high school to teach this subject—at the height of the USA-USSR Cold War. We even had an American teach part of the course, as he was pleased to visit Down Under in case the Russians dropped a nuclear bomb on the United States!

I have a sense of fulfillment in my past accomplishments, and I am not sure what I would change if I had that opportunity. I think my generation has had the best of times: post–World War II growth and prosperity, and peaceful times for many. Australia is considered "the lucky country." I think, however, it is much harder to raise children now that we are dealing with the easy availability of drugs, hard-to-regulate social media, and the proliferation of handheld digital devices.

People should make the most of what comes their way, and I have been able to do that. My husband and I have worked hard in our jobs, invested well, and are financially secure. For example, when we wanted to buy our hobby farm but not sell our apartment to do so, we borrowed half the deposit from my uncle and lived off ten dollars a week to save the rest. We have done well in the share market, with me buying my first shares as a 21-year-old and continuing to follow the market over the years.

A small regret is that in 1970 I might have been selected for the Australian softball team at the March Australian Championships. Instead, we married in early January and honeymooned in New Zealand for two weeks. I then started in my new advisory physical education role and so missed most of the team's training sessions and felt I should withdraw from the team as I was not as fit as or as committed as I usually am. Later on, I thought, "Well, maybe I could have pulled it off."

Climate change is a real global threat, and we live it here. I have had to reduce the number of cows as our rainfall declines, and with reduced rainfall and runoff comes greater wildfire danger. Only ten years ago 179 people around this area died in a horrific wildfire, and we were saved only when the wind changed. Since then we have installed a concrete fire bunker as a last resort.

I have been told I have been a good role model and a mentor for those coming behind me. I have deliberately mentored a number of female sports administrators through the Australian Womensport and Recreation Program, which I established about eight years ago. My legacy has been the associations that I established, working alongside like-minded women: the New South Wales Womensport and Recreation Association (WRNSW) and the Australian Womensport and Recreation Association (AWRA). I was the founding president of these groups and have since been made a lifetime member.

One of my legacies would have to be starting Schoolgirls Breakfasts with the Stars in New South Wales (NSW). Teenagers sat at breakfast with a sports star. The program was to have a panel of sports stars on stage for questions and answers about their careers and to have entertainment that depended on the venue I used. So, at the Sydney Olympic Pool, the entertainment was Australian divers and synchronized swimming; at the Sydney Entertainment Centre it would be gymnastics and fencing; and so on. At the Dubbo Zoo the program combined with a regional sports academy to show demonstrations by highly skilled hockey players, basketballers, and others. These became sell-out events, with over one thousand schoolgirls in attendance, and successfully raised money for WRNSW to cover basic costs of administration. More important, the breakfasts spread to other parts of NSW and to other states of Australia.

I approached breakfast food companies (for instance, Kellogg's) and market suppliers of milk and yogurt, bread, and fruit to sponsor the event and later secured a naming rights sponsor and an airline to bring the sports stars to regional centres.

WRNSW and AWRA were administered by volunteers, so much of my time was given to them as an executive president. Most weeks averaged fifteen to thirty hours of volunteer work, which I readily gave. In 2014 I was successful with a federal government grant of $50,000 to hire a part-time executive officer for AWRA which made my life easier, but my hours did not diminish, as together we worked well to cover more ground and achieve more of the policy directions and strategies of the association. Over the years I have had considerable success with government grants from the federal government, the NSW state government, and local governments.

As noted above, in NSW I was president of Manly Warringah Basketball Association, and in my time there I set up the Northern Beaches Indoor Sports Centre (NBISC) Company to build a four-court indoor sports stadium for the northern beaches of Sydney. The sports centre came together with the support of local people and organisations and took about five years of my life. A few years ago, NBISC added two more courts and is now expanding to an eight-court facility. It has been a great success. Currently I have five grandchildren and a son-in-law playing there, plus a daughter who coaches.

I was on a steering committee for the Diamond Creek Sports and Gymnastics Centre, in outer Melbourne, that was successful in building a three-court high ball multipurpose facility with an international-standard gymnastic centre attached. As with NBISC, this sports facility is sited between a primary school and a high school and allows school access during the day and community access after school. I have just completed two years on an advisory committee to upgrade and extend this sports centre. The concept plan is in place, but now we need to find the $52 million to construct it.

In 2000 I was awarded an Australian Medal for Basketball, and in 2001 I was awarded a Medal of the Order of Australia for services to women's sport and the community.

In the future I look forward to more of the same! Coming up is another visit from our Hong Kong family. Our eldest daughter and her family have lived overseas for twelve years, but their children are now starting to board at Geelong Grammar in Victoria, so we are helping as legal guardians and minders. With two children and ten grandchildren living in Sydney, we visit them and they visit us, staying on the farm.

October is the month of the Australian Masters Championships, and my team, Aussie Butterflies, is entered, as usual, in the 70-plus age group. We are probably the only team in our age group, as we were the pioneers, and we are running out of team members and opposition! So we play down, against younger women; it is getting harder as we age gracefully! But we have a lot of fun. I train with a men's club before any major competitions, as it is nearer to me and a great group, aged from 70 to 91 years.

In July 2020 there will be a Crosswhite family reunion on Maui, Hawaii, for the Australian and American branches to get together. Most likely we will have about forty Crosswhites there. From Hawaii we plan to fly to Anchorage and sail south to Vancouver to discover this part of the world. We are not normally cruise people, but this is what you need to do to see the Alaskan passage.

I will continue as communications director on the executive board of the International Association for Physical Education and Sport for Girls and Women (IAPESGW) until its next congress in Tokyo in 2021, after which I will retire. Over recent years I have been the editor of the association's monthly *International Update* newsletter, which is emailed to the membership and filed in a database. In 2016 I edited the book *Oceania Inspirational Women: Making a Difference in Physical Education, Sport, and Dance*, part of a five-continent series for the IAPESGW. This experience was quite a challenge but an enjoyable and satisfying editing job, securing the stories of eighty women from Australia, the Cook Islands, Fiji, New Zealand, Papua New Guinea, Tonga, Vanuatu, and Norfolk Island.

My passions are still the three E's—education, equality, and the environment—as well as sport and physical activity. I will continue to be active in these areas.

Rocky and I will continue to enjoy our retirement, living the best of both worlds, in the bush on the rural fringe of Melbourne—nearly always voted the most livable city in the world—and enjoying our lovely 1897 heritage city townhouse where we stay one or two nights a week to access the theater, art galleries, and downtown shopping. We will continue to be attentive parents and to provide support to our four children, their partners, and our thirteen grandchildren. Next year two granddaughters will board at

Geelong Grammar School. We are their legal guardians while they are in Australia, so we look forward to looking after them and attending many school events. Plus, as our grandchildren age, we feel it is important to be around all of them and have regular contact and some influence in their lives, which is not easy with eleven of them living interstate and in Hong Kong. We will continue to host our extended family here on the farm and to travel to them, so that we can have some grandparental influence and make a difference in their lives.

15 Fit, Fun, Forever Young

GERTRUD PFISTER

"Fit, fun, forever young": this slogan of the World Masters Games in Sydney in 2009 first drew my attention to this megasport event, and I reflected not only on my own situation as a woman in her seventies but also on the opportunities and challenges of aging women in western societies. I observed how aging women behaved in various situations, for example, when changing a tire of their car, participating in demonstrations, or sitting on a bench and feeding pigeons. I read books about "successful aging," and I talked about aging with friends, colleagues, and neighbors as well as women I met in various contexts, such as during train rides or at conferences. I also collected information about the performances and lives of extraordinary old women, like explorers, mountaineers, warriors, and athletes who clearly refuted age and gender stereotypes. In addition, I gained in-depth insights into the lives of the women and about the impact of aging on their habits, tastes, abilities, and, in general, their lives.

In this way, I detected sport and aging as a research topic, which caught my attention for several reasons. I realized that people in my environment were aware that I was not young anymore, although I did not feel old at all. They offered me a chair during a rock concert, wanted to carry my backpack during hiking trips, and advised me to select an easy-to-handle model when I was buying new skis.

Therefore, I have a personal interest in older women's opportunities and challenges not only in sport but also in everyday life. As I experimented with social constructivist approaches to gender, I found it challenging to transfer this concept to aging and sport. My central question was and is, Can age be understood as a social construction in a way similar to that of gender, and if so, how do these constructions influence engagement in sport and physical activities? As I observed aging women and their participation in sport and asked them about their practices, I became increasingly interested in their stories, their motivations, and their strategies for coping with ageism.

My own experiences and my observations of and the narratives of women over 60 show not that age is necessarily connected to a continuous decline and increasing difficulties but that one can be old and, at the same time, fit and proactive.[1] Even failing health does not prevent numerous old women and men from living active lives and participating in physical activities according to their own terms and adapted to their abilities. Important questions involve which groups of older people are physically active and what external and internal factors and processes support or prevent an active lifestyle.

It should be borne in mind, however, that aging women may have only one issue in common: their age. Their life circumstances, their aims and opportunities, and their habits and practices in general and with regard to sport and games differ considerably, depending on their situation and lifestyle but also on their social class and their ethnicity, as well as on the ascribed gender roles and relations, and the sports cultures of their countries, which influence or even determine participation. This essay focuses on sporting activities and performances of women in western countries.

As for my own case, I was born on December 12, 1945, in Eichstatt, Germany, in the state of Bavaria. My sister is four years younger. Our mother was a kindergarten teacher, and our father was a high school mathematics and physics teacher in Traunstein, Germany, where we grew up. In high school I was the only girl in my class. I was proud to be picked before less athletic boys for the soccer games in physical education class, but my experience there was not so joyful at times, because of some boys' disrespectful treatment of my father, who was not an authoritarian teacher.

I did, however, enjoy playing outside and skiing in the nearby hills, where friends and I built a ski jump. Larger ski slopes were only a train ride of thirty to forty-five minutes away. When I was a child, my family hiked and skied in the Bavarian mountains and searched for mushrooms. I also was a member of a Turner club, began playing tennis as a teenager, and even tried fencing and sailing for a while. In the summer we biked to a large lake, where we could rent sailboats. I had my own collapsible kayak as well. My love of nature and outdoor activities has persisted as I still hike, climb mountains, run, and ski when possible.

After high school I attended Ludwig Maximilian University in Munich to study Latin and physical education with the intent to become a teacher. Later, along with my boyfriend, I entered the university at Regensburg to become a medical doctor, but after my first internship at a hospital, I realized that medicine would not be a good career for me. With my love of nature and outdoor physical activities, I earned some money with the highest level of certification for a ski instructor and changed my career plans to become a physical education teacher. I continued at Regensburg to earn a doctorate in history, and then transferred to the university at Bochum, Germany, to obtain another doctorate, this one in sociology, in 1980. A year later I accepted a position at the Frei University in Berlin, where I worked for two decades. My boyfriend, Hans, accompanied me, but after twenty years of our being together, the relationship ended and I soon found a new partner. In 2001 I accepted an offer to work at the University of Copenhagen in Denmark, where I engaged in several funded research projects relative to sport.

Throughout my academic career, sport and physical activity have been a continued interest and a healthy means of recreation for me as a tennis player, skier, and runner. I have cycled and skied regularly, even heli-skiing in the country of Georgia. I have kayaked the Yukon River with friends and climbed Mount Kilimanjaro in Africa, as well as numerous mountains around the world. I tried scuba and skydiving, flew a plane, and even won a prize in a rodeo in the United States. I have run several marathons but now participate only in shorter competitions, proud that I have won some in my age group. My sports practices as well as my academic activities have taken me throughout the world, providing a wealth of knowledge and pleasure in learning about other people and other cultures. In the process I have made many friends who shared my interests.

Some of my friends were elite athletes in their youth: a handball player, Katie; a basketball player, Greta; a runner, Rosa, who set age group records; and a gymnast, Eliza, who performed in the Olympic Games. Others engaged in competitions on a local level or participated in sport on a general level rather than in elite competitions. My sister, Hildegard, cycles regularly, and my cousin, Elizabeth, is a rower. Rita, a former professor like me, played tennis and still thoroughly enjoys golf. She and the other interviewees still love to participate in sports, and all of them have developed "physical literacy," that is, they acquired the skills to enjoy even sports that require a period of learning and training such as tennis, golf, rowing, and skiing. Only two of them took part in sporting competitions: Annamarie and Lina in tennis and running, respectively.

Several interviewees expressed a connection between aging and sport activities: for example, a decrease in performance, changes in goals and tastes, and negotiations about the right way to be physically active. The interviewees also described positive feelings from doing something with others and supporting each other, but they also had experienced stereotypes about old women and their sport-related abilities and competencies.

Interviewees' Updates

I met Annamarie during a women's run in Berlin, and I played tennis with Rosa. When I started to work on this essay, I phoned or wrote to several women, whom I had interviewed several years ago, and asked if they were willing to give me an update about their lives and current activities, especially their participation in sport and their future plans for such activity. Katie had played basketball for more than half of her life, including two decades in the highest women's league of her country. The highlight of Katie's basketball career was competing with her team in the Masters Games in 2005 in Edmonton and in 2009 in Sydney. It was not easy for Katie to finance this adventure, and she started saving money two years before each event. In Edmonton, only three teams participated in her age group, and her team gained a silver medal. "I am so proud about this medal," she told me. "It was not easy at all. I am sure the other team cheated with the age. They seemed much too young for us. We had to give everything, and I felt totally exhausted after the game. But it was just great, when we all embrace in a big huddle."

"It was like the real Olympics." Katie likes to talk about the Masters Games, all the adventures during the travels, sightseeing in the host cities, the lack of training opportunities, and the people whom she came to know when she attended swimming or track events to cheer for other competitors.

She loved the game of basketball and invested not only time but also money, for example, the cost of travel to matches. In the past few years, her team, consisting of aging players, competed with younger women because there were no other teams in their age category.

Basketball is the main source of joy in Katie's life, but it is increasingly difficult for her to continue because opponents in her age group are rare and because competing against younger players means that her team loses more often. She told me that she and her teammates did not care in which league they played and that winning was not the only goal for them. They even let their coach play, although they knew that she would not contribute much to their success as she could not run anymore. But the players in their league were young, and their aggressive playing style was dangerous for older competitors. Katie described how irritating it was to have to play against women who could be their daughters or even their grandchildren. She and her teammates did not like the rough behavior and did not want to endanger their health, so some teammates stopped playing. "I miss basketball a lot; I played the game since my youth, and being a player was a part of my identity, of my life. . . . I also miss my teammates. We were not intimate friends but [were] comrades, and it was the training and the matches that brought us together. We had a special relationship."

In addition, quite a few members of Katie's team have dropped out or plan to do so for various reasons, mostly because they needed less demanding physical activities. "I am a player," she told me, answering my question about her future sport career. "I don't like running or fitness activities, and I run only if it is running after a ball; otherwise running is just boring." Currently, she and the remaining members of her team are discussing alternatives to basketball. They are convinced that they have to stay active, because otherwise they would feel useless and old. They explored other ball games, and right now it seems that badminton has a good chance of becoming the main sport in Katie's life.

Katie did not find another opportunity to play basketball. She attempted, half-heartedly, to find another sport, but being a team-oriented player, she could not force herself to train in a fitness center or to jog. But we met her former coach at a "dancing hall" in a park where many people in their fifties and sixties had a lot of fun listening to a band and dancing. Because men were a small minority, many women danced with other women. Smiles were on all faces, and we could tell the dancers enjoyed the music, the movements, and the company.

Rosa was one of my running partners when I lived in Bochum, more than thirty years ago. She was a friend of one of my students who lived near my home. I often met both of them when I was jogging, and at some point we decided to run together, as it was much more fun to exercise with a running partner than to run alone. The student also persuaded me to participate in running events such as the "city night runs" or the New Year runs that ended after five kilometers with a glass of champagne. Rosa was a far better runner than either of us. She trained systematically and steadily improved her rankings, at least on the city level, because she could run in one of the senior categories. I interviewed her several times and found out, among other things, that running and her sport club were priorities in her life.

When I searched for her many years later, I found her on the internet in record lists of long-distance running. When I contacted her again for this study, she was glad we could renew our acquaintance. She was still an avid and successful runner. Although her best performances were behind her, she still places first in her age group. She is currently considered a "world-famous athlete" on a webpage about masters athletics. As she has a lot of time, she supports her club by sitting at the "hotline," helping with the organization of events, and coaching young runners. Asked why she does not "retire," she emphasizes the numerous benefits of staying active and being in connection with her club, which she considers her family. She also emphasizes the benefits of her sport and is convinced that her training is the reason for her good health and excellent condition. "I have not been sick in years, and I am sure that running is the best sickness prevention."

In her youth, Eliza was a successful gymnast who began to exercise as a small girl in one of the many gymnastic clubs in her country. She was talented and won many championships on the national and even the international level. Study, marriage, job, and children prevented further engagement, as she had to concentrate on her new tasks. Because she wanted to share not only her life but also her interest in sports with her husband, she began to learn tennis and golf, sports she could play with family members. A major interruption in her sport career was caused by injury that required hip replacement. She emphasized in the interview that she hated to be sick, not least because her bad hip forced her to have a more sedentary lifestyle. She also described how she both liked and disliked physiotherapy: she loved the exercises, as she knew they would improve her health, but at the same time she disliked them because they were painful and the progress she gained from them was slow. The exercises were effective, however, and she took up her sports again, appreciating her ability to be active much more than before.

Rita grew up near a tennis club, so it is no surprise she became interested in the game as a child. The club was a paradise for her and other children, who hit old tennis balls against a wall and counted the hits. Sometimes they would compete; the winner was the child who could return the most balls. Later, Rita took part in tournaments, became a member of a youth team, and played competitively among the seniors. When I interviewed her for the first time, she was still playing but had considered dropping out, as training and competitions took time away from her studies. In the second interview, I learned she had moved to another city and was gainfully employed in her dream job. She planned to play tennis again but had little opportunity. Some clubs did not accept new members, others were too far from her residence; fitness training in a studio near her flat seemed to be her only opportunity to engage in physical activity. She is interested, however, in playing golf, which would provide prestige among her colleagues. Finding that membership in a club in her city is too expensive for her, she currently is investigating golf holidays and public golf courses.

When I asked in one of our talks why Rita is not interested in easily accessible games such as table tennis and badminton, she replied that they did not satisfy her desire to play a sport with an upper-class image. As golf has become her major sport interest, she can talk for hours about her experiences on the golf course. She trains often to bring down her handicap, and she believes golf will be her main or the only sport in her life as she ages.

Sara was a dedicated horseback rider; she owned a horse that took up nearly all of her free time, as it had to be regularly fed, groomed, and exercised. She talked much about this pastime in the first interview. When an increasing workload did not allow her to care for her horse properly, she sold it to someone who had more time. She was sad, but the feeling that her decision was the best one for the horse helped her accept the situation. Sara's love for horses led her to continue her equestrian activities, but she also has interests in travel, skiing, and dancing that she shares with her husband, whom she met and married while in her fifties.

Two women who reported in their first interviews about their active lifestyles that included jogging, swimming, badminton, horse riding, and sailing had to fight serious diseases that changed their lives. Both had to stop strenuous activities, and although they seem to have overcome their diseases, they did not take up their "old life." One of them was advised by her doctor, the other by a friend, to go for walks as often as possible. They did take this advice seriously and found ways to make walking more interesting. Both use portable media players to listen to music, news, and, for one of them, poetry. Thus, they forget time and exhaustion and make walking or running more enjoyable. Some of the women focused on health benefits when they started to exercise, but the more immediate incentives such as companionship, experience of nature, and relaxation were why they did not drop out even if they sometimes had to fight tiredness or pain.

Annamarie, a retired high school teacher who had loved running and biking, played tennis regularly and went skiing in the winter months. In the first narrative interview, she told me about herself and her life. She was divorced, had a grown-up son, and after some more or less successful relationships, she had become a confirmed single. She was a dedicated teacher of both English and sport at a high school, and had assumed many other functions at her school. "It is a matter of balance," she said, balance between work and relaxation, between body and mind, between meeting friends and being alone. Sport, especially running, has always played a large role in her life, and she still competes in races but also plays tennis in the summer and participates in downhill and cross-country skiing in the winter. On her holidays she often goes on hiking trips in the mountains with a group of colleagues. Now and then she also trains in a fitness center to keep her body in shape. But she cannot force herself to go there regularly.

At 60, she did not want to think about age. That everybody told her she looked so much younger than she was made her proud and helped her imagine that she would be forever young. Books about aging gracefully provided, at least for a time, guidelines for her life, especially exercising but also nutrition. Sport was a pleasure but at the same time a tool in her antiaging project. On the one hand, sporting activities helped her stay healthy and slim; on the other hand, sport, particularly good performance in running competitions, was also proof of youth and a fitness test for her.

Running with her was fun even though she was much faster than I was, and she did not have to push herself. She could tell me jokes and stories while running, whereas I had to take care not to get out of breath. "When I run, I can feel my body becoming awake and functioning. I start slowly and find my rhythm. I breathe regularly and deeply, and I feel myself getting lighter. I run faster and faster, and I know that I am good." The issue of the functioning body was of great significance for her in the following years.

"I am aging," was the first thing Annamarie said when she phoned me shortly after her sixty-second birthday. "Do I really have such large bags under my eyes? I have to talk with somebody about it." She had a new passport photo made and was frightened by the picture, which showed every trace of an aging face. In this period, she addressed the issue of her looks more often and started to discuss what she could do about it. Annamarie emphasized over and over that it was not the "others" or men she cared about but herself. She did not want to see or feel changes in her body or in her appearance. But her attitudes toward and emotions about old age were shifting and ambivalent. Mostly she seemed not to care, but at times when she was stressed at school, did not sleep well, or experienced running as exhausting, aging became a topic and a threat. Exercising and training were still a means of fighting off old age; therefore she increased her visits to the fitness club. Sport was a way to "do something and not just give in"—a phrase she often used.

But there were days when Annamarie's running lost its lightness and harmony, when she had to fight to continue. She told me, "I hate my body when I cannot do what I want. It simply resists, doesn't follow my commands. I know it before I even start running. Going down the staircase and out of my house, I can feel the tiredness in my legs. . . . I'm getting old." One way of defending her body against the attacks of aging was experimenting with supplements such as fish oil and vitamin or mineral pills. But although she took these pills, she doubted that they would help. She observed her body to trace the effects of these supplements but found no positive change; she was never sure if they really had any impact.

Annamarie talked a lot about antiaging measures: Should she buy this cream? Or even risk an operation? In one way she was totally against cosmetic surgery, but on the other hand, it had a fascination. "People should like me as I am; why should I care about others?" she said sometimes. In another conversation she mused, "Maybe I will feel better if I do something with my face . . . at least it wouldn't hurt, it can't get worse?" Before her sixty-third birthday she had an operation on her eyes, and what had caused so much discussion beforehand was no great issue afterward. She accepted, even enjoyed her new looks, but soon she took her "younger face" for granted.

Before her retirement, some of the main topics she discussed were the activities she would either take up or intensify when she stopped working. She looked forward to this change, not least because she found teaching increasingly arduous and less and less rewarding. She had many plans, but retirement was also an ambiguous event for her, an initiation, as she put it, into the last phase of her life. Using more time for sporting activities was one of her plans, and she decided to join a senior team in her tennis club and play competitions at the lowest level. Tennis and her matches now filled much of the conversations during or after running. Annamarie was ambitious, and she was very proud when she beat her opponent, especially when the "enemy" was younger. This was not only a victory in tennis but also a victory over age. But one cannot win all the time. Losing was a problem, but the negative feelings connected with losing did not last long.

Before retirement Annamarie had very seldom been ill. She used to take pills when she had a headache or a cold and tried to get back to her normal healthy state as soon as possible. When she was 65, however, a number of health problems developed, and the more she tried to ignore them, the stronger the signals got: dry eyes, a low red-blood-cell count, headaches, and a knee problem—not life-threatening diseases but disorders that required treatment. In sport, too, Annamarie tried to ignore pain; she was even proud that she managed to play tennis with her hurting knee. For her this was proof that she was a fighter and had control over her body.

It was not the "big pain" that was her problem; "in that case you just have to stop what you are doing and go to hospital to have it treated." It was the little nagging pains in her knees that come and go: "You have to force yourself; you try to think about nice things, the shower after the run, but you cannot concentrate. The only thing you concentrate on is the pain."

Annamarie found various and numerous "jobs" after retirement. She took on responsibilities in her tennis club, organized adventure holidays with friends, and started to write a crime story. Balance again became an issue during talks and interviews. Her worries concentrated not so much on her body but on her mind. "I have Alzheimer's," she said—half jokingly, half seriously—when she forgot to phone me as promised.

Sport is still her antiaging project, but she has become more relaxed. When she is doing sport, she feels herself:

> My last run was an experience—as it always is when I'm running. Problems disappear, worries become unimportant. I can relax and breathe deeply; I can feel my body and I'm aware of nature, the weather, the change of the seasons. I try to take it all in—the smell of the grass, the sun on my skin, the blue sky with some little white clouds. These are times when I listen to my body, and I like to feel my muscles working. I feel alive, time is meaningless, and I forget about aging because I'm so glad that I'm alive.

Annamarie has slowed down her pace when she runs, but I have also gotten slower, so we relax, jogging along and enjoying life.

The interviews, as well as the informal talks and observations make it obvious how Annamarie dealt with age and gender scripts, how she adopted social constructions and developed her own strategies between compliance and resistance. Her narratives also show how sport was and is integrated into her identity and used not only as a keep-fit and antiaging strategy but also as a way of resisting stereotypes, escaping the "masks of aging," transforming expectations for herself, and experiencing authentic moments of satisfaction and joy beyond gender and age.

The other team sport player among my friends is Greta, who was a member of the highest handball league in her region. She made a career not only in handball but also in sport administration and academia. In all these fields she excelled as a team player. Because of knee problems, she had to quit playing games, but she still swims and participates in fitness exercises when she finds the time.

Throughout my own life I have retained my interest in sport, engaging in jogging, cross-country skiing, biking for fun, and swimming. I particularly like that I can engage in these activities spontaneously in the local area, without depending on other people. These activities help me relax, feel and appreciate my body, and experience the environment. I have found some similar-minded women so that I now have people with whom I can share my interests. I have also found a new love life, and my husband shares my interests. I believe that sport companions are important for sharing joy in nature or achievement but also for providing support in case of an accident.

I continue to engage my lifelong curiosity in research and writing projects. While I have experienced some health issues relative to aging, particularly the need for surgery on my fingers, I do not worry about aging. My activities keep me in good health, and I remain optimistic about the future and look forward to continued travel and experiencing other cultures.

Discussion

The interviews, as well as the informal talks with and observations of all women in the project, revealed that sport was, and still is, an indispensable part of their lives. For these women, sport is a physical necessity, embedded in their identities; it is used as an opportunity for engaging in meaningful activities, experiencing success, maintaining health, and resisting the aging of the body and mind. It provides social and cultural capital and is experienced as a highlight in everyday life.

The interviewed women have developed various strategies for negotiating the social constructions and realities of gender and aging in a society that, according to Dionigi, "idolizes health, ability, and independence and that devalues aging."[2] Being active or competing in sport enabled them to defy current stereotypes about aging women. Two case studies represent two different approaches to gender and aging: Annamarie's activities could be described as a fight against aging. In keeping with Dionigi's findings, she simultaneously "mobilized and resisted aging discourses."[3] Katie's behavior, by contrast, can be interpreted as a more or less resigned acceptance of aging, at least with regard to her appearance, but a resistance against the loss of sporting abilities and opportunities. What Annamarie describes (and undertakes) as a project, that is, to remain, or at least appear, as young as possible in accordance with gendered ideals and scripts, is of minor importance to Katie, who is largely indifferent to prevailing norms and ideals and downplays gender in interactions.

It is the bodily changes that are hard to cope with for both women, not least because their sporting activities and performance are dependent on a functioning body. In addition, Annamarie is concerned about her looks and alarmed by the signs of aging, which she finds disfiguring in the light of the "forever young" mania prevalent in western societies oriented to enhancements on all levels and in all areas. Annamarie's narratives reveal how she negotiated between compliance and resistance. Sport is part of her identity and is used not only for keeping fit in the context of her antiaging strategies but also as a way of resisting stereotypes and enjoying being physically active and performing well. Both women experience sport and competition as an adventure, a source of pride, a means of gaining self-esteem and respect, and as authentic moments beyond gender and age. For both women, as for many older sportswomen, it is not the absolute performance but the participation in sport activities or competitions that counts.

Sport provides excellent opportunities not only for "doing" gender but also for "doing" age as the body and its techniques and abilities—strength, endurance, power, and aggressiveness but also flexibility, grace, and elegance as well as frailty and fatigue—are on display. Therefore, playing sport is always also "doing gender" and "doing age." In and through sport, gender- and age-related ideals and norms are not only produced but also challenged and changed. It must be emphasized, however, that for most people, sport is only one of many projects in their life course. Their choice of sports, their performance levels, and the aims and the contexts of their engagement depend not only on their sport socialization but also on their current situation and their gender identities as well as their plans and expectations for the future.

In the nineteenth century, modern sport was invented by men and for men; women were and are still—with regard to performance levels, income, and number of participants—the "second sex."[4] This second-class status is particularly true in elite sport, which attracts and rewards young men for the most part. Thus it is not surprising that the sports stars presented in and celebrated by the media are—worldwide—nearly exclusively young males.[5] Aging women have to overcome several barriers when they wish to participate and even to compete in sport. In the past few decades, however, the image of aging sports people as well as the role of sport in old men's and women's lives underwent considerable changes, especially in industrialized countries. The reasons are shifting demographic patterns, changing gender arrangements, as well as a continuous propagation of sport and exercises and their widespread use as means of health promotion, beautification, and rejuvenation.[6] Sports also provide opportunities for numerous positive experiences with other people and with oneself in the form of companionship, self-assertion, and self-presentation.

Opportunities are influenced by spaces, provisions, and significant others, among other things, and the demands refer to the capacities of sports participants, their talent, their bodily and psychological conditions, and their aims and motivations. In addition, material and immaterial rewards influence participation in sport, as do choice of activities and intensity of engagement. Furthermore, significant others and the environment, but also stereotypes about old women participating in sport, long thought of as an activity for young men, may influence the degree of engagement by individuals and groups in sports and exercises.

These dominant discourses not only have implications for the ways in which women interpret their experience of aging, menopause, and their changing bodies;[7] they also encourage individuals to engage in fitness projects and improve their health and appearance. Exercise can be seen as a form of beautification because it often can produce a slim and fit body that exudes both youth and—in particular—health.[8]

Participation in Sport and Exercises—European Trends

Worldwide, available statistics gained from surveys or memberships at sport clubs show increasing participation in sports and exercises not only among the general population but also by elderly people. This increase is especially true in industrialized countries, although opportunities to play sports vary widely among the different countries, regions, and continents.

In western countries, elite sport and successful athletes are at the center of public attention, but "sport for all," a European concept that emphasizes wholesale participation rather than elite performance, is gaining participants, not least because the ability to choose from a wide range of activities promises not only fun and relaxation but also better health, appearance, and social integration. These promises refer to current discourses, ideologies, and demands in western societies, where "healthism" and "agism" contain moral imperatives to stay young, fit, slim, and functioning.[9]

How are aging women affected by these discourses? Can they comply with the social demands if they wish to? And which sport opportunities are available to and appropriate for them? Surveys in many industrial countries provide answers and insights into the sport engagement of the population. New research in Denmark, for example, conducted by the National Research Center for Welfare, focused on older people and found that most of those surveyed were physically active and engaged regularly in walking or cycling.[10]

In Denmark the percentage of female participants in sport or physical activities is high among girls but decreases steadily as they age, from more than 80 percent of 10-to-12-year-olds to 52 percent of women aged 30 to 39. The percentage increases from that point on, however, to more than 66 percent among 60-to-69-year-olds and more than 70 percent of women over 70. Only 50 percent of the men in this age group are physically active.[11] An overview of the change since the 1960s shows a considerable increase in the sport-active population, with an above-average increase of women older than 60.

A 2010 comprehensive report to the German parliament about physical activities and sport in Germany indicated a similar tendency: 64 percent of women and men younger than 70 report that they are active in sport. Between 1990 and 2009, the percentage of active women increased from 49 percent to 66 percent, in large measure because of the greater participation by older women.

Most men and women who take part in sport and physical activities do it at the recreational level. The available information indicates only a little interest in sport competitions among the elderly. A Danish survey shows, for example, that 6 percent of men and 2 percent of women over 70 participate in competitive sports. Still, there are women 80 and older, or 0.3 percent of this age cohort, who take part in sports competitions.

Excellent indicators of the prevalence of sport and exercise among various groups of the population are membership statistics of sport organizations, such as the German Sport Confederation (Deutscher Olympischer Sportbund), which reports 23.8 million memberships, with members over 60 years of age numbering 2.6 million men and 1.8 million women.[12] Similar participation rates are reported in other countries in central and northern Europe where sport is provided by strong and centralized organizations.

A 2014 Eurobarometer report, consisting of surveys about habits, attitudes, and tastes of Europeans, focused on sport and physical activity and found that the number of people engaged in sport and exercises decreased steadily with increasing age. Forty-one percent of Europeans play sport or exercise more or less regularly. Respondents in the Netherlands (94%), Denmark (91%), France (88%), Germany (88%), Belgium (87%), the United Kingdom (86%), and Sweden (85%) reported that local sport clubs or other sport providers offer many opportunities (62). But young men, in particular, seem to make the most use of these possibilities. According to the results of this Eurobarometer survey, around 70 percent of respondents in the 55-plus age group, more women than men, never or only seldomly participated in sport and exercises despite numerous opportunities. A considerable number of Europeans, however, take part in activities such as walking and gardening, which also seem to have a positive influence on health and well-being.[13]

In many European countries, facilities for unorganized "sport for all," for example, jogging tracks, biking lanes, playing fields, and fitness equipment in parks, have been provided in big cities in the hope that people who are not physically active will use them for getting or staying fit. As more or less systematic observations in cities revealed, however, sport and fitness opportunities in informal settings are nearly exclusively used by young men.[14] This and other information on sport participation provides clear evidence that age and gender, especially their interdependencies, have a considerable influence on people's sport-related tastes, habits, and practices.

Aging Women and Sport: Narratives and Role Models

Currently, two contradictory discourses on aging influence the perception and evaluation of the engagement of older people in sport and exercises. Traditionally, aging has been and still is addressed from a medical perspective and has been identified as a problem or even a disease leading to a sedentary lifestyle. But in the past few decades, new discourses gained importance, in particular the concept of positive aging, which celebrates "later life as a period for enjoyment, good health, independence, vitality, exploration, challenge, productivity, creativity, growth, and development."[15] But staying young and healthy and finding meaning in sport and exercise demand considerable effort, depend on continuous engagement, and are matters of luck—as sickness and finally death are not avoidable. Not only training in fitness studios but also participation in competitions or involvement in adventure sports are, for many people, strategies to continue with an active life and to meet new challenges—despite aging.

Complying with the imperative of positive aging, women in particular use sport and exercise as strategies for physical beauty.[16] Following recommendations in the media, such as lifestyle journals like *Fit for Fun* and *Women's*

Health, many women work hard to get or to keep a slim figure or at least get rid of some of the "problem zones" of the aging female body.[17] The various forms of "beautification" have become a flourishing business of personal trainers, adult education institutions, and gymnastics or sport clubs, which promise their clientele will become or stay fit, slim, and "forever young." Although sport and exercise do not guarantee eternal youth, they may help one stay fit and healthy, at least for a while. Therefore, more women than ever before are physically active, and not only the numbers of older women engaging in fitness exercises but also the numbers and performances of female athletes in age categories over 60 and even over 80 are continuously increasing.

Numerous older sportswomen manage to disprove stereotypes about the aging female body and are actively redefining traditional beliefs and behavior of women their age.[18] Scholarly studies, too, point to attempts to deny or resist aging by using sport as an antiaging medicine.[19] At the same time, participants in sports and games negotiate aging processes by taking up a "positive aging discourse."[20]

There are various interrelated reasons for the increasing participation of older men and women in sport and exercise in western countries. Health messages from physicians and governments are ubiquitous, and public concern about the well-being of the aging population is growing. Healthism and ageism, the moral imperatives to be fit and functioning, are conveyed by a multitude of media that provide never-ending messages about body and beauty ideals, as well as information about "antiaging" and "beautification" strategies.[21] Sport and exercise are recommended as highly efficient means in "forever young" endeavors, which are, at the same time, effective policies and means of governmentality in western countries.[22]

For many individuals, youth, slimness and fitness, the "right" bodies, and the "right" sporting activities are elements of conspicuous consumption and contribute to one's social capital.[23] Physical activities in particular are important ingredients of the antiaging projects of women, who are affected much more than men by the beauty dictate prevailing in western cultures.[24] It would be short-sighted and simplistic, however, to ascribe the increasing interest of older women in sport and exercises only to their striving for a youthful appearance. Surveys show there are several interrelated motives, which may also vary according to the sport and the situation. They range from health and maintenance to well-being, from fun (whatever that means) to relaxation, and from being together with friends to doing something for oneself.[25] And aging women are increasingly interested in "serious" sports, intensive training, competitions, and high performance, which until recently were deemed inappropriate and dangerous for women and old people.[26] Notions of resistance, empowerment, identity, and a sense of community were found to be important in terms of understanding the role sport plays in these women's lives. Taking the women's running movement, the participation of seniors in strength and endurance sports, and the Masters Games as examples, I will demonstrate that older women, having transcended numerous barriers and refuted age as well as gender stereotypes, are entering a new sphere, one of performance sport.

It Is Never Too Late to Win—Aging Female Athletes

There are various reasons for the growing participation of older people in competitive sports, among them the sports boom of some decades ago: as athletes became older, they continued to do what they had done before, which included training and competing that rewarded them with a sense of achievement and self-respect. An interview study involving older Danish adults revealed that around one-third of them, more men than women, still participated in some forms of competitive sport. Not only the competitions, but also the training and social relations with their teams and clubs, were highlights in their everyday lives.

According to a German study, approximately 70 percent of senior sportsmen and sportswomen used to compete in sports during at least some stages of their lives.[27] This proportion may have increased in the past decade, however, because interview studies reveal that senior athletes have adopted the ideas and ideals of active aging.[28] Despite the "natural" decline in performance that occurs with age, training can have numerous positive effects not only on health but also on well-being. For women, competitive sport was for a long time controversial, and the prejudicial idea that strenuous physical activities may cause serious health problems for female athletes, especially their reproductive functions, was still widespread when today's seniors were youngsters.[29] Women formed a minority among athletes, and so it is not surprising that they are also underrepresented today among senior competitors, as the rates of male and female participants at the Masters World Games indicate.

In addition, stereotypes about health, physical capacities, and appearance affected and still affect older women and their willingness and ability to participate in sport. According to Vertinsky and Cousins, "the youthful, fertile, sensual female body is thus the 'real' woman: once past reproductive age, she becomes the 'Other,' bound for decrepitude."[30] Old women are often considered frail and weak, their health believed to be endangered by vigorous exercise or physical exertion. These stereotypes are widespread, also among the elderly, who perceive and even fear aging as a period of inevitable physical decline and sport as a privilege of youth. Consequently, older women may expect not only health problems but also negative social consequences.

Although senior women were for a long time a relatively small minority among athletes, it is astonishing that currently more and more women take part in performance sports. Among the most popular women's sports that have encouraged an increasing number of senior women to remain active was—and still is—running. Despite strong societal resistance, women managed to participate in long-distance races such as the marathon, at first unofficially. Female runners have officially taken part in the Boston Marathon since 1972, and in the Olympic marathon since 1984. In the same period, "sport for all" running events emerged and soon gained popularity among women in all age groups.[31]

Even more challenging than long-distance running is the ironman/ironwoman event—an ultralong triathlon with a 3.9-kilometer swim, 180-kilometer cycling event, and a marathon run at the end. The first long-distance triathlon, an ultimate challenge for men, was organized in 1978 in Hawaii, and since 1980 women have taken up this challenge in increasing numbers.

Masters Games

In most sports, competitions for senior athletes are growing in number and gaining in popularity. An excellent example of new ways of coping with getting old is participation in the Masters Games. Besides the quadrennial world event, Masters Games are also organized on regional and national levels. Masters Games are organized in various sports and on several levels. Held in 1985 for the first time, the games have become the world's biggest multisport event and are open to people older than 35 with varying abilities and performance levels. No other qualification is necessary, and for most competitors, participating is more important than winning. For aging elite athletes, however, the games provide the opportunity to be judged against their contemporaries: "Masters athletics provides the athletes with a structure which legitimizes and normalizes age-based attrition in performance, enabling them to retain their athletic identity."[32] Since the 1990s, more and more women have been attracted to this event, not only because of the competitions themselves but also because of the specific atmosphere of these games, where nobody is too old to be appreciated.

In 1985, 468 women and 1,220 men traveled to the first World Masters Games in Toronto.[33] At the 2002 Games in Melbourne, 38 percent of the twenty-five thousand competitors were women. And at the 2009 World Masters Games in Sydney, 41 percent of the more than twenty-eight thousand participants from ninety-five countries were women competing in twenty-eight sports. The average age of the athletes was 50 years; two participants were 100 years old. One of the stars of these games was Ruth Frith, the 100-year-old great-grandmother who set a world record in the shot-put event. She was the only competitor in the age group 100 to 104.

Participation in sports and games is beneficial not only for the athletes but also for the image of and judgments about older individuals in general. The motto of the 2009 Masters World Games, "fit, fun, forever young," addressed the new roles and positive images of seniors as well as the potential of sports to serve as a fountain of youth. This slogan conveys ambivalent messages, however, as it suggests that aging is something negative that must be avoided. The 2017 World Master Games were in Auckland, New Zealand, where more than twenty-eight thousand participants from one hundred countries competed in twenty-eight sports, and 42 percent of the competitors were women. The oldest competitor was Man Kaur, a 101-year-old woman from India, who allegedly started her sport career when she was 93 years old. She had traveled with her 79-year-old son more than thirteen thousand kilometers to compete in the one-hundred-meter and the two-hundred-meter runs as well as in javelin throwing and shot put. She won all these events and ran the one hundred meters in 1 minute 14 seconds, which was a new world record in her age group.[34]

There are various reasons for the attractiveness of the Masters Games: the social contact and the camaraderie, the fun and the challenge, the opportunity to perform and to compete with athletes of the same age—all these factors are important incentives. For many master athletes, traveling to a more or less exotic location and combining sport and holidays are additional benefits. Not only the competitions themselves but also the training for the event provide numerous opportunities for counteracting stereotypes about aging, maintaining bodily abilities, defining new goals, and maybe even giving meaning to life.[35]

Sport federations, too, offer competitions and register the performances of athletes in different age groups. In athletics, for example, there are five-year age groups for participants who are older than 34. For aging women, competitions are situations where not appearance but performance is the center of attention. Sport is thus an arena for deconstructing gender, developing an athletic identity, and gaining a sense of productivity, belonging, self-respect, and appreciation. This interpretation is supported by findings of Dionigi, Rylee, and Horter whose interviewees—twenty-three female and twenty-one male competitors, aged 56–90 years, in World Master Games—emphasized that sport helps them deal with aging processes. Some of them managed at least for a certain time to ignore aging; others intended to fight or to redefine being or getting old. Four themes emerged: "'There's no such thing as old' (a story of avoiding old age); 'Keep moving' (a story of fighting the aging process); 'Fun, fitness, friendship . . . [and] competing' (a story of redefining self and 'old age') and 'making the most of your life . . . with the capabilities that you still have' (a story of adaptation). In this way people use sport to deal—in different ways—with getting older." These stories of a "sporting later life" allow for alternative meanings to the dominant notion of aging narrative focusing on decline.[36]

Not only are aging women's records in various sports, athletics, weight lifting, and cycling astonishing, but so are their performances in risky or outdoor sports such as mountaineering, sailing, dogsledding, ultra-long-distance running, and open-water swimming, activities that are particularly demanding as the athletes find themselves often on their own and confronted with various problems such as bad weather and injuries without being able to rely on external support. Despite multiple challenges, age did not prevent women from mastering these and other adventure sports.

One of these female daredevils of retirement age is Diana Nyad, born in 1949, who swam from Cuba to Florida in 2013 and survived fifty-three hours of danger, as she did not use a protective shark cage.[37] Another adventure swimmer is Lynne Cox, born in 1957. In 1987 she swam more than a mile (1.6 km) and stayed for twenty-five minutes in the six-to-seven-degree (Celsius) cold waters of Antarctica—a world record and an adventure she described in 2004 in one of her books, *Swimming to Antarctica: Tales of a Long-Distance Swimmer*. She began her swimming career in 1971 and conducted, sometimes as the first person, numerous long-distance swims that became more and more challenging. One of her most famous swims was crossing the Bering Strait with the aim of not only setting a record in cold-water swimming but also fostering better relations between the United States and the Soviet Union during the Cold War.

Even more dangerous than long-distance swimming—as measured by the number of deaths—is mountaineering, but age did not prevent old women from climbing in the "death zone." The oldest woman to reach the summit of Mount Everest was Tamae Watanabe (born in 1938), who climbed the mountain in 2002 and again in 2012. In both cases she set a new age record for women. "It was much more difficult for me this time," she stated in 2012. "I felt I was weaker and had less power." She reached the summit from the Tibetan side on May 19 at the age of 73 years and 180 days. Watanabe still holds this record.[38]

A particularly challenging and potentially dangerous endeavor is single-handed sailing. One of the most successful women in this sport is Jeanne Socrates, who continued with long sailing trips after the death of her husband in 2003. When she was stranded because of a failing autopilot and lost her ship as well as many of her possessions, she managed to buy a new ship and to pursue her dream to sail solo nonstop around the world. She completed the journey in July 2013, after 259 days on the sea, and became the oldest woman to accomplish the feat.[39]

Another long-distance sport traditionally considered men's domain is dogsledding. The Iditarod, the world's longest dogsled race, traversing 1,850 kilometers through the Alaskan wilderness, and one of the toughest endurance competitions in the world, seemed to be too dangerous and too exhausting for the "weaker sex." But this assumption was proved wrong, as some of the most successful dog breeders and race participants were and are aging women, such as 64-year-old DeeDee Jonrowe. She reported proudly that the 2017 race would be her thirty-sixth Iditarod and that she finished among the top ten sixteen times.[40] Libby Riddles, a newcomer in 1985, became the first woman to win the Iditarod that year. One of the most successful mushers is Susan Butcher, a four-time winner and, for a time, the speed record holder in this competition. In 2016 Cindy Gallea, 64, a nurse practitioner, was the oldest female participant in the race. She had taken part in the Iditarod many times since 1999 and described her "addiction" as follows: "I have found it difficult to let go of something that is deep in my soul and that gives me the opportunity to run my dogs for days through the beauty of Alaska." Her hobbies are bicycling, hiking, outdoor activities, politics, and "my sons and granddaughter." Her two sons inherited her enthusiasm for long-distance dogsledding.[41]

Older women (and older men) engaging in these and other challenging endeavors are a small minority, but the visibility of their performances can be used as a weapon against sexism and ageism as they spread messages about the capabilities of women and seniors as well as the opportunities of "positive aging," emphasizing the positive influences of sport activities in the lives of elderly people.

A Short Conclusion

The information presented above provides convincing evidence of numerous interrelations between gender and age on the one hand and participation in sport and exercise on the other hand, meaning that sport habits change with age and the ways of aging and "doing gender" are influenced by sports and exercise. However, there is not a sudden stop of engagement in physical activities at a certain time of life but a more or less slow withdrawal from strenuous or dangerous activities.

Changes and Challenges

The growing involvement of older women in sport, the increasing performance level of female "masters athletes," and the great importance that interviewees placed on sport in their lives must be understood in the light of current developments in western countries that have had an effect on the gender order and age structure of our societies. The population in western countries is aging, but aging has changed its forms and its meaning to a certain extent, partly because of improvements in education, the economic situation, and the average state of older people's health. These changes convey new challenges but also offer new opportunities. Because of the high divorce rate and the lower life expectancy of men, many older women, including five of the ten women in my project, are single, which may imply loneliness but also freedom to choose activities and to redefine gender. As the examples of physically active women show, sporting activities allow access to male domains, provide social contacts, can be a source of well-being, and can even attract public attention to aging women, which is particularly important because older people are more or less invisible to the media and in the public sphere, where gendered stereotypes about aging prevail. In western societies, old age is often imagined as an erosion of one's physical, mental, and intellectual faculties and an adaptation of one's personality, tastes, and behavior to the "restrictions" of old age. The women described above are excellent examples of the refutation of those prophecies, even though this process may take a long time. Although the gendered scripts of society offer few attractive roles and ideals for aging women, they increasingly reject traditional roles and even write new scripts that add sport and sporting performance to the "normal biographies" of old women.

Women, more than men, are confronted with the "forever young" mania of our body-oriented and sexualized world. In her groundbreaking 1980s book, *The Beauty Myth*, American author Naomi Wolf identified striving for beauty, slimness, and youth as the fetters that kept women in their place.

Old women were, by definition, unattractive. Many, including some of my friends, have reacted to the youth mania with body and beauty projects and used sport and physical activities to gain or retain a slim body and demonstrate youth and health. Studies indicate, however, that those women who had started to take up sport only as a remedy against aging soon dropped out when they failed to find joy and satisfaction.

The narratives of my friends as well as many empirical studies on the psychological situation of older women show that while there may be crises and losses, they are mostly satisfied with their life circumstances. They learn to adapt wishes and dreams to their present situation, taking advantage of their personal and social resources. Sporting activities and performance, as well as the social capital connected with it, are important resources that may help older women cope with problematic developments and situations. Their examples provide proof that growing older is accompanied by not only losses and problems but also gains and, as the successful aging discourse suggests, a chance of being at peace with oneself. Empirical studies support this positive perspective on aging not least because seniors do not have the same aspirations, expectations, and demands as younger people. The sportswomen of my study, too, accepted their decrease in abilities and performance. Even if their circumstances deteriorate with increasing age, this happens not as a sudden stop but as a continuous process of change that enables people to adapt. Despite growing challenges, it is possible to preserve the ability to adapt and function for a long time.

Asked about the secret of her long life, Ruth Frith, the 100-year-old shot putter mentioned above, answered, "I just think each year is another year. You just enjoy each day, and let the years go by." Examples of positive aging, however, should not obscure problems and pains, the undesirability of "deep old age," and the inevitability of death.[42]

But for all the euphoria about fit and healthy seniors, we should not forget that the trendsetters are only a minority and that the life patterns and living conditions of aging people are becoming increasingly heterogeneous. Even in western countries, the gap between the well-off, healthy, and fun-oriented group of seniors on the one hand and the poor and sick on the other is steadily widening.

Women participating in sport and aiming at sporting performance profit from social changes, particularly from changes in the gender order, and they also contribute to this change. They challenge the notion of the "weak sex" and of aging as decline and make old women and their abilities more visible. Sporting activities and an athletic identity can be assets in the lives of women of all ages, providing them with self-confidence and pride, with social networks, and with aims and structures in everyday lives as well as personal empowerment. The narratives of the aging sportswomen address sport activities as a means of resistance not only to aging but also to gender stereotypes. They provide insights into the various negotiations that allow aging women to cope with gendered expectations and to be successful in a field still dominated by young men.

As I reflect on my own life, there are some pains (lost loves and loved ones) and many pleasures (finding new love, great friends, a sense of fulfillment). I have traveled throughout the world. I have gained many accolades for my research and publications, including a knighthood by the Queen of Denmark, two by the president of Germany, and presidencies of two international scholarly associations. I was even named the person who has done the most for women's sport in Europe by one scholarly organization. I established an ongoing summer school for graduate students that transmits knowledge and develops leaders for the next generation. I have been an advocate for women's sport throughout the world with the hope that such efforts will provide a better future and a positive legacy. So, I can look back on my life with a sense of pride and accomplishment that I have made some measure of difference in bettering people's lives.

NOTES

1. A. Birkeland and G. K. Natvig, "Coping with Ageing and Failing Health: A Qualitative Study among Elderly Living Alone," *International Journal of Nursing Practice* 15 (2009), 257–64.

2. R. Dionigi, "Competitive Sport as Leisure in Later Life: Negotiations, Discourse, and Aging," *Leisure Sciences* 28, no. 2 (March 1, 2006), 181–96 (quote, 181).

3. Dionigi, "Competitive Sport as Leisure," 181.

4. Gertrud Pfister, "Santé, plaisir . . . jeunesse éternelle? Les pratiques physiques de femmes âgées," *Gerontologie et Societe* 40, no. 156 (2018), 181–96.

5. T. Bruce, J. Hovden, and P. Markula, *Sportswomen at the Olympics: A Global Content Analysis of Newspaper Coverage* (Rotterdam: Sense, 2010).

6. N. Degele, "Bodification and Beautification: Zur Verkörperung von Schönheitshandeln / Bodification and Beautification: An Embodiment of Dealing in Beauty Practices," *Sport und Gesellschaft* 1, no. 3 (January 1, 2004), 244–68.

7. L. Gannon, *Women and Aging: Transcending the Myths* (London: Routledge, 1999); Lotte Hvas and Dorte Effersøe Gannik, "Discourses on Menopause, Part II: How Do Women Talk about Menopause?," *Health* 12, no. 2 (2008), 177–92; A. Hyde, J. Nee, E. Howlett, J. Drennan, and M. Butler, "Menopause Narratives: The Interplay of Women's Embodied Experiences with Biomedical Discourses," *Qualitative Health Research* 20, no. 6 (2010), 805–15; M. Lock, *Encounters with Aging: Mythologies of Menopause in Japan and North America* (Berkeley: University of California Press, 1993).

8. K. R. McGannon and J. C. Spence, "Exploring News Media Representations of Women's Exercise and Subjectivity through Critical Discourse Analysis," *Qualitative Research in Sport, Exercise, and Health* 4, no. 1 (March 1, 2012), 32–50; Jennifer Paff Ogle and Mary Lynn Damhorst, "Critical Reflections on the Body and Related Sociocultural Discourses at the Midlife Transition: An Interpretive Study of Women's Experiences," *Journal of Adult Development* 12, no. 1 (2005), 1–18.

9. R. Crawford, "Health as a Meaningful Social Practice," *Health* 10, no. 4 (2006), 401–20; T. M. Calasanti and K. F. Slevin, *Age Matters: Realigning Feminist Thinking* (New York: Routledge, 2006); Todd. D. Nelson, *Ageism* (Oxford: Blackwell, 2006).

10. "Flere aeldre er fysisk aktive og frivillige" [More elderly people are physically active and engaged in volunteerism], Institute for Population Surveys, July 14, 2014, http://www.idan.dk/nyhedsoversigt/nyheder/2014/a539_flere-aeldre-er-fysisk-aktive-og-frivillige/.

11. M. Pilgaard and S. Rask, *Danskernes motions og sportsvaner 2016* [Physical activity and sport habits in Denmark, 2016] (Copenhagen: Sports Analysis Institute, 2016).

12. "We Are Sport in Germany," German Olympic Sport Confederation [Deutscher Olympischer Sport Bund], accessed 2015, https://www.dosb.de/de/service/download-center/statistiken/.

13. Eurobarometer, 2014, https://europa.eu/eurobarometer/screen/home.

14. Pfister, "Santé, plaisir … jeunesse éternelle?"

15. Dionigi, "Competitive Sport as Leisure," 183.

16. Grit Höppner, *Alt und schön Geschlecht und Körperbilder im Kontext neoliberaler Gesellschaften* (Wiesbaden: Verlag für Sozialwissenschaften/Springer, 2011).

17. Pirkko Markula, "Beyond the Perfect Body: Women's Body Image Distortion in Fitness Magazine Discourse," *Journal of Sport and Social Issues* 25, no. 2 (2001), 158–79.

18. Jennifer Hargreaves, *Sporting Females: Critical Issues in the History and Sociology of Women's Sports* (New York: Routledge, 1994), 267.

19. B. Grant, "You're Never Too Old: Beliefs about Physical Activity and Playing Sport in Later Life," *Ageing and Society* 21, no. 6 (2001), 777–98.

20. Dionigi, "Competitive Sport as Leisure," 185.

21. J. S. Smith-Maguire, *Fit for Consumption: Sociology and the Business of Fitness* (London: Routledge, 2008).

22. M. Dean, *Governmentality* (Los Angeles: Sage, 2010).

23. Alan Warde, "Cultural Capital and the Place of Sport," *Cultural Trends* 15, no. 2–3 (2006), 107–22.

24. Degele, "Bodification and Beautification."

25. Gertrud Ursula Pfister, "Noch lange nicht zum alten Eisen—Sportbedürfnisse von Frauen," in *Ein Leben lang in Schwung: Kongress vom 4.-6. Mai 2001 in Hamburg*, ed. W. Tokarski, K. Euteneuer-Treptow, and B. Wagner-Hauthal (Aachen: Pedestal Media, 2002), 1:65–91.

26. Lee Bergquist, *Second Wind: The Rise of the Ageless Athlete* (Champaign IL: Human Kinetics, 2009).

27. A. Conzelmann, "Zur Bedeutung von Alterns- und Trainingseinflüssen für das Erreichen hoher Altersleistungen bei Seniorenleichtathleten," in *Training im Alterssport*, ed. H. Mechling (Schorndorf, Germany: Hofmann, 1998), 112–16.

28. Bergquist, *Second Wind*.

29. Gertrud Pfister and Kevin Wamsley, "Olympic Men and Women: The Politics of Gender in the Modern Games," in *Global Olympics: Historical and Sociological Studies of the Modern Games*, ed. Kevin Young and Kevin Wamsley (Oxford: Elsevier, 2005) 103–25.

30. Patricia Vertinsky and S. Cousins, "The Effects of Gender on Participation in Sport among Older Canadians," in *Sport and Gender in Canada*, ed. Kevin Young and P. White (Don Mills, Ontario: Oxford University Press, 2007), 158.

31. Emmanuelle Tulle and Cassandra Phoenix, eds., *Physical Activity and Sport in Later Life: Critical Perspectives* (Basingstoke, UK: Palgrave Macmillan, 2015).

32. Emmanuelle Tulle, *Ageing, the Body, and Social Change: Running in Later Life* (New York: Palgrave Macmillan, 2008); Vertinsky and Cousins, "Effects of Gender," 167.

33. K. N. Andersen, *Lebenslange Bewegungskultur: Betrachtungen zum Kulturbegriff und zu Möglichkeiten seiner Übertragung auf Bewegungsaktivitäten*, Theorie und Praxis der Erwachsenenbildung (Bielefeld, Germany: Bertelsmann, 2001), 57.

34. Monica Grater, "101 Year Old Wins Four Gold Medals at the World Masters Games," *Runners' World*, April 27, 2017, https://www.runnersworld.com/news /a20854017/101-year-old-wins-four-gold-medals-at-the-world-masters-games/.

35. Vertinsky and Cousins, "Effects of Gender," 167; Grant, "You're Never Too Old."

36. R. A. Dionigi, S. Horton, and J. Baker, "Negotiations of the Ageing Process: Older Adults' Stories of Sports Participation," *Sport, Education, and Society* 18, no. 3 (January 1, 2013), 370–87.

37. Matt Sloane, Jason Hanna, and Dana Ford, "'Never, Ever Give Up': Diana Nyad Completes Historic Cuba-to-Florida Swim," CNN, September 3, 2013, https:// www.cnn.com/2013/09/02/world/americas/diana-nyad-cuba-florida-swim /index.html.

38. "Climber, 73, Finally Felt Old at Summit of Everest," CBS News, May 25, 2012, https://www.cbsnews.com/news/climber-73-finally-felt-old-at-summit-of -everest/.

39. "Jeanne Socrates on S/V *Nereida*: Welcome to My Journeys," website of Jeanne Socrates, accessed September 9, 2021, https://svnereida.com/.

40. "Musher Details: DeeDee Jonrowe," Iditarod: The Last Great Race, accessed September 9, 2021, http://iditarod.com/race/2017/mushers/95-DeeDee-Jonrowe/.

41. "Musher Details: Cindy Gallea," Iditarod: The Last Great Race, accessed September 9, 2021, http://iditarod.com/race/2016/mushers/73-Cindy-Gallea/.

42. Dionigi, "Competitive Sport as Leisure," 187.

Conclusion

GERALD R. GEMS

The biographical sketches of the contributors to this volume, as well as those of their research subjects, indicate a close similarity to previous studies in that the subjects were independent, physically active individuals who followed a healthy diet, remained socially engaged, and had a sense of purpose and fulfillment in their lives.[1] In addition, twenty interviews conducted with 50-to-87-year-old users of fitness facilities at the Nanhu public park in Changchun, China, March 29–31, 2019, augment the international data provided by the contributors in their autoethnographies.[2]

As evident in the contributed essays, race, ethnicity, social class, education, gender, and income remain factors in successful aging. In 2016 in the United States, more than 19 percent of African Americans and more than 18 percent of Hispanic residents lived in poverty, while less than 9 percent of non-Hispanic white residents faced such a dilemma. People without substantial financial resources face greater stress and are more likely to live without a proper diet, necessary medication, and a safe living environment. Older women were more likely to experience such setbacks than elderly men.[3] A recent study showed that 41 percent of the elderly are in danger of running out of money before they die. As a remedy, many in the baby boomer generation are now working longer and retiring at later ages than their predecessors did.[4]

A study of the role of social class in quality of life in Ireland also showed that poverty and financial strain contributed to stress and poor health among more than 25 percent of the population. For those over the age of 70, poor health and safety issues became most prominent for working-class respondents beset by multiple problems.[5]

Among the Chinese participants at the Nanhu Park in Changchun, interviewees represented a spectrum of social class and occupations, from doctors, an engineer, and an architect to factory workers, farmers, and a coal worker. At this point in their lives, all had become urban dwellers and, under the communist welfare system, access to health care did not pose a problem for them. Perhaps more so than in western cultures, they also enjoyed the support of family and friends as they aged. This is an especially important factor for the elderly. In Asian societies, children and grandchildren are expected and even required by law to care for their familial elders.[6]

Among the contributors to this book, none faced poverty or great financial strain in later life, although several were born into the lower ranks of society and worked diligently to improve their social and economic capital. While all experienced the normal stresses of life, they enjoyed the support of family and friends. The best-selling book *Tuesdays with Morrie* provides insight into the importance of family, particularly for those suffering from terminal illness. Family photos, stories, and visits prompt good memories of one's past, reminiscences about youthful follies and later successes, a sense of pride and appreciation, and a reliving of the joys of parenting, things that garner a sense of fulfillment in one's life.[7]

The benefits of higher education and the income derived from such obtainment provided a comfortable retirement for most. All but one of the contributors and at least five of the Chinese interviewees had obtained college degrees, most of which were advanced. All have the leisure time to pursue an active lifestyle. The contributors continue to engage in physical activity that keeps them relatively healthy, while thirteen of the twenty Chinese interviewees pursued physical activity daily for a period of one to five hours. Although not as active now as they were in their youth, these respondents engage in regular exercise that has proved to be a boon in maintaining their health.

Neuroscientist Daniel Levitin contends that engaging in physical activity is the most important factor in successful aging in that it promotes better health and consequent longevity. Group activities enhance social relations and help prevent the isolation, despair, and loneliness that lead to premature death.[8]

Social class influences one's perceptions relative to the value of physical activity. French philosopher Pierre Bourdieu determined that the social class in which one was raised influenced world view and that such a disposition was difficult to change, just as one may acquire a predilection for certain ethnic foods early in life. He called such a mindset one's habitus.[9]

Many working-class people, who generally possess less education, less income, and less social status, esteem physical prowess. Sports such as boxing, American football, and soccer enable participants to publicly display such abilities, and an interest in sport may become a lifelong pursuit. The middle and upper classes, with access to more social and economic capital, may favor different sports, such as tennis and golf, and pursue such lifetime activities to maintain physical health.[10] The type of physical activity is not as important as the actual practice. Just walking is beneficial to the elderly.

The Chinese users of the Nanhu Park facility all professed awareness of the health benefits of regular exercise, but some expressed a working-class habitus relative to sport. Dr. Lei, at 80 years old, fondly recalled his days as an interscholastic athlete on basketball, track-and-field, volleyball, and table tennis teams. Mr. Hu, another 80-year-old and a former teacher, reminisced about his days as an ice hockey player. Mrs. Sun, a 53-year-old company worker, played both basketball and volleyball on school and company teams; while 66-year-old Mrs. Li, an engineer, engaged in volleyball, badminton, and equestrian events. Others took great pride in demonstrating their great flexibility and still prominent gymnastic skills on the high bar and parallel bars.[11]

Among the contributors to this book, several with working-class roots detail their continued attraction to sports such as running, weightlifting, baseball, and soccer that attracted them during their youth. Others pursued more middle-class activities such as tennis, golf, and skiing or adapted

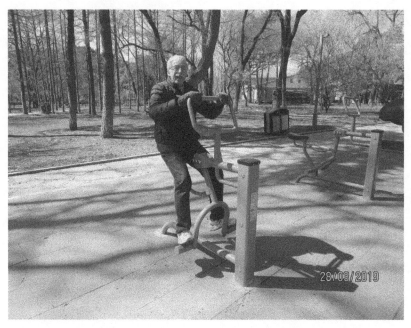

The author/editor at Nanhu Park in Changchun, China. Photo by Gertrud Pfister.

their leisure activities to other interests as they aged, but all remain active to some degree.

A study begun in 1995 by the National Institutes of Health tracked the physical activity of more than 315,000 people, aged 50 to 71. Subjects, who differed by gender, race, ethnicity, and educational level, lived in six states across the United States and two urban centers, Atlanta and Detroit. Fifty-eight percent of the subjects were men. Even those who had been inactive and resumed physical activity between the ages of 40 and 61 had a 32–35 percent lower risk of mortality, similar to those who had been exercising their entire lives. Those who exercised also decreased their chances of getting cancer or heart disease. A study published in *Preventive Medicine* in 2017 claimed that those who exercised enjoyed a nine-year aging advantage over sedentary persons.[12] Spanish researchers found similar benefits for subjects who began exercising later in life. They followed 2,836 subjects over the age of 60 for two years and found that those who engaged in moderate exercise decreased the risk of developing cardiovascular disease by 25 percent and those who engaged in vigorous activity dropped their risk by 58 percent.[13]

Regular exercise that increases heart rate provides additional benefits as one ages. The American Heart Association recommends 150 minutes of regular and moderate exercise per week and 75 minutes of more vigorous exercise per week.[14] Exercise has been shown to be a "powerful intervention for greater immunity and [to] improve health in the elderly, the obese, patients with cancer, and [people with] viral infections."[15]

Maintenance of one's flexibility decreases the chance of injuries due to falling, and strength training lessens bone loss and fractures.[16] See the remarkable videos of older adults engaging in modified forms of parkour, a form of running combined with gymnastics that began evolving in France in the 1970s.[17] Other videos show older women, some in their seventies, still performing on gymnastic rings and a trapeze.[18] A recent study followed skateboarders in their forties and fifties.[19] It is during midlife when "individuals tend to revaluate [sic] their sense of identity and confront issues of bodily decline, morbidity, and death."[20] Group exercise or team sports provided the additional benefits of sociability, a positive change in self-concept and psychological well-being, a reduction in depression, and greater cognition in the elderly.[21]

Many of the Chinese participants in the park activities clearly enjoyed socializing with friends, often exercising in groups. Mrs. Sun stated that "doing physical exercise is not only for keeping in better physical condition but also for improving mental health." Another respondent, an 80-year-old doctor, came to the fitness site in the afternoon and again in the evening, as he believed that exercise kept him "mentally refreshed, energetic, and vigorous."[22] Such activity need not be competitive in nature, nor physically demanding, as demonstrated by those who partake in regular dancing.[23]

In South Korea the government provides community dances for seniors over the age of 60. Lee Do-sun, the director of a welfare care center in Seoul, claims that "freestyle dancing helps seniors move muscles they wouldn't normally use, and participating in mass sing-alongs can be effective in preventing Alzheimer's." One of the dancers, 78-year-old Byeon Jeong-ja,

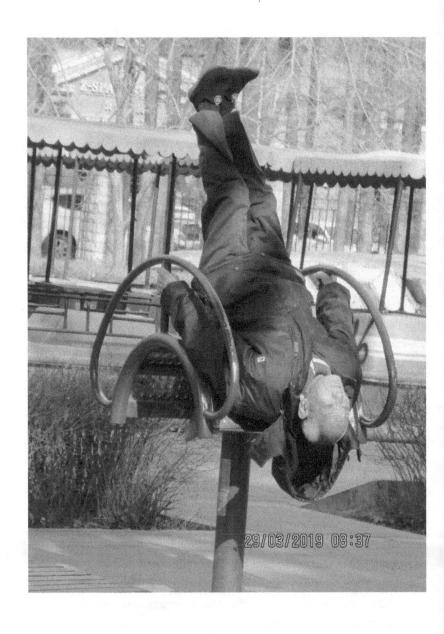

Elderly fitness adherent at Nanhu Park in Changchun, China. Photo by Gerald Gems.

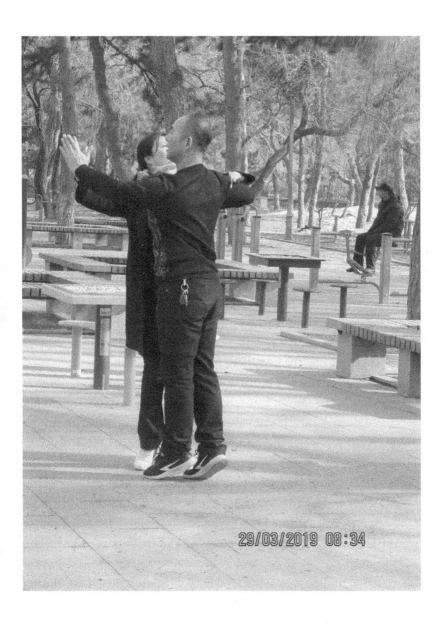

Ballroom dancing at Nanhu Park in Changchun, China. Photo by Gerald Gems.

stated, "I can't even describe how great this program is, both mentally and physically. It's good for my health and I get to relieve my stress." Another female participant, 75-year-old Cho Sun-bun, said that the dances made her feel "twenty years younger." The senior disco parties not only led older adults to make new friends but also diminished "distrust and hostility that existed [between] people of different socioeconomic backgrounds," providing both individual and social benefits.[24]

The closing of gyms and fitness centers during the global COVID pandemic resulted in less physical activity for many, and as people quarantined themselves, their level of socialization was diminished. Such conditions increased symptoms of gloom and depression. It has been shown that exercise boosts the immune system and contributes to the improvement of both mental and physical health.[25]

The choreographer Twyla Tharp offered her perspective on the benefits of dancing. At age 78, she performs regular exercises but also works on dance routines for two hours daily. She subscribes to a different perception of aging, stating that the body does not diminish but alters and changes. "An astute person changes with it rather than fights against it.... You have to be willing to change.... You don't want to have a goal that you cannot accomplish. You want one that will continuously pull you along to the next discovery."[26] A positive mental outlook is essential to successful aging. Though the body may be more restricted in its physical capabilities, the brain is still capable of new learning and new pleasures.

One study, in which a survey was offered randomly to more than a thousand respondents, both men and women aged 18–40, showed that people who disliked physical education classes in school maintained that feeling and did not engage in exercise later in life, while those who enjoyed physical education continued to be active later in life.[27] Some schools have already changed their curricular offerings to lessen competitive activities and offer more electives, such as dancing and yoga.

Other countries have taken an active role in trying to engage the elderly in productive physical activity. In China, municipalities provide free public exercise facilities in parks as well as in apartment complexes. Tai chi classes are conducted in the parks and in public plazas early every morning, and

Chinese families reinforce the study of martial arts training over generations. Tai chi is particularly useful in that it allows for individual interpretations of movement at a slow speed. It is not goal oriented and is inclusive.[28]

Rural dwellers, however, do not have easy access to such facilities, a primary requirement for regular usage. Free access to fitness machines is available at some parks in the United States but is not yet the norm. Outdoor gyms appeared in London in 2009, but frequent use by youth and young children discouraged the elderly from participation. Denmark has taken a proactive measure to provide more possibilities for activity by older people. While skateboard parks and parkour playgrounds attract the young, activity centers for adults aged 65 and older in Copenhagen allow members to determine their activity program offerings by consensus. Seated flexibility and strength exercises accommodate the more infirm; while such games as floorball, similar to floor hockey, allow for somewhat greater exertion. For the more competitive individuals, there are regular running events and age-group soccer leagues for men and women aged 50 and older.[29]

Contributors to this book largely matched those in other research studies relative to their diet consisting of fiber, fruits and vegetables, beans, nuts and seeds, and limited amounts of sweets and fried foods.[30] Healthy eating adds years to one's life. The long-lived residents of blue zones eat substantial amounts of beans and eat meat only once per week. In addition, the Mediterranean diet, which consists of fruits and vegetables, olive oil, fish, legumes such as peas and beans, and whole grains like wheat, oats, corn, and rice, has been shown to decrease cognitive impairment as people age, a safeguard against the onset of dementia.[31]

The oldest contributor in this study shows no sign of cognitive impairment, and her lifestyle fits that of the studied centenarians. She eats sparingly, mostly salads, fruits, and vegetables, and cooks with olive oil. She drinks water, coffee, and an occasional glass of wine, beverages consistent with that of centenarians. Gianni Pes, an epidemiologist who studies centenarians, cautions that the spouses of centenarians live longer than siblings of centenarians, which may indicate that one's lifestyle is more important than one's genetic makeup.[32]

Most of the contributors to this book benefited from higher education, and all had found their purpose in life. Many were teachers, with or without teaching credentials, such as grandparents who helped to raise grandchildren and great-grandchildren. "When older adults share experience and knowledge with the young, they gain emotional satisfaction and feelings of fulfillment, according to a Stanford Center for Longevity report."[33] As stated in *Tuesdays with Morrie*, aging should not be perceived as a period of decline. "As you grow, you learn more. . . . Aging is not just decay . . . it's growth."[34]

Julia "Hurricane" Hawkins, the 103-year-old track star noted in the introduction, stated the importance of continuing to persevere as one ages. "I just like the feeling of being independent and doing something a little different and testing myself, trying to get better." Anna Mary Robertson, better known as Grandma Moses, didn't start painting until the age of 75 and continued doing so at 101. George Shultz, a secretary of state under President Ronald Reagan, published his eleventh book at age 97. Before he died in February 2021, he worked out regularly with a Pilates instructor.[35] Musician Judy Collins continues to write music and perform at the age of 80. She admonishes others to "never stop growing. Never stop being curious."[36] Successful aging requires intellectual growth.

Regardless of social class origins, almost all the contributors to this study managed to improve their socioeconomic status by virtue of their education. They have chosen careers that are both fulfilling and satisfying, and can reflect on their successful achievements. They are independent yet engaged with the larger culture. They are cheerful optimists who care for others. They have demonstrated that they are resilient and able to persevere in times of adversity or hardship. They are resourceful and train both the body and the mind, and all seem to have found their purpose in life.

Neenah Ellis interviewed numerous centenarians for her book *If I Live to Be 100*. On the whole, she found them to possess similar qualities. They were positive thinkers, who persevered through difficult times, "curious and generous, with open minds and open hearts."[37] They exhibited independence, passion, serenity, and fulfillment in their old age. Anna Wilmot, a former basketball player, still enjoyed skinny-dipping at 100. Abraham Goldstein never married but found contentment as a teacher for 70 years, still tutoring students at 100. Margaret Rawson, an expert on dyslexia, wrote a book at age 96, while Marion Cowen continued to work on a novel at 101. Sadie and Gilbert Hall still danced and played shuffleboard together beyond the century mark. Similarly, Ruth Ellis started a self-defense class at 80, and still danced and bowled at 99. Helen Boardman remarried at 97, to a man of 78. Ray Stamper also remarried, to his fourth wife, at age 103. They did not lose their zest for life and reveled in new opportunities.[38]

Old age inevitably results in reflection, and it is important to remember not only the past, which created one's identity, but also the present, in which a new identity is formed. Sport sociologist Liz Pike stated that "ageing does not have to be experienced as a deficit or heroic, but an everyday sense of acceptance of who one is."[39] Other scholars agree that acceptance of one-self, as well as active engagement, close personal relationships, happiness, and enjoyment are keys to successful aging.[40]

As stated by Professor Morrie Schwartz in *Tuesdays with Morrie*, "you have to find what's good and true and beautiful in your life as it is now."[41] As one approaches his or her inevitable end, there is solace in knowing that "we can die without really going away. All the love you created is still there. All the memories are still there. You live on in the hearts of everyone you have touched and nurtured while you were here."[42] That sentiment can be appreciated by all regardless of their station in life.

One divergence from previous studies of successful aging was the lack of importance placed on religion. While contributors espoused a variety of religious beliefs, as well as atheistic convictions, none expressed an overriding influence of religion in their lives.[43] This finding is consistent with an increase in secularization over the past century.

I suggest that the process of aging should be reconceptualized according to the wellness paradigm of psychologist Abraham Maslow, which permits older adults to negotiate and challenge negative conceptions of aging and resist the dominant discourses and power relations that create such stereotypes.

As noted in chapter 1, Maslow proposed his hierarchy of physical, emotional, and social needs as early as 1943 and refined it thereafter in a pyramid model. The physiological needs of food, shelter, and clothing that form the base of the pyramid are followed by safety, and then emotional needs, such as love. The fourth level is esteem, and the top of the pyramid is self-actualization, or reaching one's full potential in life. Maslow contended that only 6 percent of individuals reached that point. Among the contributors to this study the majority might be judged to have accomplished that goal, as they have excelled across the criteria.[44] The contributors to this study also indicated the value of team sports or group activities in promoting socialization and inclusion.

Although sport need not be a requirement in any stage, clearly those engaged in the masters competitions and sport clubs, like many of the contributors to this study, experience a sense of community and camaraderie in physical activity. A 2013 study showed that masters athletes accepted the aging process and adapted to redefine the typical "declining body" narrative.[45] A more recent study of Canadian masters athletes ascertained that they not only achieved greater levels of health and fitness but also made more friends and had lower stress levels. Negotiating the aging process became positive and empowering.[46]

The perils of the heroic model portrayed by the masters athletes have been previously noted. Not everyone can reach that level of self-actualization, which is based on an ethnocentric standard of worth and value and might better be termed a sense of fulfillment. In that sense, all should be able to reach the level of esteem at which they feel valued and respected as they age gracefully.

For the more educated and economically secure upper classes, such levels of Maslow's hierarchy are more easily achieved. They are more likely to engage in sport or some form of physical activity for good health. Many working-class people, however, engage in sport to acquire esteem through their physical prowess, which inevitably decreases as one ages. Among the contributors to this study who came from working-class origins, all but one managed to improve their socioeconomic status, yet all remained engaged in physical activity, supporting Bordieu's concept of habitus. While the Masters Games competition provided such outlets for some, training and travel require financial expenditures well beyond the budgetary means of many.[47]

Relative to the other steps in Mazlow's hierarchy, all contributors could meet their basic physiological needs such as adequate food and safety. As for psychological and emotional needs, all had gained a measure of love from family, spouses, partners, and friends. Almost all had reached Mazlow's epitome of the self-actualized person by virtue of their widespread recognition as scholars, teachers, administrators, and athletes. For the few younger contributors who have not yet achieved such goals, it is clear that they are taking the steps to reach such acclaim. The oldest contributor, Frances Gems, was unable to reach her aspirations. Her father, an illiterate Sicilian shepherd who stowed away on a ship to America, met his future wife on the voyage, a motherless girl raised by nuns. They produced eleven children, only six of which survived to adulthood. Gifted with musical talent, Frances was denied the opportunity to pursue her ambitions due to the ethnic, social class, and gender norms to which her father subscribed. Upon her high school graduation, he deemed it necessary for her to seek immediate employment to meet the family needs. Upon marriage she assumed the traditional role of the domestic housewife and nurturing mother but won the esteem of neighbors for her charitable works. She extended that communal service to her parish church and school, where she helped cook a daily meal for fifteen hundred students. Fellow parishioners elected her to preside over a large mothers' club, and enrollment reached a record number under her administration. Her limited musical ambitions were expressed in the parish's annual theater productions. Although self-actualization in Maslow's sense eluded her, she clearly enjoyed the esteem of her contemporaries. As her story indicates, in old age she served as the family matriarch, thoroughly involved in the child-rearing of her great-grandchildren as a master teacher, extolling the wisdom gained in nearly a century of existence.

While aging is an inevitable and progressive process, it occurs at different rates in individuals, and some aspects, such as one's resting heart rate and personality, do not change unless the latter is afflicted by dementia. A positive state of mind can make the process an enjoyable one. Philosopher Seymour Kleinman stated that "the experience of activity should become an increasingly qualitative one for us as we age. It should provide and enable us to reach a level of maturity, self-knowledge, and enlightenment to which the young can only aspire."[48] Aging should be perceived not as a period of decline but as a unique developmental stage. The elderly have more wisdom, derived from a lifetime of maturation that brings a greater perspective relative to tolerance and understanding, which can be shared with younger generations.[49]

Neuroscientist Daniel Levitin states, "Older adults live differently than younger adults, spending more of their available time doing things they like." He states that happiness increases after the age of 54.[50] Aging should thus be perceived as an enjoyable and welcome stage of life rather than a negative experience, and we should all aspire to a well-lived existence.

NOTES

1. John Withington, *Secrets of the Centenarians: What Is It Like to Live for a Century and Which of Us Will Survive to Find Out?* (London: Reaktion Books, 2017), 97–100, 198–203; Dan Buettner, *Blue Zones: The Science of Living Longer* (Washington DC: National Geographic Society, 2016), 8–9; Elizabeth C. J. Pike, "Physical Activity and Narratives of Successful Aging," in *Physical Activity and Sport in Later Life*, ed. Emmanuelle Tulle and Cassandra Phoenix, 21–31 (Basingstoke, UK: Macmillan, 2015); Matthew Carroll and Helen Bartlett, "Aging Well across Cultures," in *Routledge Handbook of Cultural Gerontology*, ed. Julia Twigg and Wendy Martin, 285–92 (London: Routledge, 2015).

2. Interviews were conducted with the assistance of graduate student "Dolores" Li Jiaqi of the Northeast Normal University in Changchun, China. The twenty interviewees were among sixty persons who frequented the fitness site regularly. In addition to those engaged in use of the exercise and gymnastic equipment, nighttime brought an additional nine couples, as well as nearly a dozen independent dancers who practiced their ballroom steps to music provided with a boom box.

3. American Psychological Association, "Fact Sheet: Age and Socioeconomic Status," accessed July 31, 2019, https://www.apa.org/pi/ses/resources/publications/age; Kerstin Gerst Emerson and Jennifer Gay, "Physical Activity and Cardiovascular Disease among Older Adults: The Case of Race and Ethnicity," *Journal of Aging and Physical Activity* 25, no. 4 (October 2017), 505–9.

4. Judith Graham, "Boomers in the Next Decade: Working Longer, Living Better," Kaiser Health News, January 16, 2020, https.abcnews.go.com/Business/boomers -decade-working-longer-living/story?id=683319514&cid=clicksource_4380645 _12_hero_headlines_headlines_hed.

5. Economic and Social Research Institute, "Quality of Life Problems Differ by Age Group and Social Class," accessed July 31, 2019, https://www.esri.ie/news /quality-of-life-problems-differ-by-age-group-and-social-class.

6. Sarah Lamb, "Beyond the View of the West: Ageing and Anthropology," and Alfred C. M. Chan and Carl H. K. Ma, "Ageing Trends in the Asia-Pacific Region," both in Twigg and Martin, *Routledge Handbook of Cultural Gerontology*, 37–44, and 428–37, respectively.

7. Mitch Albom, *Tuesdays with Morrie: An Old, Man, a Young Man, and Life's Greatest Lesson* (New York: Doubleday, 1997), 90–95. See Zoe Lake, Ashley Riegle, Mack Muldofsky, and Anthony Rivas, "Town Square Senior Daycare Center in San Diego Treats Dementia Patients by Helping Them Relive the 1950s," ABC News, August 30, 2019, https://abcnews.go.com/US/town-square-senior-daycare -center-san-diego-treats/story?id=65299324&cid=clicksource_4380645_null _bf_related, on the use of reminiscence therapy for patients with dementia.

8. Daniel J. Levitin, *Successful Aging: A Neuroscientist Explores the Power and Potential of Our Lives* (New York: Dutton, 2020), 165, 179, 281–85.

9. Pierre Bourdieu, *Outline of a Theory of Practice* (Cambridge: Cambridge University Press, 1977).

10. Victoria J. Palmer, "Keeping It in the Family: The Generational Transmission of Physical Activity," in Tulle and Phoenix, *Physical Activity and Sport in Later Life*, 69–80, relates the inculcation of a love for hiking across three generations of a Scottish family as evidence of an ingrained habitus of shared beliefs and practices.

11. "Dolores" Li Jiaqi interviews, in author's possession.

12. David C. Nieman and Laurel M. Wentz, "The Compelling Link between Physical Activity and the Body's Defense System," *Journal of Sport and Health Science*, November 16, 2018, https://www.sciencedirect.com/science/article.pii /S209524618301005; "New to Exercise? Benefits Are Big, Study Reveals," *AARP Bulletin* 60, no. 4 (May 2019), 4; *Preventive Medicine* cited in Mike Zimmerman, "99 Ways to Add Healthy Years to Your Life," *AARP Bulletin*, January–February 2019, 10–16, (citation, 11); Pedro F. Saint-Maurice, Diarmuid Coughlan, Scott P. Kelly, Sarah K. Keadle, Michael B. Cook, Susan A. Carlson, Janet B. Fulton, and Charles E. Matthews, "Association of Leisure-Time Physical Activity across the Adult Life Course with All-Cause and Cause-Specific Mortality," *JAMA* 2, no. 3 (2019), doi: 10.1001/jamanetworkopen.2019.0355.

13. Sara Higueras-Fresnillo, Pilar Guallar-Castillón, Verónica Cabanas-Sanchez, Jose R. Banegas, Fernando Rodríguez-Artalejo, and David Martinez-Gomez, "Changes in Physical Activity and Cardiovascular Mortality in Older Adults," *Journal of Geriatric Cardiology* 14, no. 4 (2017), 280–81.

14. "American Heart Association Recommendations for Physical Activity in Adults and Kids," American Heart Association, accessed February 1, 2021, https://www.heart.org/en/healthy-living/fitness/fitness-basics/aha-recs-for-physical-activity-in-adults#:~:text=Recommendation.

15. Richard J. Simpson, Hawley Kunz, Nadia Agha, and Rachel Graff, "Exercise and the Regulation of Immune Functions," in *Progress in Molecular Biology and Translational Science*, ed. Claude Bouchard, 135 (Burlington MA: Academic Press, 2015), 355–80 (quote, 356). Also see R. Andrew Shanely, David C. Nieman, Drew A. Henson, Fuxia Jin, Amy M. Knab, and W. Sha, "Inflammation and Oxidative Stress Are Lower in Physically Fit and Active Adults," *Scandinavian Journal of Medicine and Science in Sports* 23 (2013), 215–23.

16. Zimmerman, "99 Ways," 11–12; Bonnie Field, Tom Cochrane, Racel Davey, and Yohannes Kinfu, "Walking Up to One Hour Per Week Maintains Mobility as Older Women Age: Findings from an Australian Longitudinal Study," *Journal of Aging and Physical Activity* 25, no. 2 (April 2017), 269–76, followed more than ten thousand women aged midseventies to late eighties over a twelve-year period.

17. Jeffrey L. Kidder, *Parkour and the City: Risk, Masculinity, and Meaning in a Postmodern City* (New Brunswick NJ: Rutgers University Press, 2017), 18–46. Sincere thanks to Damien Puddle of the University of Waikato in New Zealand for providing access to the following videos, both accessed July 24, 2019: http://www.pkmove.org/pk-silver.html and http://www.westcoastparkour.co.uk/london-seniors.

18. "Movement of Bones: Strong and Active for Life," See and Do, accessed July 24, 2019, http://see-do.com/portfolio/movement-of-bones-2/.

19. Paul O'Connor, "Beyond the Youth Culture: Understanding Middle-Aged Skateboarders through Temporal Capital," *International Review for the Sociology of Sport* 53, no. 8 (December 2018), 924–43.

20. Rylee A. Dionigi and Chelsea Litchfield, "The Mid-life 'Market' and the Creation of Sporting Sub-cultures," in *Sport and Physical Activity across the Lifespan: Critical Perspectives*, ed. Rylee A. Dionigi and Michael Gard (Palgrave, 2018), 283–300 (quote, 287).

21. Anne-Marie Elbe, Stine Nylandsted Lyhne, Esben Elholm Madsen, and Peter Krustup, "Is Regular Physical Activity a Key to Mental Health? Commentary on 'Association between Physical Exercise and Mental Health in 1.2 Million Individuals in the USA between 2011 and 2015: A Cross-Sectional Study,' by Chekroud et al., Published in *Lancet Psychiatry*," *Journal of Sport and Health Science*, November 22, 2018, accessed January 15, 2019; Yu-Kai Chang, Yu-Hsiang Nien, Chia-Liang Tsai, and Jennifer L. Etnier, "Physical Activity and Cognition

in Older Adults: The Potential of Tai Chi Chuan," *Journal of Aging and Physical Activity* 18, no. 4 (October 2010), 451–72; Claire R. Jenkin, Rochelle M. Eime, Hans Westerbeek, and Jannique G. Z. van Uffelen, " Sports for Adults Aged 50+ Years: Participation Benefits and Barriers," *Journal of Aging and Physical Activity* 26, no. 3 (July 2018), 363–71. Michael Ego, "Sport, Dementia, and Alzheimer's Disease: Cause, Cure, and Compassion?," August 21, 2018, https://www.blogs .hss.ed.ac.uk/sport-matters/2017/01/10, presents some innovative programs in Scotland and the United States that employ recollections of soccer and baseball to promote socialization among elderly with dementia.

22. "Dolores" Li Jiaqi with Mrs. Sun and unidentified doctor on March 31, 2019. See Maria Priscila Wermilinger Ávila, Jimilly Capto Corrêa, Alessandra Lamas Granero Luchetti, and Giancarlo Luchetti, "The Role of Physical Activity in the Association between Resilience and Mental Health in Older Adults," *Journal of Aging and Physical Activity* 26, no. 2 (May 2018), 248–53.

23. Cecilie Thogersen-Ntoumani, Anthony Papathomas, Jonathan Foster, Eleanor Quested, and Nikos Ntoumanis, "Shall We Dance? Older Adults' Perspectives on the Feasibility of a Dance Intervention for Cognitive Function," *Journal of Aging and Physical Activity* 26, no. 4 (October 2018), 553–60; "Footloose," *AARP: The Magazine*, June–July 2019, 38, details the nearly two dozen dance halls in Chongqing, China, frequented by the elderly, where a partner is not a necessity. I observed similar ballroom dancers on March 31, 2019, in a public park in Changchun, China, where both partnered and independent dancers practiced their steps to music emanating from a boom box.

24. Hansol Park, "Modeling, Freestyle Dancing: South Korea's Creative Solutions to Keep Its Rapidly Aging Population Young," ABC News, November 2, 2019, https://abcnews.go.com/International/modeling-freestyle-dancing-south-koreas -creative-solutions-rapidly/story?id=66685974.

25. Arti Sahu and Waqar M. Naqvi, "Quarantine Exercises in the Time of Covid-19: A Review," *Journal of Evolution of Medical and Dental Sciences* 9, no. 26 (2020), 1922–27.

26. Twyla Tharp, "People Are Terrified of Change, Period," *AARP Bulletin*, March 2020, 32.

27. Gretchen Reynolds, "How You Felt About Gym Class May Impact Your Exercise Habits Today," *New York Times*, August 22, 2018.

28. Junyu Deng, "A Case Study of Family Intergeneration Transmission of Chinese Martial Arts," presented at the 2019 World Congress of the Sociology of Sport, University of Otago, Dunedin, New Zealand, April 26; Gary Kenyon, "Physical Activity and Dementia: Tai-Chi as Narrative Care," in Tulle and Phoenix, *Physical Activity and Sport in Later Life*, 92–100.

29. Jinyua Lin, "Research on the Social Support of Elderly Migrant Women's Sport Participation in China," presented at the 2019 World Congress of the Sociology of Sport, University of Otago, Dunedin, New Zealand, April 26; Alistair John, "Outdoor Gyms: An Analysis of Public Leisure Spaces in London," presented at the 2019 World Congress of the Sociology of Sport, University of Otago, Dunedin, New Zealand, April 25; Adam B. Evans, Anne Nistrup, and Gertrud Pfister, "Active Ageing in Denmark; Shifting Institutional Landscapes and the Intersection of National and Local Priorities," *Journal of Aging Studies* 46 (2018), 1-9. Gertrud Pfister and Verena Lenneis, "Aging Women Still Play Games: (Auto) ethnographic Research in a Fitness Intervention," in Tulle, and Phoenix, eds. *Physical Activity and Sport in Later Life*, 149-60, indicated that the noncompetitive (no score kept) floorball games produced enthusiasm and a sense of joy, as the women stated that they "felt like a child again" (157) as they perceived the physical activity as fun rather than work.

30. Buettner, *Blue Zones*, 8-9, 12-17, 23-29, 33, 40-4, 46-50; Hyung Wook Park, *Old Age, New Science: Gerontologists and Their Bisocial Visions, 1900-1960* (Pittsburgh: University of Pittsburgh Press, 2016), 129-69; Monique Tello, "Healthy Lifestyle: 5 Keys to a Longer Life," *Harvard Health Blog*, March 25, 2020.

31. Zimmerman, "99 Ways," 12; Hallie Levine, "Is It Alzheimer's . . . or LATE?," AARP online, May 10, 2019, https://hssm.semel.ucla.edu/longevity/news/it -alzheimersor-late.

32. Dan Buettner, "Foods to Live By," *National Geographic*, January 2020, 104-21.

33. Levine, "Is It Alzheimer's . . . or LATE?,"16.

34. Albom, *Tuesdays with Morrie*, 118.

35. Levitin, *Successful Aging*, 23 (quote), 24, 117-18.

36. Levitin, *Successful Aging*, 135.

37. Neenah Ellis, *If I Live to Be 100: Lessons from the Centenarians* (New York: Three Rivers Press, 2004), 7.

38. Ellis, *If I Live to Be 100*.

39. Elizabeth C. J. Pike, "Outdoor Adventurous Sport: For All Ages?," in Dionigi and Gard, *Sport and Physical Activity*, 309.

40. Kelly Carr, Kristy Smith, Patricia Weir, and Sean Horton, "Sport, Physical Activity, and Aging: Are We on the Right Track?," in Dionigi and Gard, *Sport and Physical Activity*, 317-46.

41. Albom, *Tuesdays with Morrie*, 120.

42. Albom, *Tuesdays with Morrie*, 174.

43. Joanna Malone and Anna Dadswell, "The Role of Religion, Spirituality, and/or Belief in Positive Ageing," *Geriatrics* 3, no. 2 (June 2018), https://www.ncbi.nlm .nih.gov/pmc/articles/PMC6319229/; Helen Lavretsky, "Spirituality and Aging,"

Aging Health 6, no. 6 (2010), 749–69; Lindanor Jaco Chaves and Claudia Aranha Gil, "Older People's Concepts of Spirituality Related to Aging and Quality of Life," *Ciencia & Saude Coletiva* 20, no. 12 (December 2015), http://www.scielo .br/scielo.php?pid=S1413-81232015001203641&script=sci_arttext&tlng=en.

44. Abraham H. Maslow, "A Theory of Human Motivation," *Psychological Review* 50, no. 4 (1943), 370–96.

45. R. A. Dionigi, S. Horton, and J. Baker, "Negotiations of the Ageing Process: Older Adults' Stories of Sports Participation," *Sport, Education, and Society* 18, no. 3 (2013), 370–87.

46. Jordan Deneau, Rylee Dionigi, and Sean Horton, "The Benefits of Masters Sport to Healthy Aging," Sport Information Resource Center, March 21, 2020, https:// sirc.ca/blog/the-benefits-of-masters-sport-to-healthy-aging/.

47. Dionigi and Litchfield, "The Mid-life 'Market' and the Creation of Sporting Sub-cultures," in Dionigi and Gard, *Sport and Physical Activity*, 288–95; Carr, Smith, Weir, and Horton, "Sport, Physical Activity, and Aging," 325–28.

48. James S. Skinner, "Biological, Functional, and Chronological Age," and Seymour Kleinman, "Aging and a Changing View of the Body," 62–65 (quote, 64), both in *American Academy of Physical Education, Physical Activity and Aging: Sixtieth Annual Meeting, Kansas City MO: April 5-6, 1988* (Champaign IL: Human Kinetics, 1989). Thanks to Susan Bandy for bringing this source to my attention.

49. Levitin, *Successful Aging*, xii–xxii.

50. Levitin, *Successful Aging*, 370–72 (quote, 371), 400.

APPENDIX

AGING PROJECT SURVEY

1. Provide a historical sketch of your life: date of birth, gender identity, ethnic or racial ancestry, social class, any religious affiliation, education, sports participation.
2. Have you experienced any prejudice, discomfort, et cetera due to any of these characteristics? Please explain.
3. How have these or other factors affected your sense of identity?
4. What are your hobbies and/or interests?
5. At what age are people considered to be elderly in your culture? What government services are offered to assist the elderly in their social, medical, financial needs, et cetera?
6. How do you perceive your aging body?
7. What strategies or coping mechanisms are applicable to the aging process? Dietary changes, social life, et cetera? Is sport or physical activity involved? If so, please explain.
8. What do you consider to be your successes or achievements thus far? Do you feel a sense of pride or self-esteem in your past? What personal qualities have enabled you to reach such accomplishments?
9. What are the particular joys and fears in aging? Does age bring greater wisdom?

10. Have you experienced personal setbacks? Have you experienced any bouts of depression? Any health problems? How have you coped with such episodes?

11. Would you characterize yourself as an optimist or a pessimist, resilient or complacent? Do you engage in nostalgia?

12. How important has friendship and love been in your life?

13. Do you have any regrets, or do you have a sense of fulfillment?

14. Have you thought about your legacy? How would you like to be remembered?

15. How do you look toward the future? What is left for you?

CONTRIBUTORS

A retired professor from the University of Birmingham, United Kingdom, **TANSIN BENN** had a long career in teaching, lecturing, and research in the fields of physical education, dance, and sociocultural topics. Her insights come from reflecting on a lifetime of movement as a significant part of her identity and the ways that it influenced her understanding of opportunities and challenges faced by others in the field of human movement.

JAMES R. COATES JR. is a retired university professor at the University of Wisconsin, Green Bay. His work focuses on teaching, cultural studies, and sport, leisure, and recreation in the African American community. He has lectured, consulted, presented, and published articles and essays on sport, education, and African American history. Coates was an educator for forty-four years.

JANICE J. CROSSWHITE is a retired physical education teacher, education consultant, lecturer, executive officer, sports administrator, sports consultant, and recreation planner. The Australian has worked across commonwealth, state, and local government levels as well as operated her own consultancy. Janice has demonstrated a high level of volunteer commitment to community organizations across education, sport, and the environment. She was awarded an Australian Sports Medal in 2000 for services to basketball, and the Order of Australia Medal in 2002 for services to the community and women's sport.

MAHA EBEID'S education, scholarly achievements, and administrative abilities gained her election to the position of dean of faculty at Women's University in Alexandria, Egypt. She is the founder of the *International Sport Science Alexandria Journal*.

FRANCES GEMS found her life's purpose in community service and family, raising three generations of children. She has a curious nature and likes to spend her leisure time reading, gardening, cooking, and conversing with her extended family.

GERALD R. GEMS is a past president of the North American Society for Sport History, a past vice president of the International Society for the History of Physical Education and Sport, and a Fulbright scholar. He has presented his research in thirty-six countries and is the author of more than 250 publications, including twenty-eight books. In 2016 he was awarded the Routledge prize for scholarship.

M. ANN HALL is an author and a retired professor who taught for over thirty years in the Faculty of Kinesiology, Sport, and Recreation at the University of Alberta in Canada. She has published extensively on gender and sport, and on the history of Canadian women's sport. Her latest book is *Muscle on Wheels: Louise Armaindo and the High-Wheel Racers of Nineteenth-Century America*. Her current research project is about the evolution of physical education and kinesiology within the Canadian context.

TONY KALETH is a retired junior high school teacher, a musician, a craftsman, and an avid runner. A devoted sports fan, he reads and runs daily with his wife.

KOHEI KAWASHIMA teaches at Waseda University, School of Sport Sciences, in Japan as a professor of the history of sport, anthropology of sport, and American history, and serves as a visiting professor to the International Research Center for Japanese Studies. His recent publications include a chapter in *Touchdown: An American Obsession* and the article "We Will Try Again, Again, Again to Make It Bigger: Japan, American Football, and the Super Bowl in the Past,

Present, and Future," in a 2017 issue of the *International Journal of the History of Sport*. He frequently presents papers at annual conferences of the North American Society for Sport History.

LUCIANE LAUFFER, a PhD candidate in management at Macquarie University, Sydney, Australia, was born and raised in Brazil, where she worked as a journalist for almost a decade, and has also lived in Berlin, Germany, and Vancouver, Canada, as well as Australia. Her writing interests include women studies, football, and travel.

GARY OSMOND lectures and performs research in sport history in the School of Human Movement and Nutrition Sciences at the University of Queensland. His research focuses on the experiences of Aboriginal people and Torres Strait Islanders in Australia during the twentieth century and on new approaches to investigating and reframing those pasts.

GERTRUD PFISTER is a former professor at the University of Copenhagen. She is a past president of the International Society for the History of Physical Education and Sport and a past president of the International Sport Sociology Association. Called the person who has done the most for women's sport in Europe, she has been knighted three times, once by the Queen of Denmark and twice by the president of Germany. She has published more than three hundred works, including over forty books.

SAMUEL O. REGALADO was a professor of history at California State University, Stanislaus. He is a musician and songwriter; a well-known historian whose research centers on U.S. sport, ethnicity, and law; and the author of many articles and several books, including the acclaimed *Viva Baseball! Latin Major Leaguers and Their Special Hunger*.

ELSE TRANGBÆK, a professor emeritus at the University of Copenhagen, has researched women and sports and written books and articles on the subject. A longtime volunteer leader in sports, she was also an elite athlete and a participant in the 1968 Olympics in artistic gymnastics. In 2020 she was awarded the International Olympic Committee's Women and Sports Award for Europe for her many years of work in the world of sport and her writing on women and sport.

CHIA-JU YEN is an adjunct assistant professor, teaching sport history and sociology of sport at National Taiwan Sport University. Her research interests include sport history, sociology of sport, sport anthropology, body culture, and sport philosophy. She worked as a librarian for thirty years before transferring to academic affairs as a chief of the registration section.

INDEX

AARP (American Association of Retired People), 27

Abdul-Jabbar, Kareem, 2

Aborigines (Indigenous Australians), 196–201

Adelaide, 240

Africa, 18, 107, 109, 139, 248

African Americans, 5, 9, 72–95, 120, 220, 277

Alaska, 43, 167, 244, 268–69

Albæk, Morten, 213, 228

Alberta, 163–65, 167, 169, 171

Alcott, William, 20

Ali, Muhammad, 26, 116, 118, 122

ALS (amyotrophic lateral sclerosis), 160

Alzheimer's disease, 144–45, 255, 281

American Association of Retired People (AARP), 27

American Heart Association (AHA), 281

Anchorage, 244

Antarctica, 9, 268

anthropology, 99

archery, 85

Aristotle, 17

Arizona, 88, 99, 117

art, 85, 89, 95, 125, 130–32, 134, 137, 139–40, 146

Ashby, LeRoy, 125–27

Asia, 6, 18, 22, 96–115, 128, 129, 140, 279

Atlanta, 280

Atlas, Charles, 207

Auckland, 235, 266

Australia, 3, 150, 155–56, 158, 169, 191, 192, 194–210, 229–45

Australian football, 229, 230

Austria, 69, 150

autoethnography, 9–10

backpacking, 88

badminton, 98, 174, 252, 253, 279

Bahrain, 150

Baltimore, 19

Bannerman, Christopher, 138

Barcelona, 237

Barnes, Auntie Alice, 199

Barreto, Ed, 5

Barrett, Ann E., 210

baseball, 29, 30, 87, 90, 124, 128, 162, 178; in Alaska, 43; in Canada, 161–62; coaching, 92; interscholastic, 76–77, 84–85, 119–21, 202; in Japan, 181; players, 2, 116, 118, 120, 121, 123, 127, 130; professional, 118, 131; as recreation, 77, 130–33; and women, 23, 161; youth, 39, 45, 75–76, 99, 118–19, 161

basketball, 91, 162, 178, 251; coaching, 82, 92, 231; college, 82, 88, 163–64, 236; facilities, 71, 242; interscholastic, 45, 82, 202, 279; Olympic, 229, 236, 237; players, 1–2, 122–23, 240; professional, 229, 237; as recreation, 87, 106; and women, 5–6, 23, 230, 234–37, 242–44, 249–50, 286; youth, 47, 75–77, 99, 181

Bavaria, 247

beauty, 262–63, 269–71

Belgium, 261

Belichick, Bill, 83

Bell, James "Cool Papa," 120

Bergquist, Lee, 5

Berlin, 248, 249

Birmingham, England, 137, 140, 142, 144, 165

Black Power, 220

Blanda, George, 1, 29

blue zones, 7–8, 208, 285

Boardman, Helen, 287

bocce, 91

Bochum, Germany, 248, 251

Bosnia, 150

Boston, 19, 21, 192, 265

Bourdieu, Pierre, 28–29, 140, 279, 288

Bowden, Bobby, 82

bowling, 40, 145, 231, 287

boxing, 2, 23, 29, 43, 76, 122, 178, 279

Brady, Tom, 1

Braxton, Toni, 87

Brazil, 150, 153–56, 159, 219

Brisbane, 235

Broesamle, John, 124, 125–26

Brown, H. Rap, 83

Brown v. Board of Education, 78

Butcher, Susan, 269

California, 5, 7, 116, 124, 125, 128–31

Canada, 3, 150, 158, 160–75, 191, 192, 194, 203, 209, 236, 288

Canberra, 236–37

cancer, 3, 7, 8, 99, 103, 108, 113, 135, 174, 281

canoeing, 161, 166–67, 170–71, 196

cardiorespiratory disease, 7, 8

Carlos, John, 220

Carlson, Janet, 148

Carter, Vince, 2

Castle, Irene, 23

Catholics, 20, 35, 44–45, 97, 118, 121, 153

centenarians, 3, 4, 5, 7, 97, 285, 286, 287

Center for Disease Control and Prevention, 7

Chaline, Eric, 207

Changchun, China, 277, 278

Charleston, 19

Chavez, Cesar, 120

Chelios, Chris, 2

Chicago, 35, 44, 46

Child, Lydia, 20

China, 18, 96, 112, 143, 150, 278, 281, 284–85

civil rights, 83, 118, 120, 122, 196–201

Civil War, 19, 22, 96

Clay v. United States, 118, 122

Clemens, Roger, 2

Cleveland, 117

climate change, 242

Cole, Thomas, 26
Collins, Judy, 286
Colón, Bartolo, 2
Colorado, 26
Communism, 216, 279
Confucius, 96
Copenhagen, 215, 218, 221, 222, 248, 285
Costa Rica, 7, 150
Cousins, Sandra, 265
Cousy, Bob, 2
COVID-19, 6, 284
Cowen, Marion, 287
Cox, Lynne, 268
crafts, 231-32
Croatia, 70, 103
Cuba, 2, 116, 267
culture, 110, 177-78, 188, 191, 192, 201, 204, 210, 227, 248, 279; African American, 85, 92; Asian, 96-97, 100-101, 103-5, 278; in Australia, 196, 203, 206; counterculture, 24-26; in Denmark, 222-25; differences in, 7, 61-65, 93, 140-41, 158; ethnic, 35-43, 140, 154-56; in Germany, 101-2; gym, 207; Latino, 133, 155-56, 159; in Middle East, 58-60, 139-40; multicultural, 89-90; and perspective, 9-10; working class, 29-30, 35-43, 48-49, 132, 135; youth, 23-25, 38-39, 49, 118-19, 122, 270-71
cycling, 168, 169, 206, 215, 249, 257, 262; competitive, 107, 182, 267-69; female, 3, 64, 253; in Germany, 102-3, 248; male, 187, 202; as recreation, 91, 106, 205, 207, 260; youth, 38, 248
Czechoslovakia, 220

dance, 7, 36, 37, 98, 134, 154, 231, 235, 253, 281, 293; as exercise, 251, 281,

283, 284, 287; as inspiration, 101-2, 116; schools, 135, 137-38; teaching, 135-52; in youth culture, 23-25, 155
Danish Sports Association (DIF), 218, 224-25
Davis, Howard, 85, 87
Davis, Willie, 120
dementia, 3, 7, 8, 107, 110, 144, 151-52, 183, 285, 289
Denmark, 6, 28, 213-28, 248, 260, 264, 272, 285
depression, 37, 42, 46-53, 94, 110, 184, 201, 239, 281, 284
Detroit, 280
diabetes, 7, 8
diet, 18, 23, 106, 139, 189, 192, 208, 277; deficiencies, 8; in Newfoundland, 205; successful aging and, 7, 17, 40, 70, 89, 109, 175, 205, 235, 285; therapy, 185; training, 4, 50, 89; vegetarian, 25
DIF (Danish Sports Association), 218, 224-25
Dionigi, Rylee, 258, 267
disability, 10, 19, 104, 105, 106, 107, 109, 143, 183, 234
disc golf, 72, 91
discrimination, 72-95, 122, 196-201, 224; and age, 104-5, 110-12, 142, 180; ethnic, 124, 129, 178-79; and gender, 57-71, 155-57, 163, 214, 225-26, 230-31; racial, 72-95; and social class, 179-80
Ditzel, Meta, 216-17
divorce, 5, 10, 28, 44, 56, 99, 107, 156, 270
DNA, 153-54
dogsled racing, 268-69
Do-sun, Lee, 281

Douglass, Frederick, 73
Dubai, 150
Dubček, Alexander, 220
Duncan, Tim, 2
Duran, Roberto, 2
Dykes, Gene, 4

economy, 26, 214; American, 24; in China and Taiwan, 103–4; in Denmark, 204; digital, 196; in England, 144; in Japan, 177–80; national, 20; premodern, 21
Edinburgh, 239
Edmonton, 164, 168–69, 172, 174, 235, 249
education, 35, 85, 214, 244, 277, 279, 280, 288; Catholic, 121–22; domestic, 154; elementary, 36, 38–39, 45, 96–97, 112, 117–18, 216–17; graduate, 58, 98–100, 157, 169, 177–78, 203, 221; higher education, 25–29, 46, 52–53, 57–58, 79, 85, 87, 92–93, 97, 103, 121, 124–27, 134–39, 146, 200, 241, 278, 285–86; lack of, 36, 91, 143, 192, 229; in Middle East, 59–70; in nineteenth century, 21–22; political, 218–20
Egypt, 18, 56–71, 140, 150
Ehrenreich, Barbara, 174–75
Eichstatt, Germany, 247
Elizabeth I, Queen of England, 18
Ellis, Neenah, 286
Ellis, Ruth, 287
England, 18, 19, 44, 63, 135, 164–65, 229
environment, 37, 167, 170, 244, 257, 299
equestrianism, 21, 168–73, 199, 234–35, 248, 253, 279
ESPN, 2, 5
ethnicity, 6, 9, 35–43, 117–18, 126, 139, 178, 247, 277, 280, 289
Europe, 20, 21, 23, 28

family, 10, 21, 72, 96–97, 110, 135, 176–77, 192, 215–16, 229, 235–36; adoptive, 153–54; biological, 160; ethnic, 35–43, 117–18, 178; importance of, 18, 40–42, 56, 91–92; responsibility for, 18, 44–46, 49–50, 96, 104–7, 144–46, 193–94, 239; as social support, 8, 9, 42, 50–52, 56–57, 91–92, 147, 208–9, 226–27; and working class, 29
farming, 19, 21, 96, 176, 230, 232–33, 236, 237, 238, 239–40, 243, 279
feminism, 22–23, 24, 61, 137, 159, 165–68, 218, 231
fencing, 21, 248
field hockey, 85, 229–30, 242
Fields, Sarah K., 130
fighting, 75, 76, 94
figure skating, 161–62
Fiji, 156, 244
Finland, 213
fishing, 21, 91, 170–71, 193, 205, 206
Flood, Curt, 123
Florida, 2, 82, 267
Flutie, Doug, 1
football, 30, 87, 132, 279; Australian rules for, 229; coaching, 92; college, 84; history of, 1; interscholastic, 74–82, 84–85, 121; in Japan, 178; players, 1–2, 29; professional, 94; as recreation, 87; semipro, 39, 78; youth, 39, 45, 47, 75–76
Foreman, George, 2
Foundation of Olympic and Sport Education, 61
France, 19, 21, 61, 70, 153, 184, 188, 190, 207, 261, 281
Franco, Julio, 2
Frank, Arthur, 10
Freeman, Cathy, 210

friendship, 8, 9, 42, 54, 93, 131, 146, 158, 188–89, 195, 209–10, 235, 267

Frith, Ruth, 3, 4, 266, 271

Fukushima, Japan, 183

Galen, 17

Gallea, Cindy, 269

gambling, 186

gardening, 3, 39, 42, 91, 106, 232, 262

Geard, David, 7

gender, 6–7, 9, 19–20, 48, 139, 165–68, 188, 213, 217, 225, 246–79, 280, 289; bias, 155, 196; femininity, 22, 49, 137, 167, 215, 218–20, 222–23, 225, 230–32, 259; masculinity, 23, 49, 155–56, 178, 191, 196, 201–4

Georgia, 177

Germany, 4, 20, 21, 68, 100–102, 150, 153, 169, 172, 184, 188, 190, 214, 215, 219, 247, 248, 261, 272

gerontology, 10, 25

Gibson, Josh, 120

Gillard, Julia, 156

Goldstein, Abraham, 286–87

golf, 2, 40, 45, 72, 91, 106, 188, 189, 190, 249, 252–53, 279

Graham, Martha, 149

Graham, Sylvester, 25

Grant, Madison, 23

Great Britain, 20, 61, 62, 65, 165, 201

Greece, 7, 17, 61, 69, 150

Green, Darrell, 2

Grierson, Bruce, 26

Guam, 99

Gubrium, Jaber F., 191

Gumber, Clayton, 210

Guttmann, Allen, 126

gymnastics, 80, 110, 136, 146, 148, 213–28, 249, 252–63, 279, 281, 282; clubs,
141–42, 213, 217, 224–25, 242, 248, 252; coaching, 141–42, 225; in nineteenth century, 21; in Olympics, 218–21; as recreation, 106; in schools, 81, 85, 154, 241; youth, 76, 153

Halas, George, 29

Hall, Gilbert, 287

Hall, G. Stanley, 23

Hall, Sadie, 287

handball, 58, 71, 77, 106, 249, 257

Hawaii, 4, 99, 244, 265

Hawkins, Julia "Hurricane," 4, 286

Hawthorne, Nathaniel, 19

Hays, Guy, 92

Haywood, Spencer, 122

heart disease, 8, 280

Herodotus, 17

Hershey, Milton S., 114

Herzegovina, 150

hiking, 89, 91, 106, 174, 178, 227, 246, 248, 254, 269

Hill, Grant, 2

Hindu, 140

Hispanics. See Latinx

history, 48, 70, 71, 121–23, 178, 195–96, 202, 241; of aging, 1, 6, 10, 17–34; of education, 124–30; of Olympics, 23, 161–62, 181, 210, 218–20, 227, 236, 265; social, 10, 126; of sport, 1–6, 91, 103, 119–21, 126–30, 164–65, 181, 191, 197–201, 203, 207, 218, 221–23, 227; teaching, 92, 128, 132–33, 190, 197–201, 239–40

hockey, 161–62

Hofmann, Annette, 70, 101–3

Holstein, James A., 191

Holt-Lunstad, Julianne, 208

Hong Kong, 243, 245

horse racing, 2
horseshoes, 36, 72, 75, 91
Hoshi, Hyuma, 181
Howard, Alf, 201
Howe, Gordie, 2
Huang, Dan, 113
Hult, Joan, 92
Hume, Richard, 127
Hungary, 216, 217
hunting, 125, 193

IAPESGW (International Association
    of Physical Education and Sport for
    Girls and Women), 60–61, 136–37,
    146, 231, 244
ice hockey, 2, 5, 202, 279
Iceland, 195
ice skating, 164, 193, 202, 206
Iditarod, 269
Ikaria, 7
Illinois, 128, 129
Inada, Hiromu, 4
India, 18, 139, 140, 143, 150, 266
insurance, 20–21, 25, 39, 104–5, 183, 214,
    226, 234
International Association of Physical
    Education and Sport for Girls and
    Women (IAPESGW), 60–61, 136–37,
    146, 231, 244
International Society for the History
    of Physical Education and Sport
    (ISHPES), 60, 69–70, 103, 222
Iran, 150
Iraq, 150
Ireland, 277–78
ISHPES (International Society for the
    History of Physical Education and
    Sport), 60, 69–70, 103, 222
Islam, 139–40

Italy, 3, 7, 35, 63, 117, 235, 289

Jackson, Michael, 176
Jágr, Jaromír, 2
James, LeBron, 1
Japan, 4, 7, 112, 130, 150, 176–90, 240
Jeong-ja, Byeon, 281, 284
Johnson, Lyndon, 20
Johnson, Randy, 2
Jonrowe, DeeDee, 269
Jordan, Michael, 2
journalists, 26, 84, 127, 224

Kai-shek, Chiang, 96
Kajiwara, Ikki, 181
karate, 181
Kaur, Man, 266–67
Kawakami, Tetsuharu, 181
kayaking, 167, 171, 248
Kelly, Edward, 113
Kennedy, John F., 118
Khan, Nasrullah, 165
Kidd, Jason, 2
King, Martin Luther, Jr., 120
Kingston, Canada, 162, 166–68
Kiraly, Karch, 2
Kissinger, Henry, 123
Kleinman, Seymour, 289–90
Kotelko, Olga, 3, 4
Kowalski, Stanislaus, 4
Ku Klux Klan (KKK), 93

Laban, Rudolf, 137
lacrosse, 76, 77, 83
Lamm, Richard, 26
Larrimore, Al, 78, 80–81
Las Vegas, 99
Latin America, 18, 147–48, 156
Latinx, 117–34, 277

leisure, 6, 8, 94, 182–83, 215, 221, 226, 228, 280; cycling, 39; goals, 190; in Japan, 178, 181; senior, 108; serious, 100; time, 99, 182, 216, 224, 232, 278

Levitin, Daniel, 279, 290

Libya, 140

Lieberman, Nancy, 2

life expectancy, 8, 18, 20, 22, 104, 108–9, 183, 195, 200, 213, 233–34, 270

lifestyle, 6–8, 18, 24–26, 35, 247, 252–53, 262, 278, 285

Lillehammer, 238

Lindroth, Jan, 221

Loma Linda CA, 7

London, 61, 135, 285

Los Angeles, 99, 117, 124, 125, 127

Lou Gehrig's disease (ALS), 160

Ma, Yingjiu, 107

Macfadden, Bernarr, 23, 25

Malone, Karl, 2

Mamby, Saoul, 2

Manchester, England, 239

marathon, 3, 4, 5, 26, 106, 107, 182, 187, 248, 265

Marshall, Bobby, 1

Maryland, 72–73, 78, 84, 88, 92, 126

masculinity, 120, 133, 137, 176–90, 191, 196, 201–4, 207, 260

Maslow, Abraham, 27–28, 287–89

Masters Games, 3–5, 7, 26, 28, 230, 235, 244, 246, 249–51, 264–67, 270, 288

Mauritius, 158

Mawson, Douglas, 201

Mays, Willie, 120

McCormick, Harold, 25

McGovern, George, 123

McGuire, Mark, 129–30

McHugh, Betty "BJ," 3

McIntosh, Peter, 164

McNelly, Don, 5

media, 93, 107, 118, 235, 249–51, 264–67, 270, 288; digital, 105, 209, 241; print, 23–25, 142, 244, 246; radio, 38; sports, 5, 190, 220; television, 142

Meiji era, 176

Melbourne, 201, 229, 230, 236, 237, 239–40, 244, 266

menopause, 184

Mexico, 63, 117, 121, 125, 127, 133, 218, 220

Middle East, 18, 140

Minneapolis, 5

Miñoso, Minnie, 2

Montreal, 162, 229

Morocco, 150

Moscow, 229

mountaineering, 247, 248, 268

Mount Everest, 268

Mount Kilimanjaro, 107, 248

Moyer, Jamie, 2

Muenster, Germany, 101–2

Murphy, Willie, 6

music, 24, 36, 48, 55, 118, 137, 170; concerts, 145; ethnic, 36; jazz, 25; love of, 45, 116, 139, 251; organ, 119; playing, 49, 51, 116, 123–25, 130–33, 148–49, 152, 253; reading, 148; singing, 37–38, 289; soul, 95; teaching, 39, 146; as therapy, 53, 112, 151; writing, 286

Muslim, 67, 139

Muslim Brotherhood, 67

Mutombo, Dikembe, 2

NAACP (National Association for the Advancement of Colored People), 91, 93

Nash, Steve, 2

NASSH (North American Society for Sport History), 126, 127–28
National Association for the Advancement of Colored People (NAACP), 91, 93
Native Americans, 18, 22, 117
Navratilova, Martina, 2
Nesser, John, 1
netball, 136
Netherlands, 261
New South Wales, 158, 231, 242
New York, 5, 6, 19, 21, 62, 120, 173, 192
New Zealand, 201, 241, 244, 266
Nicoya, Costa Rica, 7
Nixon, Richard, 122, 123
Norman, Greg, 2
North American Society for Sport History (NASSH), 126, 127–28
North Carolina, 93, 229
Northern Ireland, 239
Norway, 150, 213, 225, 227
nutrition, 4, 7–8, 17, 18, 23, 25, 70, 143, 144, 205, 254
Nyad, Diana, 2, 267

Oakland CA, 1
obesity, 7, 8, 143
Okinawa, 7
Olympics, 3, 23, 61, 172, 181, 205, 210, 224, 242, 249, 250, 265; and Australian Olympic Committee, 236; books about, 223, 227; and Canadian team, 161–62; and Egyptian Olympic Committee, 71; and International Olympic Committee, 238; participation in, 218–21, 229, 237; and United States team, 87, 237; Winter, 238
Oman, 58–59, 64, 140, 150
Ontario, Canada, 162–63, 166–67, 170, 171–72

optimism, 30, 42, 53–54, 96, 106–7, 142, 158, 197, 257, 286
Ortiz, David, 2
Ottawa, Canada, 160–61, 163
Oyama, Masutatsu, 181

Paige, Satchel, 2, 116, 120, 121, 133
Pakistan, 165
Papua New Guinea, 244
Paris, 21, 123, 207
Parish, Robert, 2
Pennsylvania, 126
Perth, 169
Pes, Gianni, 285
Pfister, Gertrud, 60
Philadelphia, 19, 21, 123
Phillips, Murray, 197
physical education, 76, 135, 141, 146, 241, 244; in Denmark, 221; in higher education, 56–61, 65–70, 84–85, 100, 138, 161–65, 248; in Japan, 178; and research, 62; in schools, 75–77, 80, 84, 136–37, 139, 161–62, 215, 231, 236, 247, 284; standards for, 65
physiology, 3, 7, 28, 221, 222, 226, 287–89
pickleball, 174
Pike, Elizabeth, 287
Pilates, Joseph, 173–74, 286
Plato, 17
Player, Gary, 2
Poland, 28, 44
politics, 17, 26, 116, 216, 269, 279; American, 122; in China, 96; Cold War, 216, 241, 267–78; in Denmark, 217–20; international, 232; issues concerning, 30; and legislation, 20–21, 27; local, 93; national, 96, 232; in Taiwan, 103–4
Portland, 235

psychology, 3, 5, 8, 22, 23, 27–28, 53, 99, 110, 134, 165, 208, 260, 287–89

Qatar, 70
Qigong, 103, 105, 106, 108, 110
Quebec, 163

race, 9, 26, 72–95, 120, 122, 125, 196, 220, 277, 280
racquetball, 164
Raschker, Philippa, 4
Rawson, Margaret, 287
reading, 39, 46, 48, 53, 120, 155, 167, 184, 210, 232, 246, 254
Reagan, Ronald, 286
Reed, Pam, 4
Reeve, Jim, 5
Regensburg, Germany, 248
religion, 7–8, 9, 19–20, 35, 37, 44, 72, 91, 139–40, 153, 177, 229, 287
retirement, 95, 114, 131, 183, 210, 222, 227, 244, 251, 254; activities, 147–49; contemplation of, 94, 190; early, 171, 196–97; history of, 20; planning, 238–39; regrets in, 113; in Taiwan, 105–6; in United Kingdom, 134, 141–43
Rice, Jerry, 1
Riddles, Libby, 269
Rio de Janeiro, 219
Robertson, Anna Mary (Grandma Moses), 286
Robinson, Jackie, 120
rock climbing, 100
Rodriguez, Alex, 2
roller skating, 36
Ross, Edward Alsworth, 23
rowing, 231, 249
rugby, 23

running, 53, 161, 166, 178, 180, 231, 262, 281; competitive, 249, 254, 285; as exercise, 55, 72, 75–76, 88–89, 106–7, 154, 164, 187, 227, 248–49, 251–53; and identity, 46–50; and seniors, 3–5, 249, 250–51, 253–57, 264–65; sprinting, 30, 38, 220; ultra-long-distance, 268
Russia, 241
Ryan, Nolan, 2

sailing, 76, 77, 248, 253, 268–69
Samuel, Lawrence, 6
samurai, 176
San Diego, 5
Sandow, Eugene, 207
San Francisco, 99, 116, 118, 129–30
Sansonetti, Ugo, 3
Sardinia, 7
Saudi Arabia, 59
Scharenbrock, Ray, 5
Schultz, George, 286
Schwartz, Morrie, 287
Scott, Barbara Ann, 161–62
Scully, Vin, 126
Sears, Eleanora, 2
Seattle, 123
Seoul, 177, 281
Sertich, Mark, 5
Sherman, S. R., 210
Shieh, Chih-Mou, 100
Shizuoka, Japan, 184
Shoemaker, Willie, 2
shuffleboard, 287
Singh, Fauja, 4
skateboarding, 285
skiing, 3, 101, 164, 166, 167, 202, 205, 227, 247–48, 253–54, 257, 279
Smith, Gina, 172

Smith, Ron, 126
Smith, Tommie, 220
soccer, 23, 47, 101, 155, 157, 181, 247, 279, 285
social class, 8, 9, 28–38, 117–18, 126, 135, 143, 178–80, 182, 247, 286, 289; and aging, 6–7; middle class, 28–29, 161, 176, 279–80; upper class, 28–29, 176, 288; working class, 22–23, 26, 29–30, 35–43, 45–47, 73, 91, 117, 214, 277–79
Social Security, 20–21, 25
sociology, 9, 23, 164, 165, 248, 287
Socrates, 17
Socrates, Jeanne, 268–69
softball, 3, 47, 72, 84, 92, 106, 131, 229–30, 231, 240–41
Sosa, Sammy, 129–30
South Africa, 143, 150
South Korea, 240, 281
Soviet Union, 219–20, 268
Spain, 106
squash, 2, 164, 165, 166, 231
Squires, Lee Walling, 23
Stamper, Ray, 287
St. Louis, 119, 123
Stockton, John, 2
stress, 8, 97, 103, 131, 133, 157, 172, 184, 254, 277, 278, 284, 288
Struna, Nancy, 92
sumo wrestling, 178, 181
Sun-bun, Cho, 284
Suzuki, Ichiro, 2
Sweden, 220, 221, 225, 261
swimming, 7, 136, 139, 202, 220, 227, 250; benefits of, 205; distance, 182, 268; facilities, 69, 91, 233; and family, 87, 98–99, 206; female, 2, 57, 88, 98; interscholastic, 229; masters, 4; Olympic, 3; as recreation, 106, 187, 196, 206–7, 233, 253, 257, 286; senior, 40, 196, 233; synchronized, 242; teaching, 64, 161
Switzerland, 153
Sydney, 3, 155, 210, 235, 236–38, 242, 246, 266
Syria, 140, 150

table tennis, 69, 98, 106, 110, 174, 252, 279
tai chi, 110, 284–85
Taipei, 96–97, 111
Taiwan, 96–115
Talbot, Margaret, 61, 63, 65
Tanaka, Hirofumi, 7
tennis, 125, 174, 181, 279; competitive, 1, 2, 25; as exercise, 3, 233, 253, 255; facilities, 91; as recreation, 23, 77, 106, 227, 248–49, 252; teaching, 164
Texas, 117
Thailand, 99, 158
Tharp, Twyla, 284
theory, 9–10, 28–29, 120, 126, 127, 152, 162, 165, 247, 288
Tibet, 268
Tóibín, Colm, 201–2
Tokyo, 176, 180, 181, 183, 235, 244
Tonga, 244
Toronto, 160, 162, 163, 167, 266
Torres, Dara, 3
track and field, 136, 230, 250, 253, 272; interscholastic, 47, 76, 92, 162, 229, 241; masters, 3–4, 266–67; Olympic, 219
Trason, Ann, 4–5
Traunstein, Germany, 247
travel, 49, 55, 158, 225, 250; for education, 39, 48, 106, 155; international, 61–62, 71, 99, 111, 140, 143, 155, 159,

192, 253, 260–67, 272; local, 90, 95, 163, 245

triathlon, 4, 107, 187

Trump, Donald, 116

Tulle, Emmanuelle, 5

Tunisia, 69

Turin, 235

Turkey, 150

United Kingdom, 137, 139–40, 142–43, 146, 149, 150, 234, 261

United Nations, 108, 213, 217

United States Naval Academy, 77, 80, 82, 83

Valenzuela, Fernando, 127, 133

Vancouver, 125

vegetarians, 7, 25

Venezuela, 150

Vertinsky, Patricia, 265

Victoria, 240, 243

Vietnam War, 118, 122–23

Vinatieri, Adam, 1

Virginia, 19, 90, 91

volleyball, 2, 64, 91, 154, 162–63, 181, 230, 279

volunteering, 40, 91, 93–94, 136–40, 142, 145–46, 150, 155, 166, 224, 230, 243, 289

Von Willebrand disease, 239

walking, 5, 28, 39, 40, 190, 227, 232; as exercise, 8, 106, 110, 224, 253, 260, 262, 279; as recreation, 205; speed, 112, 187; trails, 168

Ware, Bronnie, 113

War of 1812, 19

Washington (state), 125, 127, 133

Washington DC, 62, 90

Watanabe, Tamae, 268

Webster, Marsh, 5

weight training, 3, 6, 23, 26, 50, 72, 76–77, 82, 87–88, 93, 207, 267–68

Weston, Edward Payson, 5

Whitelock, Anna, 18

whiteness, 6, 8

Whitlock, Ed, 4

Wilhelm, Hoyt, 2

Williams, Serena, 1

Wills, Maury, 120

Wisconsin, 46, 93, 94

Wolf, Naomi, 270

women, 27, 115, 155–58, 165–68, 186, 208, 245; as athletes, 1, 5–6, 24, 157, 163–65, 196, 235, 264–69, 271; friendships of, 153, 166–67, 246–75; history of, 19–23, 126, 259, 270–71; as leaders, 166–67, 213, 230–31, 233, 236–37, 242, 272; and research, 9, 166; social status of, 19–23, 156–58, 230, 260, 263; as teachers, 134–52

World Health Organization, 9

World War I, 23, 25, 173

World War II, 25, 41, 44, 96, 117, 130, 135, 177, 214, 241

wrestling, 76, 85, 178

yachting, 21, 182

Yale University, 25

YMCA (Young Men's Christian Association), 87

yoga, 3, 40, 70, 91, 106, 110, 173, 284

youth, 21–24, 26–27, 76, 258, 262, 278; and appearance, 18, 27, 260; attributes of, 5; emphasis on, 23–24, 49, 158, 263, 270–71; rebellion, 26, 215, 218

Yukon River, 248

CPSIA information can be obtained
at www.ICGtesting.com
Printed in the USA
LVHW020252190422
716595LV00003B/348

9 781496 231611